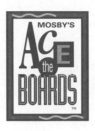

Pharmacology

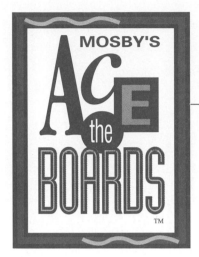

MOSBY'S USMLE step 1 REVIEWS

Pharmacology

S. J. Enna
Ph.D., Professor and Chairman

Michael A. Gordon
Ph.D., Associate Professor

Thomas L. Pazdernik
Ph.D., Professor

Department of Pharmacology, Toxicology, and Therapeutics,
University of Kansas Medical School,
Kansas City, Kansas

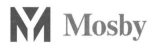

St. Louis Baltimore Boston Carlsbad Chicago Naples New York Philadelphia Portland
London Madrid Mexico City Singapore Sydney Tokyo Toronto Wiesbaden

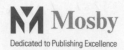

Vice President and Publisher *Anne S. Patterson*
Editor *Emma D. Underdown*
Developmental Editor *Christy Wells*
Project Manager *Dana Peick*
Production Editor *Jeffrey Patterson*
Manufacturing Supervisor *Tony McAllister*
Book Designer *Amy Buxton*
Cover Designer *Stacy Lanier/AKA Design*

Printed in the United States of America
Composition by Graphic World, Inc.
Printing/binding by R. R. Donnelly

Mosby–Year Book, Inc.
11830 Westline Industrial Drive
St. Louis, Missouri 63146

Library of Congress Cataloging in Publication Data

Enna, S. J.
    Mosby's USMLE step 1 reviews—pharmacology/S. J. Enna, Michael Gordon, Thomas Pazdernik.
        p.   cm.—(Ace the boards)
    Includes index.
        1. Pharmacology—Outlines, syllabi, etc.   2. Pharmacology-
-Examinations, questions, etc.   I. Gordon, Michael, 1949-
II. Pazdernik, Thomas.   III. Title. IV. Series.
        [DNLM: 1. Pharmacology—examination questions.   2. Pharmacology-
-outlines. QV 18.2 E59m 1996]
    RM301.14.E56   1996
    615.1′076—dc20
    DNLM/DLC
    for Library of Congress   95-47218
                                                          CIP

    ISBN 0-8151-3112-7   (IBM)
    ISBN 0-8151-3152-6   (MAC)

96   97   98   99   00   /   9   8   7   6   5   4   3   2   1

CONTRIBUTORS

In addition to the editors, all of the following are, or were, members of the faculty at the University of Kansas Medical School during the preparation of this work. Except for Dr. Pelling, who is in the Department of Pathology and Laboratory Medicine, the contributors are from the Department of Pharmacology, Toxicology, and Therapeutics.

Richard H. Alper, Ph.D.
Associate Professor

Timo M. Buetler, Ph.D.*
Assistant Professor

Ruben D. Buñag, M.D.
Professor

Curtis D. Klaassen, Ph.D.
Professor

Beth Levant, Ph.D.
Assistant Professor

Sara Antonia Li, Ph.D.
Associate Professor

M. Helen Maguire, Ph.D.
Professor

Andrew Parkinson, Ph.D.
Professor

Jill Pelling, Ph.D.
Research Associate Professor

Allan M. Poisner, M.D.
Professor

Gregory A. Reed, Ph.D.
Associate Professor

*Current address: Medical Research Department, F. Hoffmann-La Roche Ltd., CH-4002, Basel, Switzerland

PREFACE

The clinical relevance of information gained in other science courses is most evident in pharmacology. That is, to fully appreciate the actions and uses of drugs there must be some understanding of human physiology, biochemistry, anatomy, and pathology, as well as a working knowledge of microbiology, neuroscience, and basic chemistry. While the integrative nature of pharmacology is one of its more popular features, the level of detail can be overwhelming. Most troublesome is the seemingly endless list of drugs with arcane names that must be committed to memory. Ideally, a variety of approaches are used in a pharmacology course to provide varying experiences that facilitate understanding of both the integrating concepts and factual details. A grasp of the *basic principles* of the discipline, and an appreciation of the *primary agents* in each drug class, including an understanding of their pharmacokinetics, pharmacodynamics, adverse effects, and clinical uses, is necessary for clinical training and success on board exams. This text was designed specifically to reinforce the fundamentals of pharmacology and to highlight those drugs most important for the practice of medicine.

Mastery of the principles is crucial to appreciate and properly use drugs developed in the future, as well as for understanding and recalling the drugs of choice encountered in the clinic. To this end, the subject matter has been distilled to provide instruction and to aid in the recall of basic information that may have been learned earlier. As designed, this offering will benefit those who have already been exposed to the subject, but in addition, the text and diskettes will be of value as a study guide in pharmacology courses or could serve as a primary source of information.

PEDAGOGICAL FEATURES

To facilitate review, information is prioritized by means of a bulleted (●) colorized format. In addition, the layout allows for notes to be readily inscribed on the page where a topic is mentioned. While key issues and facts are distinguished in the narrative portion of the text, they are reinforced and condensed further in illustrations, tables, lists, and charts. Icons are used to guide the reader in locating particular topics.

In addition to these aids, each section contains a series of multiple choice or matching questions designed to reinforce important principles, drugs, or drug classes. A greater number of questions is contained on the computer diskette, which provides an immediate indication of areas requiring additional study. Because explanations are given as to why a particular response is, or is not, correct, the questions and answers provide a level of instruction not normally encountered in practice exams.

Thus, a significant effort has been made to incorporate various modes of instruction in a single text. The narrative provides sufficient information to give context to the subject for those who learn best in this way. Others may choose to focus on the highlighted material as an outline of the topic. The tables, charts, and figures will be favored by those who require only an organized listing of the drugs and their actions. All should benefit from the questions, which are designed to test knowledge and to instruct at the same time. With the aid of this volume, the reader should be able to acquire the fund of knowledge required to meet the challenges presented by national examinations and clinical training.

ACKNOWLEDGMENTS

Portions of this text are taken from teaching materials developed over the past three decades. During this time, the faculty has drawn from, and been inspired by, many excellent published works in pharmacology and toxicology. Primary sources used over the years deserving special recognition are Goodman and Gilman's *The Pharmacological Basis of Therapeutics* (Pergamon); *Basic and Clinical Pharmacology* (Appleton & Lange); Cassarett and Doull's *Toxicology: The Basic Science of Poisons* (Pergamon); *Human Pharmacology: Molecular to Clinical* (Mosby); *Applied Therapeutics: The Clinical Use of Drugs* (Applied Therapeutics); *Principles of Drug Action: The Basis of Pharmacology* (Churchill Livingstone); *Principles of Medical Pharmacology* (University of Toronto); *Drill's Pharmacology in Medicine* (McGraw-Hill).

We thank all of the other faculty in the Department of Pharmacology, Toxicology, and Therapeutics at the University of Kansas Medical School, and Dr. Pelling in Pathology and Laboratory Medicine, who labored with us in preparing this volume. We are also indebted to Ms. Rosa Meagher and Ms. Maxine Floyd for their administrative support, Laszlo Kereesen, M.D., for technical assistance and advice and to Ms. Emma Underdown, Ms. Christy Wells, and their colleagues at Mosby for their guidance and suggestions. Acknowledgment is also extended to the following medical students who carefully reviewed the text and provided excellent suggestions for improvements:

Joy Mockbee
University of Arizona College of Medicine
Yung Chen
Temple University School of Medicine

S. J. Enna, Ph.D.
Michael Gordon, Ph.D.
Thomas Pazdernik, Ph.D.

Test-Taking Strategies

Suzanne F. Kiewit, M.Ed.

To perform well on the USMLEs, it is imperative that you begin with a **plan.** Preparation time is at a premium, so you will want to be as efficient and effective as possible by planning well.

MONTHS AHEAD OF THE EXAM

- Sit down with a blank calendar and block in your commitments: classes, final exams, scheduled events.
- Include time for activities of daily life: eating, sleeping, exercising, socializing, banking, maintaining your home, and so forth.
- The remaining time is available for study/review.
- Determine an orderly approach to the material you need to cover that fits your particular set of needs (e.g., subject-by-subject approach, systems approach, pathologic state approach).
- Assign the remaining time to content areas. This is done in various ways: material covered freshman year first, easiest first, least comfortable material first, detailed subjects last, whatever. Your plan should reflect your goal: to maximize your score.
- Establish a warm-up, which may consist of breaking the tension in major muscle groups (neck rolls, shoulder rolls, etc.), a quick visualization of you performing successfully, or a brief meditation. Practicing this warm-up routine before each of your study sessions will make it a familiar activity that helps you learn effectively, as well as take exams effectively.
- Designate time at the end of your study period for panoramic review. Depending on your needs, that might be a week or just several days before the exam.
- Plan for feedback on your efforts. Schedule time for answering questions on the material you are reviewing and for taking at least one mock comprehensive exam.
- Do the comprehensive exam midway through your study period so that you can refine your efforts to reflect the degree of your performance.

DAYS AHEAD OF THE EXAM

- Divide each day into thirds: morning block, afternoon block, and evening block.

- Consider the time of day that is most productive for you and do the most difficult or least favorite material at that time.
- Assign more blocks of study to those areas requiring the most review to reach a comfortable knowledge level.
- A popular way to use blocks is to pair subjects or materials. For instance, pair strong content with weaker content so that you are not always in the position of not knowing material (which would invite negative feelings or ineffectiveness). Or pair a conceptual subject with a detail subject, such as physiology with anatomy, so that you are not always doing the same kind of thinking (this invites positive effort).
- Use your most productive blocks of time for actual study/review. Use the nonpeak times for reinforcement of material covered or feedback by answering questions on material that you have covered.

Planning the Blocks

- Once you determine time allocations for each content area and an orderly approach that fits your needs and goals, you want to specify what you plan to do during each block.
- Be specific as to content area, material to study, and task; for example, MICRO: review chart on viruses; PHYS: answer questions on renal; and so forth.
- Each study block will last approximately 3 to 4 hours. To be most efficient and effective, plan to take a 5- or 10-minute break every hour. If you are having difficulty getting into the study mode, plan to study for 25 minutes, then take a 5-minute break. Reserve longer breaks for switches between subjects. Get up and move around on breaks.

BEFORE THE EXAM

Knowing about the USMLEs helps demystify them. In general, the USMLE exams are a 2-day, four-book examination. Approximately 3 hours are allotted per exam book. Each day you will complete one book of about 200 items in the morning and another book in the afternoon.

In each exam book, questions are organized by question type, not content. Specific directions precede each set of questions. Only two question formats are used: one-best-answer multiple choice items (which typically come first on the exam) and matching items (toward the end of the exam). Students have reported that one-best-answer items make up the bulk of the exam (70% to 75%) and negatively stemmed items make up only 10% to 15% of the questions.[1] Matching sets, which make up about 15% to 20% of the items, may include short leading lists or long leading lists of up to 26 items from which to choose.

From year to year there may be variations in the organization and presentation of both content and item formats. It would be wise to read the National Board of Medical Examiners' *General Instructions* booklet, which you will receive when you register. This booklet contains descriptions of content, item format, and even a set of practice items. Be certain you read this booklet and familiarize yourself with the questions.

You can further maximize exam performance by taking control. Adults tend to perform better when they feel that they have a measure of control. For the USMLE it is easy to feel out of control. You are told what time to arrive, where to go, what writing instrument to use, when to break the seal, and so on. You want to assume control of as many aspects as possible to maximize your performance:

STUDY   Follow the sage advice of planning your work and working your plan to maintain satisfactory preparation with regard to study.

SLEEP   Get a good night's rest. Sleep needs vary, but 6 hours is usually minimum. Try to get the appropriate amount of sleep that you require.

NUTRITION   Maintain proper nutrition during both study time and exam time. Eat breakfast. Choose foods that help keep you on an even energy level. Eat light lunches on exam days. If you have a favorite food and can take it with you, treat yourself.

MEDICATION   It may be cold, flu, or allergy season. Take no medications that may make you drowsy.

CLOTHING   Heating and cooling systems are rarely balanced enough to suit everyone. Wear articles of clothing that can be added or removed as necessary. Strive for personal comfort.

READINESS   Develop physical, mental, emotional, and psychologic readiness for the exam. Keep your thoughts about the exam and your preparation efforts running positively. You must believe that *you can do this!*

ARRIVAL   Plan to arrive as close to the designated time as possible and still allow yourself sufficient time to check in. Keep to yourself so that other people's anxieties will not affect you. Take care of personal needs. Find your seat.

ACCLIMATION   Settle in and get comfortable. Take several deep breaths. . . RELAX. A relaxed mind thinks better than a tense one—it's that old "fight-or-flight" syndrome. Do your warm-up routine to help you relax.

ATTENTION   Pay attention to the proctor. Complete all identification material as required. Read all instructions carefully. Ask for clarification as needed. Do not open your booklet until told to do so. After you are told to break the seal, quickly glance through the whole test to see how it is set up and how questions are organized. Again, you want to take control of the situation. A quick review eliminates surprises and allows you to develop a plan.

DURING THE EXAM

Plan Your Approach

There are numerous approaches to answering questions. Answer questions in the order that appeals to you. Doing the easier ones first may give a psychologic boost; however, the ones you skip may stay on your mind and cloud your thinking.

Another approach is to answer each question in sequence. Start with the first one in the section with which you begin and fill in an answer for each question. Do not leave any blanks! The theory behind this is that if you spend any time at all on an item, you should mark your best response at that time and go on. If you are not certain of your choice, mark "R" in the test booklet for review and return to it later as you have time.

Some students plan to do the matching items first. Matching items are the last set of questions in the booklets. If you prefer matching items, this is a reasonable plan because it helps you get started with items about which you feel confident. It is also reasonable because matching items are not good items on which to guess if you run short of time. **You** must decide the order in which you want to do the questions.

Complete the Bubble Sheet or Answer Card Carefully

There are two schools of thought on this matter. One is to fill in the bubble sheet **item by item** as you go. This method minimizes transcription errors. The other method is **block transfer.** Complete a logical chunk of questions in the test booklet (one or two pages) and then transfer responses to the bubble sheet. Be sure that the last question number on the page is the last numeral you blacken. This method saves time and offers a mini-mental break at the end of each block. Such minibreaks help decrease fatigue during a long exam. Choose the method that will work for you and *practice* it as you take prep questions.

Budget Your Time

If only the allotted time and the number of questions were considered, you would have approximately 54 seconds per question. Obviously, some questions may go more quickly and balance out the ones that take longer. To keep track, you need a pacing strategy. A good strategy is to establish checkpoints at 30-minute intervals. When you overview the booklet, circle the numerals corresponding to where you should be at 30 minutes, 60, 90, 120, and so on. For example, if you have 200 questions on a 3-hour exam, you should be at question number 33 at 30 minutes. As you complete the exam, check your time at the circled items. This technique keeps you from watching the clock too much, yet permits multiple opportunities to adjust your pacing.

If you find yourself spending too much time on any one question, select your best choice at that time, mark an answer, and "R" it for later review. The point is to keep going. Laboring too long on one question limits you from responding to other items you may know well. Remember, controlling your time helps you maximize your points.

ANSWERING THE QUESTIONS

- **Read and *understand* the stems and alternatives.**
  The most frequent error made on exams is misreading or misinterpreting the various aspects of a question. The **stem** is the introductory question or statement. The **alternatives** are the options from which you select the one best response. To encourage reading and understanding, use a process.
- **Follow a process to answer questions.**
  1. Quickly read the stem.
  2. Quickly read the options. (Combined, the first two steps create a preview of the item.)
  3. Carefully read, underline, and mark the stem in a timely fashion.
     - Selectively underline key words and phrases.
     - Pay attention to nouns, verbs, and modifiers.

- Circle age and gender.
- Note data in telescopic form (e.g., ↑ BP).
- Graphically represent material if it helps you to understand (e.g., diagram the renal tubule to answer a question about reabsorption).
  4. Carefully read each alternative. Mark as appropriate.
- **Consider each alternative as one in a series of true, false, or not sure (?) statements.**
  Read each alternative. Rather than slashing out the ones you eliminate, work with each one and designate it as **true, false,** or varying degrees of **true/false/?.** This marking strategy requires you to make judicious decisions about alternatives relative to the stem. It also provides a record of your original thinking, which will save you re-thinking time if you need to reconsider a question. Practice this strategy on preparation questions so it becomes second nature.
- **Avoid premature closure.**
  Sometimes you may read a question and anticipate a response. Such a reaction helps focus your attention. However, be sure to read *all* the options so that you are selecting the *best* response. In one-best-answer multiple choice questions, there is one *best* and several *likely* responses. Avoid being misled; consider all the alternatives.
- **Be leery of negative stems.**
  Negative stems require shifting to a negative thinking mode to determine which alternatives are not correct. You can avoid this shift by using this strategy:
  - Circle such words as *except, least, false, incorrect, not true* to raise your awareness of them.
  - Cross out the negative and read the stem as though it were a positive.
  - Mark each option as T/F/?. The F option will then be the appropriate choice.
- **Keep your original answers.**
  To change or not to change answers is a difficult decision. The answer depends on a person's previous history. If you are the kind of student who, if you change answers, changes them from wrong to right, then selectively changing answers may be worthwhile. If, on the other hand, your past experience has been to change right answers to wrong answers, selectively changing answers is probably not a good idea. Good performers change answers, but only if they have reason, such as acquired insight or discovery of misreading or misinterpretation.

- **Maintain an even emotional keel.**
  If a question upsets you, calm yourself. Take several deep breaths. Tell yourself, "I can do this!" Give yourself a mental or physical break. Pay special attention to the next two or three questions after a bout of emotional uneasiness. It is possible to miss items when attention is diffused.

THINKING THROUGH QUESTIONS

- **Use logical reasoning and sound thinking.**
  - Read the item carefully. After careful reading, ask "What is this question really asking?" Restate it so that you know what is being asked.
  - Engage in a mental dialogue with the question. Talk to yourself about what you do know. Always start with what **you** know. Verbalize your thinking.
  - If a diagram or graphic representation is included, orient yourself to it **first** so that the options do not lead your thinking.
- **Use information found within the questions themselves to help you answer others.**
  There will not be "gimmes" on a nationally standardized exam. However, there may be items or graphics that trigger remembrances.
- **Create a diagram, chart, map, or graphic representation of given information.**
  Material that is visually presented usually helps clarify thinking. Use selective, quick sketching as warranted.
- **Reason through information like a detective.**
  - Sift through the details (preview).
  - Determine the relevant information (selectively mark).
  - Put the clues together as in solving a puzzle (reason).
- **Read carefully and note key descriptors.**
  - Note words such as *chronic, acute, greater than, less than, adult, child.*
  - Attend to prefixes such as hyper-, hypo-, non-, un-, pre-, post-.
- **Analyze base words and affixes.**
  Studying a question at the word level may help you remember salient information. Look for base words or related words. Determine Latin or Greek word parts and use their meanings to assist you.
- **Consider similar options equally.**
  If you mark one alternative as "false" for a particular reason and another option is qualified for the same reason, it's probably "false" as well.
- **Trust the questions.**
  The questions are designed to determine if you

have a working knowledge of the material. They are not written to trick you. You need to believe that your medical school curriculum and your study efforts prepared you for most of the questions.

- **Meet the challenge of clinical vignettes.**
  Longer, vignette items challenge you to discern the relevant from the irrelevant material. In doing so, you are given multiple clues to consider. To effectively handle the vignette item, follow this strategy:
  - Scan the stem and read the first several lines.
  - Skip to the end of the stem and read the last several lines.
  - Check the alternatives to narrow your focus.
  - Now that you know what the question is about, go back to the stem; read and mark what's important to your informed decision making.
  - Make good T/F/? decisions.
- **Reread your underlines and markings when you are down to two choices, at 50/50.**
  By the time you work through a stem and numerous alternatives, it is easy to lose the gist of the question. Checking your focus by rereading only the underlines ensures that you are answering the question being posed.

ANSWERING MATCHING ITEM SETS

Matching items are used to measure your ability to distinguish among closely related items. They require knowledge of specific sets of information. As you study, be alert to potential material that could be tested in this way.

Matching items can be formatted in two ways. **Short leading list matching** items include a set of five, lettered options followed by a lead-in statement and then several numbered stems. **Long leading list matching** items include a set of up to 26 lettered options, followed by a lead-in statement and then several numbered stems.

To efficiently deal with a short leading list item, consider it as an upside-down multiple choice item with the same repeated options. To handle it effectively, do the following:

- Scan the list; determine the topic.
- Read the lead-in statement; determine the focus.
- Quickly read the stem; then read and mark key words.
- In the left margin, create a grid with A, B, C, D, E at the top.

- Make good T/F/? decisions about each stem, marking them in the grid. In this way you can see the pattern of your responses. Similarly, a grid with the item numbers can be drawn beside the leading list and responses marked there.

Handling long leading list matching items effectively requires some modifications in the process. It is not efficient to make T/F/? decisions about each option, so follow this strategy:

- Scan the list; determine the topic.
- Read the lead-in; determine the focus.
- Read a stem and generate your own response.
- Narrow the focus. Put a check mark by those related options in the long list.
- Read and mark specifics in the stem to differentiate among those alternatives you marked.
- Make good T/F/? decisions.

For each stem, mark the narrowed-list options with a different symbol (star, dash, etc.). Items are listed in logical order, alphabetically or numerically. When looking for an option such as "xanthinuria," do not start at the beginning of the list. Looking in the appropriate place saves valuable seconds.

TEST WISENESS

How a question is worded can often influence your response to it. Most clues about "test psychology" are a function of the way in which a question is worded—test constructors cannot rename body parts, drugs, diseases, and so forth. Being aware of the psychology behind the wording can often help you answer the test question.

Using techniques of test psychology to arrive at a correct answer has limited value on standardized exams because those who construct the exams are well aware of the use of these techniques. Nonetheless, being wise to these techniques of test psychology may add another point or two to your score, and they can also enhance your sense of control. Knowing these techniques provides additional strategies to employ should the question temporarily stump you.

The best way to take any exam is to be totally prepared with a strong knowledge base and personal test confidence. The following techniques should be used only if you have exhausted your knowledge base, eliminated all distractors, and cannot come up with the answer even with logical thinking and sound reasoning. Such techniques are **not** a substitute for knowledge, nor are they foolproof.

- **Identify common ideas or themes within the options and between the stem and options.**

- Circle repeated words in the options.
- Select the option with the most repeated words or phrases.
- Circle words repeated in both stem and options.
- Select the option that contains key words or related words from the stem. This is a stem/option repetition.

- **Beware of words that narrow the focus or are too extreme because they tend to be incorrect.**
  Circle such words as **all, always, every, exclusively, never, no, not, none.**

- **Options that are look-alikes are good candidates for exclusion.**

- **Note qualifiers that broaden the focus because they may be correct.**
  Circle words such as *generally, probably, most, often, some, usually.*

- **Identify antonyms or two opposing statements as potentially correct options.**
  Test constructors may use pairs of opposites, so this tip may lose its effectiveness.

- **Select the most familiar-looking option.**
  Always go from what you know. Alternatives with unknown terms may be likely distractors.

- **Select the longest, most inclusive answer.**
  This would include "All of the above" as a strong potential response.

- **In numerical items, knock out the high and low alternatives and select one in the middle that seems most plausible.**

- **In negatively stemmed questions, categorize responses; the one that falls out of the category is a likely candidate.**

- **Mark the same alternative consistently throughout the test if you have no best guess and cannot eliminate distractors.**
  Before the test, decide which letter (A, B, C, D, E) will be your choice. In this way, if you have given a question your best effort and cannot decide, mark your favorite response and move to questions that cover more comfortable material.

AFTER THE EXAM

- **Between sessions and overnight:**
  - Take a well-deserved break. Eat nutritionally.
  - If you feel the urge to study, study material that is comfortable, from a source with which you are familiar (e.g., personally developed study cards or your annotated review book).
  - If you discovered a recurring "theme," you might desire to consult that set of information.

- Do something pleasurable. Relax. Get a good night's rest.
- **After the final booklet:**
  - Recognize that this exam is a measure of what you know on a given day for a given set of information at a given point in time. Keep a reasonable perspective.
  - **Celebrate!**

References

Bushan V, Le T, Amin C: First aid for the USMLE Step 1, ed 5, Norwalk, Conn, 1995, Appleton & Lange.

MONEY-BACK GUARANTEE

We are confident that ACE THE BOARDS will prepare you for passing the USMLEs. We are so sure of this, that we'll offer you a money-back guarantee should you fail the USMLE. To receive your refund, simply mail us a copy of your failed USMLE report, plus the original receipt for this product. Mail these materials to:

Marketing Manager, medical textbooks
Mosby–Year Book, Inc.
11830 Westline Industrial Drive
St. Louis, MO 63146

CONTENTS

PART 1

Biochemical and Physiologic Basis of Drug Action

Chapter 1

General Principles of Pharmacology

OVERVIEW

The information contained in this text is a review of the pharmacologic principles and essential facts necessary to prescribe medications in a manner that will maximize the desirable and minimize the undesirable effects. This chapter covers basic pharmacology, pharmacokinetics, pharmacodynamics, adverse effects, and pharmacotherapeutics.

SECTION 1.1 INTRODUCTION

Medical pharmacology deals with the role of chemicals to cause, prevent, diagnose, and treat diseases. The science of pharmacology includes an understanding of pharmacokinetic, pharmacodynamic, toxicologic, and pharmacotherapeutic principles.

- **Pharmacokinetics** Pharmacokinetics is the branch of pharmacology that deals with issues reflecting the presence of a drug in the body over time. This includes the processes of absorption, distribution, localization in tissues, biotransformation, and excretion.

- **Pharmacodynamics** Pharmacodynamics is the branch of pharmacology concerned with the mechanism of action of drugs on living systems.

- **Toxicology** Toxicology is the branch of pharmacology relating to the diagnosis and treatment of the adverse effects of drugs and other chemical agents.

- **Pharmacotherapeutics** Pharmacotherapeutics is the branch of pharmacology covering the clinical use of drugs to diagnose and treat diseases.

- **Chemistry of Drugs** To master the principles of pharmacology it is important to understand the physical and chemical properties of drugs, such as their solubility, degree of ionization, binding characteristics, functional groups, and so forth. One should not attempt to learn the structure of every drug, but it is important to become acquainted with general structural features or functional groups of major drug classes. This will result in understanding the pharmacologic actions of drugs.

- **Ionization Properties of Drugs** Knowledge of ionization properties is necessary to understand what determines the ability of a drug to penetrate cell membranes, to distribute throughout the body, and to interact with biologic receptors. At physiologic pH, drugs can be classified as follows:

  - **Neutral compounds** Neutral compounds are un-ionized, uncharged, or nonpolar compounds that are usually more soluble in lipid than in aqueous environments (Fig. 1.1).

● **Permanently charged compounds** Permanently charged compounds are ionized, charged, or polar compounds that are usually more soluble in aqueous than in lipid environments. Many permanently charged quaternary ammonium compounds are used as drugs. *Study hint:* Quaternary ammonium compounds often end in *ium* (Fig. 1.2).

● **Weak organic acids** A weak organic acid is a compound that gives up a proton in its un-ionized form. Conversely, the conjugate base of a weak organic acid is the ionized form, which accepts a proton. Thus a weak organic acid can exist in both a lipid-soluble and a water-soluble form, which is determined by its pK_a and the pH of its environment (Fig. 1.3).

● **Weak organic bases** A weak organic base is a compound that accepts a proton in its un-ionized form. Conversely, the conjugate acid of a weak base is a compound that donates a proton. Like weak organic acids, a weak organic base may exist in both a water-soluble and lipid-soluble form, depending on its pK_a and the pH of its environment (Fig. 1.4).

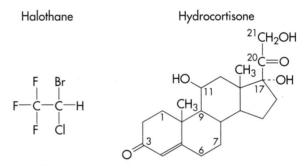

Halothane

Hydrocortisone

Fig. 1.1 Structures of neutral compounds.

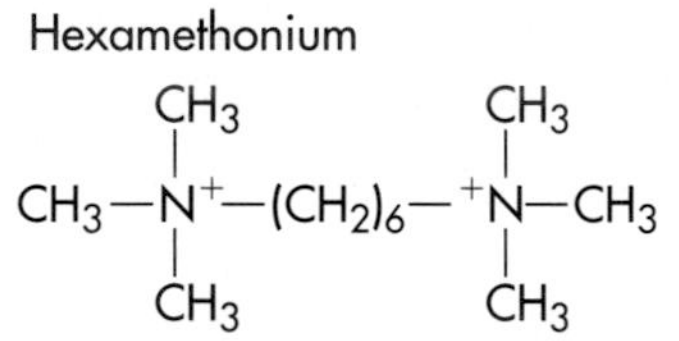

Hexamethonium

$$CH_3-\overset{\overset{\displaystyle CH_3}{|}}{\underset{\underset{\displaystyle CH_3}{|}}{N^+}}-(CH_2)_6-\overset{\overset{\displaystyle CH_3}{|}}{\underset{\underset{\displaystyle CH_3}{|}}{^+N}}-CH_3$$

Fig. 1.2 Structure of hexamethonium.

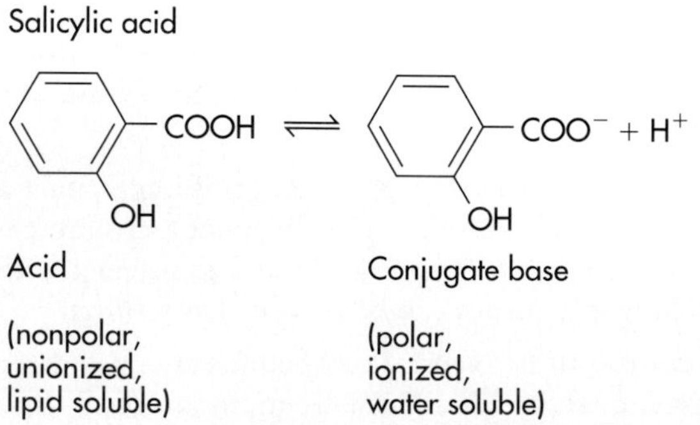

Salicylic acid

Acid

(nonpolar,
unionized,
lipid soluble)

Conjugate base

(polar,
ionized,
water soluble)

Fig. 1.3 Ionization of a weak organic acid.

Amphetamine

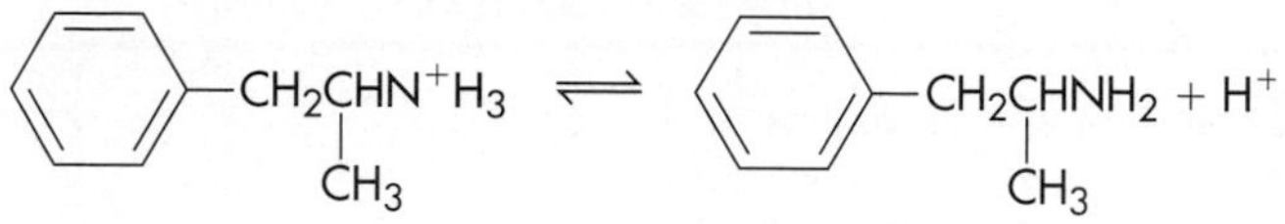

$$\underset{\underset{\text{CH}_3}{|}}{\text{CH}_2\text{CHN}^+\text{H}_3} \rightleftharpoons \underset{\underset{\text{CH}_3}{|}}{\text{CH}_2\text{CHNH}_2} + \text{H}^+$$

Conjugate acid   Base

(polar,   (nonpolar,
ionized,   unionized,
water soluble)   lipid soluble)

Fig. 1.4 Ionization of a weak organic base.

Many drugs are weak organic acids or bases because it is advantageous for a drug to have the potential to exist in both a water-soluble form when it is ionized (polar) and a lipid-soluble form when it is un-ionized (nonpolar) to facilitate diffusion through aqueous environments (body fluids) and lipid environments (biologic membranes). Weak organic acids are best at traversing biologic membranes at acidic pH, whereas weak organic bases penetrate membranes best at basic pH.

■ **Calculation of Ionized Versus Un-ionized Compounds** The degree of ionization is a function of the pK_a of the molecule and the pH of its environment.

The pK_a is a measure of the acidity of a drug or its ability to donate a proton. The lower the pK_a, the more acidic the drug.

When a drug is exposed to a pH equal to its pK_a, 50% of the molecules will be in the ionized form and 50% in the un-ionized form.

The percentage of drug molecules existing in the ionized and un-ionized forms can be calculated using the Henderson-Hasselbalch equation (Box 1.1) or as exemplified using the simplified rules presented in Boxes 1.2 and 1.3.

Box 1.1

HENDERSON-HASSELBALCH EQUATION
$\log \dfrac{\text{(protonated form)}}{\text{(unprotonated form)}} = pK_a - pH$

Problem: What percentage of phenobarbital (pK_a = 7.4), a weak organic acid, exists in the ionized form in the urine at pH 6.4? Simple solution in Box 1.2.

Problem: What percentage of cocaine (weak base; pK_a = 8.5) exists in the unionized form in the stomach at pH 2.5? Simple solution in Box 1.3.

■ **Binding Forces in Drug Interactions**

● **Covalent bond** Covalent bonds are uncommon for drugs because these types of bonds are very stable (100 kcal/mol) and therefore produce a prolonged and perhaps irreversible response. Normally a transient response is sought because it can be regulated. However, some drugs do form covalent bonds.

● **Hydrogen bonds** Relatively weak hydrogen bonds (2.5 kcal/mol) form between hydrogen and nitrogen or oxygen. Hydrogen bonds are common in water-soluble drugs.

● **Ionic bonds** Either cationic or anionic, ionic bonds are about twice as strong as hydrogen bonds (5 kcal/mol).

Covalent Bonds

phenoxybenzamine—
  alkylating
neostigmine—acylating
paraoxon—phosphorylating

Box 1.2

SIMPLE SOLUTION

Write the equation for a weak acid:

$$HA \rightleftharpoons A^- + H^-$$

Acid   Conjugate base
un-ionized   ionized

Find the absolute difference between pK_a and pH.

$|pK_a - pH| = \Delta$

$|7.4 - 6.4| = 1$

Take antilog of difference (Δ) = magnitude of ratio between the ionized and un-ionized forms of the drug.

antilog of Δ

antilog of 1 = 10

If pH = pK_a then HA = A^-.

If pH is less than pK_a, the acid form (HA) will **always** predominate.

If pH is greater than pK_a, the basic form (A^-) will **always** predominate.

Because the pH (6.4) is less than the pK_a (7.4), the acid form of phenobarbital will predominate.

Thus the ratio of

$$\frac{HA}{A^-} = \frac{10}{1}$$

% ionized =

$$\frac{A^-}{A^- + HA} \times 100$$

$$= \frac{1}{1 + 10} \times 100 \cong 9\% \text{ ionized}$$

Box 1.3

SIMPLE SOLUTION

Write the equation for a *weak base* as the *conjugate acid*:

$$HB^+ \rightleftharpoons B + H^+$$

Conjugate acid   Base
ionized   un-ionized

We will always use pK_a in this text:

$pK_a + pK_b = 14$

Find the absolute difference (Δ) between pK_a and pH.

$|pK_a - pH| = \Delta$

$|8.5 - 2.5| = 6$

Take antilog of difference (Δ) = magnitude of ratio between the ionized and un-ionized forms of the drug.

antilog of Δ

antilog of 6 = 1,000,000

If pH = pK_a then HB^+ = B.

If pH is less than pK_a, the acid form (HB^+) will **always** predominate.

If pH is greater than pK_a, the basic form (B) will **always** predominate.

Because the pH (2.5) is less than the pK_a (8.5), the acid form will predominate.

Thus the ratio of

$$\frac{HB^+}{B} = \frac{1,000,000}{1}$$

% un-ionized =

$$\frac{B}{HB^+ + B} \times 100$$

$$\cong 1 \times 10^{-4}\%$$

- **Weaker bonds** Weaker bonds include dipole-dipole interactions and van der Waals forces. These bonds are approximately 0.5 kcal/mol and occur only when chemical agents are in close proximity with one another, that is, the van der Waals forces vary with the seventh power of the separating distance. Although these bonds are weak, the summation of several groups in a molecule exhibiting such forces could be considerable.

- **Hydrophobic interactions** Refers to the degree of attachment resulting from the exclusion of water molecules by nonpolar groups (not strictly bonding).

■ **Drug Permeation** Relates to the movement of drug molecules into the body from the site of administration (absorption), their movement among organs and tissues (distribution), and their elimination (excretion). Because the body is protected from the outside environment and is itself internally compartmentalized by membrane barriers, permeation of drug molecules across biologic membranes plays a role in determining their clinical action.

Drug Permeation
Filtration
Passive diffusion
Active transport
Facilitated diffusion
Pinocytosis

- **Aqueous diffusion or filtration** Drugs enter or exit cells through small aqueous pores in membranes. In most membranes (e.g., the epithelial lining of the surfaces of the body, such as the cornea, intestine, and bladder), cells are connected by tight junctions, and therefore only very small molecules (molecular weight [MW] < 100 to 150; e.g., Li^+, methanol) are able to pass by this mechanism. In contrast, most capillaries have large pores between cells that allow molecules as large as MW 20,000 to 30,000 to cross. Although most capillaries in the brain lack these pores (blood-brain barrier) areas such as the pituitary and pineal glands, the medium eminence, the area postrema, and the choroid plexus are vascularized by capillaries with pores large enough for many molecules to transverse. The largest pores exist in the endothelial cells of the kidney glomeruli. Thus glomerular filtration is an important excretory pathway for drugs.

- **Lipid diffusion or passive diffusion** Most drugs cross biologic membranes by directly passing through the lipid bilayers, a process driven by a concentration gradient. This is a relatively slow, nonsaturable process. A high degree of lipid solubility relative to aqueous solubility (often quantitated as the octanol/water or olive oil/water partition coefficient) favors this mode of permeation. Inasmuch as drugs must first be in aqueous solution to gain access to the lipid membrane, too little water solubility is also undesirable. Recall that weak organic acids are best at crossing lipid membranes in acidic environments, whereas weak organic bases cross lipid membranes most easily in basic environments.

- **Active transport** Characteristics of active transport include substrate selectivity, competitive inhibition by chemical congeners, a requirement for energy, saturability, and movement against an electrochemical gradient. Active transport is responsible for the movement of some drugs across neuronal membranes, the choroid plexus, renal tubular cells, and hepatocytes. This is rapid but is of limited capacity because there is a limited number of carrier molecules. Transport molecules are also a site of drug interactions.

- **Facilitated diffusion** Facilitated diffusion is a carrier-mediated process that does not require energy; therefore movement of chemicals cannot occur against a concentration gradient. This process is responsible for the transport of sugars, amino acids, purines, pyrimidines, and other water-soluble solutes across most cell membranes. This process differs from active transport in that it is slower, is not energy dependent, and cannot transport a solute against a chemical gradient.

● **Pinocytosis** Drugs of exceptionally large size (MW over 1000) enter cells only by pinocytosis, a process whereby the cell engulfs extracellular material within membrane vesicles. This is of importance for only a few chemicals, most of them proteins (e.g., botulinum toxin).

Absorption
Solubility
Dissolution
Concentration
Circulation
Surface
pH
Contact time
Route

SECTION 1.2 PHARMACOKINETICS

The pharmacokinetic properties of a drug relate to its absorption, distribution, biotransformation, and excretion and the relationship of these processes to the intensity and duration of the clinical responses (Fig. 1.5).

■ **Absorption** Absorption is the process whereby a drug gains entry into body fluids, usually blood, that distribute it throughout the organism.

● **Factors that modify absorption** Factors that influence the absorption of drugs include solubility, dissolution, concentration, circulation, surface, pH, contact time, and route.

— *Solubility* Drugs administered in aqueous solution are absorbed more readily than those in oily solution, suspension, or solid form because the former mixes more readily with the aqueous phase at the absorptive sites.

— *Dissolution* Drugs administered in solid form (tablets) must dissolve in the aqueous environment before they can be absorbed. The rate of dissolution depends on the formulation itself and the patient, and therefore there is variation in the rate of absorption among patients and among products formulated by different manufacturers. For drugs given orally, factors affecting the dissolution rate include aqueous solubility, particle size, crystalline form, salt form, rate of disintegration of the tablet or capsule, and gastrointestinal pH, motility, and content.

— *Concentration* Drugs administered at high concentrations are absorbed more readily than dilute agents.

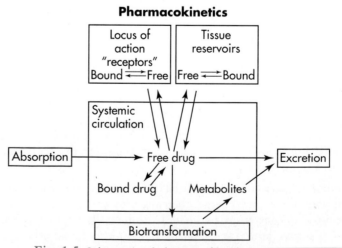

Fig. 1.5 Schematic of pharmacokinetic processes.

— *Blood flow* Increased blood flow at the absorbing surface brought about by massage or heating enhances absorption. Decreased blood flow, such as that caused by vasoconstrictors (e.g., epinephrine used with topical anesthetics), shock, cold compresses, or disease, slows absorption. Because the blood supply to subcutaneous tissues is usually lower than to muscle, the rate of absorption from a subcutaneous site is usually slower than from an intramuscular site.

— *Absorbing surface* This is one of the most important determinants of the rate of absorption. Drugs are absorbed rapidly from organs with large surface areas, such as the lung and intestine. This is also why drugs are absorbed more completely from the duodenum than the stomach.

— *pH* The pH determines the relative amount of drug in the ionized or un-ionized forms for weak acids and bases, which, in turn, affects their solubility in lipid and aqueous environments.

— *Contact time* The longer a drug remains in contact with tissues, the greater the amount absorbed. Because of its length and surface area, drugs stay in contact with the small intestine longer than other areas of the gastrointestinal system.

● Routes of administration

— *Oral (enteral, PO)* This is the most common method of drug administration. It is also the safest, most convenient, and most economical. Disadvantages include emesis as a result of irritation to the intestinal mucosa, destruction by enzymes present in the gastrointestinal system (e.g., peptide and proteins) or by low pH (e.g., some penicillins), irregularities in absorption as a result of gastrointestinal contents or disease, and the necessity for cooperation by the patient. Also, drugs administered through the gastrointestinal tract may be metabolized by the intestinal flora or by enzymes present in intestinal mucosa or the liver before gaining access to the general circulation. Orally administered drugs travel to the peripheral venous circulation almost exclusively by way of the hepatic portal system. Thus the absorbed drug is exposed to the liver during the first pass through the body and may be extensively metabolized. This phenomenon, termed the first-pass effect, can significantly decrease systemic bioavailability.

First-Pass

Morphine
Imipramine
Propranolol

— *Gastric emptying time* This is another important factor in the rate and amount of drug absorbed. Anything that slows gastric emptying delays absorption because the drug resides for a longer time in the poor absorptive environment of the stomach before it reaches the intestine (Box 1.4).

Box 1.4

GASTRIC EMPTYING	
Slowed	**Faster**
Fats	Fasting
↓ pH	Hunger
Bulk	↑ pH
Anticholinergics	Anxiety
Hypothyroidism	Hyperthyroidism
Aluminum hydroxide	

— *Binding to food* Most drugs are absorbed more readily when administered on an empty stomach.

— *Slow release* The so-called time-released, sustained-released, or prolonged-action preparations are designed to produce slow, uniform absorption of the drug for 8 hours or longer. Potential advantages include a reduction in the frequency of administration (thereby improving patient compliance), maintenance of a therapeutic effect, and a decreased incidence of undesirable effects because concentration of drug in the blood is maintained. Unfortunately, absorption is often irregular and erratic with these products.

— *Parenteral routes* When drugs must be given by injection, several options are available.

Intravenous Intravenous injection is the most direct route of administration, bypasses the absorption barriers, and is the easiest to titrate the dose. This mode of administration is the preferred route for emergency use and is suitable for large volumes and for irritating substances, if properly diluted. Intravenous injection is not suitable for oily solutions or suspensions. There is also a significant risk of adverse effects caused by high drug concentrations immediately after injection.

Intramuscular Drugs in aqueous solution are usually absorbed fairly rapidly when injected into muscle. Depot injection of drugs in oil can be used to provide a slowly absorbed reservoir of drug. Some preparations provide significant blood levels of drugs for weeks after a single injection. Drugs that produce severe pain or tissue damage at the site of injection should not be given intramuscularly. Intramuscular administration of drugs may interfere with certain diagnostic tests (e.g., creatinine phosphokinase).

Subcutaneous Drugs injected subcutaneously are usually absorbed more slowly. Irritating substances are painful when given by this route, and large volumes should not be administered subcutaneously unless they contain hyaluronidase, an enzyme that facilitates the spread of the injected solution through the tissue. Subcutaneous injection is often used for implantation of some solid pellets (e.g., Norplant, a progestin implant for long-term contraception).

— *Intraperitoneal* The peritoneal cavity offers a large absorbing surface. However, drugs administered into the peritoneum must first pass into the portal vein, and therefore first-pass metabolism is possible. Intraperitoneal (IP) injections are seldom used clinically because of danger of infection, lesions, and pain.

— *Intraarterial and intrathecal* These routes are used to achieve high drug concentrations in specific organs.

— *Inhalation* Inhalation is used for gaseous anesthetics, agents that readily vaporize (e.g., amyl nitrite), and drugs administered by aerosols. Because of the large surface area of the alveolar membranes and the high blood flow through the lungs, drugs administered by this route are absorbed rapidly. In some cases the airway itself is the target of drugs such as those used in asthma, with aerosols routinely used to deliver agents to the bronchi. Inhalation is an important route of entry for toxic substances. Local and systemic reactions to allergens may occur after inhalation.

— *Topical* This includes the application of drugs to the skin, eye, nose, throat, or vaginal surfaces, usually for local effects. Systemic absorption is also achieved by this route. For example antidiuretic hormone is administered through the nasal mucosa.

— *Skin* Most drugs do not readily penetrate the intact skin. Absorption through this tissue is proportional to the surface area exposed and the lipid solubility of the drug because the epidermis behaves as a lipid barrier. The dermis is freely permeable to many drugs; therefore absorption occurs more readily through abraded or denuded skin. Inflammation and conditions that increase cutaneous blood flow enhance absorption by this route.

— *Transdermal* Transdermal application of drugs is typically used as a means of obtaining systemic effects. Special formulations are available that enhance the rapid and controlled permeation of many substances through the skin. An example is the administration of nitroglycerin via a transdermal tape formulation with the dose regulated by the length of the tape applied. Patches containing scopolamine, placed behind the ear, provide protection against motion sickness. A transdermal preparation of clonidine that reduces blood pressure for 7 days after a single application is now available.

— *Eye* Ophthalmic drugs are often applied topically for their local effects.

— *Buccal or sublingual* This route is important for drugs that must be self-administered but are extensively degraded by the first-pass effect (e.g., nitroglycerin). Blood flow through the buccal mucosa is high and venous drainage is into systemic veins, not the portal circulation.

— *Rectal* This route is useful when oral ingestion is precluded by vomiting or when the patient is unconscious. In addition, absorbed drug does not pass through the liver before entering the systemic circulation. However, rectal absorption is often irregular and incomplete, and many drugs irritate the rectal mucosa.

■ **Distribution** Once a drug has entered the circulation, it is usually distributed to different physical compartments in the body (Fig. 1.6).

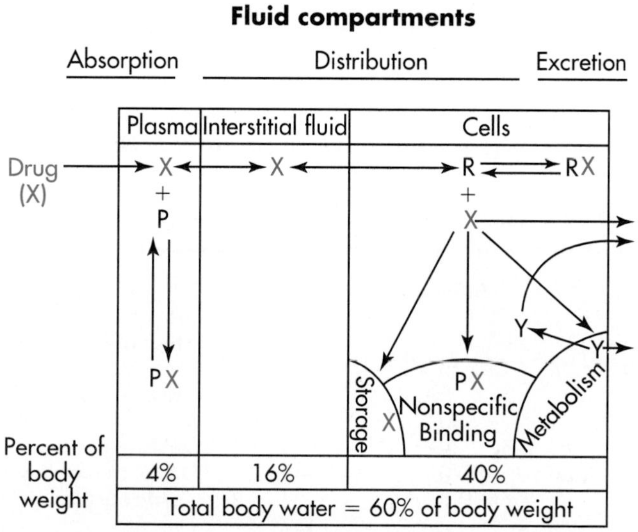

Fluid compartments

	Absorption	Distribution	Excretion
	Plasma	Interstitial fluid	Cells	

Drug (X) → X + P ⇌ P X

Storage · Nonspecific Binding · Metabolism

R ⇌ R X

Percent of body weight	4%	16%	40%	
	Total body water = 60% of body weight			

Fig. 1.6 The fluid compartments in the body. *P*, protein; *R*, receptor; *X*, drug; *Y*, metabolite.

- **Compartmentalization** Some regions in the body are physical compartments that determine the volume of distribution (Table 1.1). Factors such as gender, age, edema, and body fat influence the size of these compartments. Most drugs do not totally dissolve in these fluid compartments because they also bind to cells and intracellular macromolecules. The fluid compartment in which a drug seems to distribute is the *apparent volume of distribution (V_d)*. V_d is calculated as shown in Box 1.5, where C_0 is the extrapolated concentration of drug in plasma at time zero after equilibration.

- **Storage depots of drugs** Numerous sites in the body accumulate drugs and act as reservoirs, decreasing plasma levels and prolonging half-lives.

  — **Fat** Drugs that are highly lipid-soluble (e.g., thiopental, chlorinated insecticides such as DDT) accumulate in fat. General anesthetics are lipid-soluble compounds, which may make it more difficult to anesthetize obese individuals because their fat stores must first be saturated before circulating levels of the drug become significant.

  — **Tissues** Many drugs bind reversibly to various components. When the tissue mass is large, as with skeletal muscle, it may represent a sizable reservoir. A number of drugs accumulate in the liver. For example, the concentrations of quinacrine (Atabrine) is 22,000 times greater in the liver than in the plasma. Drugs normally attach to tissue components such as proteins, phospholipids, or nucleoproteins through electrostatic or hydrogen binding. Such binding is readily reversible.

  — **Bone** Because tetracyclines have chelating properties they are deposited in calcium-rich regions (bones and teeth) and therefore are not usually administered to children whose teeth are still developing. Not only will the deposition of tetracyclines discolor the teeth, it may also delay bone growth. Inasmuch as tetracyclines cross the placental barrier, they can also affect the skeletal development of the fetus. Lead, radium, and fluoride also concentrate in bones.

  — **Plasma protein binding** Drugs that have a high degree of plasma protein binding accumulate in plasma water and thus usually have low V_d, high plasma concentrations, and prolonged half-lives.

  — **Transcellular reservoirs** Drugs may accumulate in transcellular reservoirs such as the gastrointestinal tract. In this case the gastrointestinal

Box 1.5

VOLUME OF DISTRIBUTION
$V_d = \dfrac{\text{Amount of drug (IV)}}{C_0}$

Sites of Concentration

Fat
Tissue
Bone
Plasma protein
Transcellular

Table 1.1 *Body Compartments in Which Drugs May Distribute*

COMPARTMENT	VOLUME L/KG	LITERS IN 70 KG HUMAN	EXAMPLES
Plasma water	0.045	3	Strongly plasma-protein bound drugs and very large drugs; **heparin**
Extracellular water	0.20	14	Large water-soluble drugs; **mannitol**
Total body water	0.60	42	Small water-soluble drugs; **ethanol**
Tissue concentration	>0.70	>49	Drugs that avidly bind to tissue; **chloroquine** (115 L/kg)

tract serves as a reservoir for drugs that are slowly absorbed or undergo
enterohepatic circulation.

- **Sites of drug exclusion**   There are a number of fluid compartments that
  are more difficult for drugs to enter.

- **Plasma protein binding of drugs**   Many drugs in the vascular compartment bind reversibly with one or more plasma proteins, most typically albumin or orosomucoid (α_1 acid glycoprotein) (Table 1.2). Changes in
  plasma protein binding account for many drug interactions that lead to toxicity. Displacement is of greatest importance when drugs are highly bound
  to plasma protein because a small decrease in binding—98% reduced to
  92%—increases the concentration of free drug fourfold. Changes in the
  dose or disease (e.g., hyperalbuminemia, hypoalbuminemia, uremia) or administration of other drugs can change the concentration of free drug in
  plasma.

- **Placental transfer of drugs**   During the first trimester, when many
  women are unaware of the pregnancy, the fetus is most vulnerable to the
  teratogenic effects of drugs. The study of this phenomenon is call teratol-
  ogy. The most notorious example of a teratogenic effect was the thalidomide
  disaster. The fetus is most at risk during the first trimester because this is
  the period of organogenesis. There is little information concerning which
  drugs may be teratogenic, in part because there is poor correlation as to the
  susceptibility to teratogenic effects between laboratory animals and humans.

- **Mammary transfer of drugs**   The transfer of drugs into breast milk can
  have significant consequences for nursing infants and for individuals consuming milk obtained from cows receiving medications.

    Drugs enter into the milk by passive diffusion. Because more acidic than
  plasma, basic drugs tend to accumulate in this fluid. Tetracyclines, which
  chelate calcium, also accumulate in milk. Lipid-soluble drugs also accumulate in milk because of its high fat content.

- **Redistribution**   Several forms of redistribution may occur, but the
  most clinically relevant is observed with highly lipid-soluble agents. For
  example, when thiopental is administered intravenously, it is initially distributed to areas of highest blood flow such as brain, liver, and kidneys. Following this, the drug is redistributed to and stored in muscle and adipose
  tissue, decreasing plasma concentrations. As the plasma levels fall, thiopental
  diffuses out of the sites of initial accumulation, decreasing the brain levels
  and terminating the clinical effect. Ultimately, most of the thiobarbiturate is
  localized in fat, from which it is slowly released, metabolized, and excreted.

- ■ **Biotransformation or metabolism**   Individuals are exposed daily to a wide
  variety of foreign chemicals, or *xenobiotics*. This exposure may be unintentional

Sites of Exclusion

Cerebral fluid
Ocular fluid
Endolymph fluid
Fetal fluid
Pleural fluid

Table 1.2 *Plasma Protein Binding*	
ALBUMIN	**OROSOMUCOID**
↓ with many diseases	↑ with inflammation
Phenytoin	Quinidine
Salicylates	Propranolol

(via food, drink, or environment) or intentional (drugs). Some xenobiotics themselves provoke biologic responses, whereas others must be biotransformed to an active agent. Some xenobiotics are readily eliminated from the body by renal excretion or by another means, especially those of low molecular weight or those that possess polar characteristics such as functional groups that are fully ionized at physiologic pH. Most xenobiotics, including drugs, do not possess such physicochemical properties and therefore must be biotransformed to be excreted.

When drugs are metabolized, whether by oxidation, reduction, hydrolysis, or conjugation, they are usually converted to more polar substances, which are more readily excreted. Without biotransformation, many drugs could not be used because their half-lives would be measured in months.

Most metabolic biotransformations occur some time between absorption of the drug and its renal or biliary excretion. Some drugs are metabolized in the intestinal lumen or intestinal wall. In general, all of the chemical reactions are classified as either *Phase I* (functionalization) or *Phase II* (synthetic or conjugation) (Fig. 1.7).

● **Phase I reactions** Many drug-metabolizing enzymes are located in the lipophilic membranes of the smooth endoplasmic reticulum of the liver and other tissues. When the liver is homogenized, these lamellar membranes form vesicles called microsomes that can be isolated by fractionation techniques. Microsomes are rich in enzymes responsible for oxidative drug metabolism, the most important of which are mixed function oxidases (MFO) or monooxygenases. Microsomal drug oxidations require cytochrome P-450, cytochrome P-450 reductase, NADPH, and molecular oxygen (Fig. 1.8). The cytochrome P-450 actually consists of a family of isozymes that can oxidize numerous lipophilic drugs and chemicals with diverse structural features.

Selected oxidative Phase I reactions are given in Table 1.3.

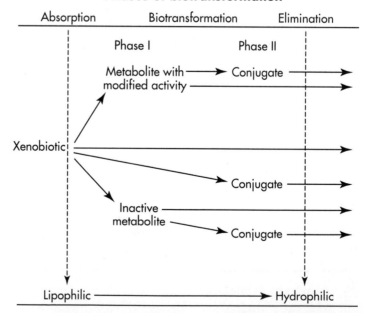

Phases of biotransformation

Fig. 1.7 Diagrammatic illustration of how Phase I and Phase II biotransformations affect the elimination of drugs.

Cytochrome P-450 cycle

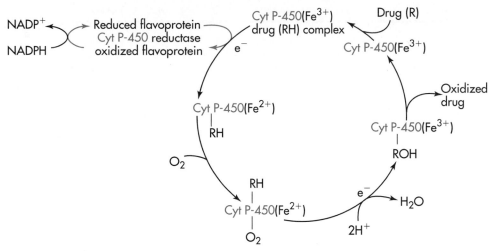

Fig. 1.8 The cytochrome P-450 cycle for drug biotransformation.

Table 1.3	*Phase I Oxidative Reactions*	
REACTION	STRUCTURAL CHANGE	EXAMPLE
Aromatic hydroxylation	H-Ar $\rightarrow$ Ar-OH	Phenytoin
Aliphatic hydroxylation	R-CH$_3$ $\rightarrow$ R-CH$_2$-OH	Pentobarbital
N-dealkylation	RNHCH$_3$ $\rightarrow$ RNH$_2$ + CH$_2$O	Diazepam
O-dealkylation	ROCH$_3$ $\rightarrow$ ROH + CH$_2$O	Codeine
S-dealkylation	RSCH$_3$ $\rightarrow$ RSH + CH$_2$O	6-Methylthiopurine
N-oxidation	R$_2$NH $\rightarrow$ R$_2$N-OH	Acetaminophen
S-oxidation	R$_2$S $\rightarrow$ R$_2$S = 0	Chlorpromazine
Desulfuration	R$_2$P = S $\rightarrow$ R$_2$P = 0	Parathion

Selected reductive Phase I reactions are given in Table 1.4.
Selected hydrolytic Phase I reactions are given in Table 1.5.

● **Phase II reactions** In Phase II reactions a conjugate is formed with a
high-energy intermediate and the parent compound, or a Phase I metabolite by way of a transfer enzyme. Such enzymes may be located in the
microsomal or cytosolic fractions of a cell. Conjugation transferases located
in the microsomal fraction, such as glucuronyltransferases, are inducible
by some drugs (phenobarbital, phenytoin). In contrast, cytosolic transferases
are not inducible (Table 1.6).

— *Glucuronide conjugation* This is one of the most common conjugation reactions for drugs and endogenous chemicals such as steroids and
bilirubin. Glucuronide transferase activity, which is inducible, is localized in the endoplasmic reticulum, mainly in the liver. However,
significant activity is also found in the kidney, intestine, skin, brain,

Table 1.4   *Phase I Reductive Reactions*

REACTION	STRUCTURAL CHANGE	EXAMPLE
Azo	$RN = NR' \rightarrow RNH_2 + R'NH_2$	Prontosil
Nitro	$RNO_2 \rightarrow RNO \rightarrow RNOH \rightarrow RNH_2$	Chloramphenicol
Carbamyl	$R\text{-}CO\text{-}R' \rightarrow RCH(OH)\text{-}R'$	Naloxone

Table 1.5   *Phase I Hydrolytic Reactions*

REACTION	STRUCTURAL CHANGE	EXAMPLE
Esters	$R\text{-}CO\text{-}OR' \rightarrow R\text{-}CO\text{-}OH$ $+ R'OH$	Cocaine Aspirin Succinylcholine
Amides	$R\text{-}CO\text{-}NHR' \rightarrow R\text{-}CO\text{-}OH$ $+ R'NH_2$	Lidocaine

and spleen. Glucuronyltransferase activity is extremely low at birth, but it increases significantly during the first week of life. Because of this, drugs such as chloramphenical, which are predominantly metabolized by glucuronidation, should not be given to the newborn. Phenobarbital is an effective inducer of glucuronyltransferase. Many glucuronide conjugates are readily secreted by active transport processes in the kidney and liver.

Conjugation reactions usually make compounds more water soluble and thus more excretable. In some cases, however, as with methylation or acetylation, reactions often make drugs less water soluble. Thus the acetylated products of sulfonamides tend to precipitate in acidic tubular urine, resulting in crystalluria.

● **Drug interactions at the site of biotransformation**   Many drug interactions occur at the site of metabolism. Important enzyme inducers and enzyme inhibitors are shown in Box 1.6.

Box 1.6

DRUG INTERACTIONS

Inducers	Inhibitors
Phenobarbital	Cimetidine
Phenytoin	Ketoconazole
Polycyclic aromatics	Chloramphenicol
Glucocorticoids	Disulfiram
Chronic alcohol	Erythromycin
	Acute alcohol

Table 1.6 *Phase II Conjugation Reactions*

Type of Conjugation	Endogenous Reactant	Transferase (Location)	Substrates	Examples
Glucuronidation	UDP-glucuronic acid	UDP-glucuronyl-transferase (microsomes)	Phenols, alcohols, carboxylic acids	Morphine, acetaminophen, diazepam, chloramphenicol
Acetylation	Acetyl-CoA	N-acetyltransferase (cytosol)	Amines, hydrazines	Sulfonamides, isoniazid, p-aminosalicylic acid
Glutathione conjugation	Glutathione	GSH-S-transferase (cytosol, microsomes)	Epoxides, arene oxides, nitro groups	Ethacrynic acid
Sulfate conjugation	Phosphoadenosyl phosphosulfate	Sulfotransferase (cytosol)	Phenols, alcohols, aromatic amines	Methyldopa, morphine, acetaminophen
Methylation	S-adenosylmethionine	Transmethylase (cytosol)	Catecholamines, phenols, amines	Dopamine, epinephrine, histamine, morphine
Glycine conjugation	Glycine	Acyl-CoA Glycine Transferase (mitochondria)	Carboxylic acids	Salicylic acid, benzoic acid, nicotinic acid

● **Diseases affecting drug metabolism** Acute or chronic disorders that affect liver architecture or function decrease the metabolism of drugs. Such disorders include fat accumulation, alcohol hepatitis, active or inactive alcoholic cirrhosis, hemochromatosis, chronic active hepatitis, biliary cirrhosis, acute viral or drug hepatitis, liver tumors, and drug-induced liver damage. Also, there is a general reduction in liver metabolism in the elderly.

● **Genetic polymorphisms influence drug effects** Genetic factors can influence enzyme levels and thereby influence the pharmacologic or toxic effects of drugs (Table 1.7).

● **Formation of reactive intermediates** Metabolism of xenobiotics does not always lead to detoxification and elimination. *Reactive intermediates* are sometimes responsible for adverse responses, including mutagenic, carcinogenic, and teratogenic effects, as well as specific organ-directed toxicities.

■ **Excretion** Excretion is the process whereby xenobiotics or their metabolites are eliminated from the body. The major excretory organs for xenobiotics are the kidney (most important), liver, gastrointestinal tract, and lungs. Minor routes of excretion are sweat, glands, ducts, breast milk, and skin. The amount of drug excreted by any process per unit time depends on the rate of elimination for that process and the concentration of the drug in plasma. Because the drug concentration in plasma is inversely related to the volume of distribution, it

Reactive Metabolites

Acetaminophen-induced hepatoxicity
Isoniazid-induced hepatoxicity
Phenacetin-induced nephrotoxicity
Benzene-induced aplastic anemia
Aflatoxin- and benzo(a)pyrene-induced tumor induction

Table 1.7 *Genetic Polymorphisms and Drug Metabolism*

PREDISPOSING FACTOR	DRUG	CLINICAL EFFECT
Glucose-6-phosphate dehydrogenase deficiency	Primaquine, sulfonamides	Acute hemolytic anemia
Slow-*N*-acetylation	Isoniazid	Peripheral neuropathy
Slow-*N*-acetylation	Hydralazine	Lupus syndrome
Ester hydrolysis	Succinylcholine	Prolonged apnea
Oxidation	Tolbutamide	Cardiotoxicity
Oxidation	Ethanol	Facial flushing

logically follows that a drug with a large volume of distribution is eliminated more slowly than a drug with a lower volume of distribution.

● **Kidney** Drugs are excreted by the kidneys by two processes: glomerular filtration and tubular secretion.

— *Glomerular filtration* All drugs with MW <5000 are completely filtered from the plasma into the urine as they pass through the glomerulus, whereas drugs with MW of 5000 or 100,000 are only partially filtered. Because only the drug not bound in plasma is filtered, those that are highly protein bound are more slowly eliminated. Drugs that are not protein bound and not reabsorbed after filtration are excreted at a rate approximately equal to the creatinine clearance (125 ml/min).

— *Tubular secretion* Some drugs are actively secreted by special transport mechanisms located in the middle segment of the proximal convoluted tubule. There are two transport systems, one for acids (anionic) and one for bases (cationic). Drugs that are highly ionized at plasma pH are preferentially excreted by this process. Tubular secretion of drugs has all the characteristics described earlier for active transport. Because this is a rapid process, drugs that are eliminated by secretion and not reabsorbed (e.g., penicillin) are cleared at a rate approaching renal plasma flow (660 ml/min). In fact, an organic acid, p-aminohippuric acid (PAH), which is actively secreted, is used to measure renal plasma flow. Unlike glomerular filtration, both the free and bound form of the drug are available for tubular secretion. Therefore high plasma protein-binding favors excretion of drugs that are secreted because the V_d is lower and more drug is retained in the plasma and available for secretion. Because tubular secretion is a saturable process, the transporters are sites of many drug interactions. A classic example is the inhibition of penicillin secretion by probenecid, an interaction that was used to clinical advantage when supplies of penicillin were scarce. Examples of compounds secreted by anionic and cationic transport systems are shown in Box 1.7.

— *Reabsorption* Not all drugs that enter the kidney tubules by filtration or secretion are eliminated immediately. Once in the tubular urine, the drug is exposed to the lipid membrane of the nephron, across which lipid-soluble drugs can be reabsorbed. This accounts, in part, for the relatively long half-lives of lipid-soluble agents. In fact,

Box 1.7

TUBULAR SECRETION	
Acids (Anionic)	**Bases (Cationic)**
p-Aminohippuric acid	n-Methylnicotinamide
Penicillins	Procaine
Cephalosporins	Quinine
Salicylates	Tetramethylammonium
Thiazide diuretics	Tetrethylammonium
Ethacrynic acid	Hexamethonium
Uric acid	Neostigmine
Glucuronide	Pyridostigmine
conjugates	

most drugs are not eliminated until they are metabolized to more polar substances. Weak organic acids and bases can be trapped in the ion form (ion-trapping) by changing the urinary pH, thereby enhancing their elimination. Excretion of weak organic acids (e.g., phenobarbital, salicylates) is facilitated by alkalinization of the urine, usually with sodium bicarbonate. Excretion of weak organic bases (e.g., amphetamine) is fostered by acidification of the urine, usually with ammonium chloride.

● **Liver** The liver has three systems for the secretion of xenobiotics into the bile: an organic acid system (anions), an organic base system (cations), and a system for neutral compounds. In general, larger chemicals (MW > 325) are more likely to be secreted into bile. Drugs secreted into bile are not always excreted but often go through the *enterohepatic cycle* (Fig. 1.9).

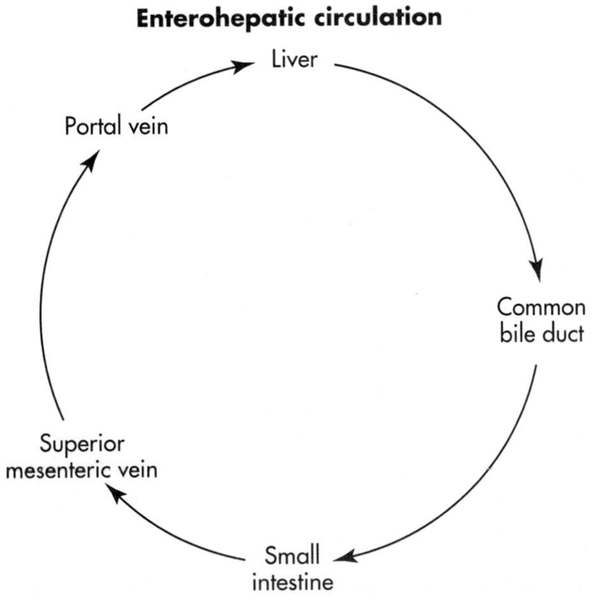

Enterohepatic circulation

Fig. 1.9 The enterohepatic cycle.

Drugs that enter the enterohepatic cycle often have long half-lives. Some glucuronides that are secreted into the bile are cleaved by glucuronidases in the small intestine, releasing the parent drug for reabsorption. Excretion is enhanced by agents that bind drugs in the intestine (e.g., charcoal, cholestyramine). Examples of drugs eliminated by biliary secretion are shown in Table 1.8.

- **Gastrointestinal tract** The walls of the stomach and intestine constitute a large lipid membrane across which drugs can be transferred from blood into the lumen. This passive diffusion process can be of importance when, for example, a weak organic base is present at high concentration in the blood. Thus, after intravenous administration of a large dose of morphine, the drug is found trapped in the ion form in the acidic environment of the stomach.

- **Lungs** Although the lungs are the most important route of excretion of gaseous anesthetics, they are relatively unimportant for most other agents. However, even the excretion of small amounts of drug in the expired air can be used for analytical purposes, such as with breath-analyzers for determining plasma alcohol levels.

■ **Kinetic Processes** The goal when administering any drug is to optimize the beneficial effects and minimize the adverse effects. The pharmacotherapeutic utility of a drug is highly dependent on the rate and extent of three pharmacokinetic processes—INPUT, DISTRIBUTION, and LOSS (Fig. 1.10). Before addressing the basic pharmacokinetic processes of drug absorption, distribution, metabolism, and elimination, it is necessary to understand the difference between *zero-order* and *first-order* kinetic processes.

- **Zero-order kinetics** In zero-order kinetics the rate of a process (e.g., absorption, distribution, metabolism, or excretion) remains constant and is independent of the concentration or amount of drug (Box 1.8).

  — *Important characteristics of zero-order processes* The biological system (e.g., alcohol dehydrogenase) is a rate limiting, or saturable, process.

    The rate of absorption or elimination (e.g., 10 ml/hr) is independent of drug concentration.

    The pseudo-half-life ($t_{1/2}$) is proportional to the dose.

    When presented graphically, drug concentration versus time yields a straight line with a single slope of -K.

- **First-order kinetics** In first-order kinetics the rate of the process is directly proportional to the concentration or amount of drug present at that time (Box 1.9). With first-order kinetics, the concentration of drug changes by a constant fraction per unit time.

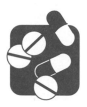

Box 1.8

ZERO-ORDER KINETICS
$\dfrac{-dC}{dt} = K = \text{constant}$

Box 1.9

FIRST-ORDER KINETICS
$\dfrac{-dC}{dt} = K[C]$

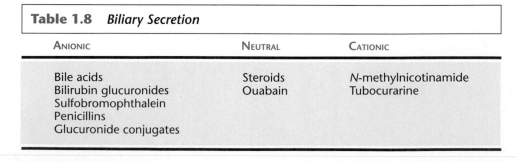

Table 1.8 *Biliary Secretion*

ANIONIC	NEUTRAL	CATIONIC
Bile acids	Steroids	*N*-methylnicotinamide
Bilirubin glucuronides	Ouabain	Tubocurarine
Sulfobromophthalein		
Penicillins		
Glucuronide conjugates		

Dose-effect relationships

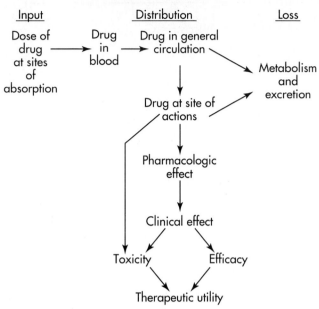

Fig. 1.10 The dose-effect relationships among pharmaco-kinetics, pharmacodynamics, and adverse effects determine the therapeutic utility of the drug.

— *Important characteristics of first-order processes* Drug concentration is rate limiting (i.e., the rate depends on drug concentration).

The drug concentration changes by some constant fraction per unit (e.g., $0.1 \ hr^{-1}$).

The half-life ($t_{1/2}$) is constant (i.e., independent of dose).

Most pharmacokinetic processes are described by first-order kinetics.

Graphically, a semilogarithmic plot of drug concentration versus time yields a straight line with a slope of $-K_{el}/2.303$.

The time course of drug concentration (C) is described by the equation shown in Box 1.10 or a semilogarithmic plot of drug concentration versus time, which yields a straight line, as shown in Fig. 1.11.

Box 1.10

FIRST-ORDER EQUATIONS
$C = C_0 e^{-K_{el} \cdot t}$ $\ln C = \ln C_0 - K_{el} \cdot t$ $\log C = \log C_0 - \dfrac{k_{el}}{2.303} \cdot t$ K_{el} = elimination constant C_0 = extrapolated concentration at time zero

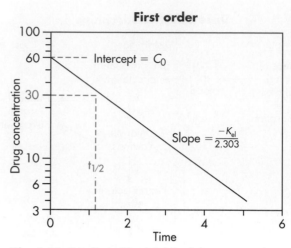

First order

Fig. 1.11 Semilogarithmic plot of drug concentration versus time for a first-order process.

Box 1.11

ELIMINATION RATE CONSTANT
$K_{el} = K_m + K_{ex}$

Box 1.12

HALF-LIFE
$t_{1/2} = \dfrac{\ln 2}{K_{el}} = \dfrac{0.693}{K_{el}}$

Box 1.13

AMOUNT OF DRUG IN BODY
$X_b = V_d \times C$

● **Elimination** Most drugs disappear from plasma in a semilogarithmic fashion, indicating first-order kinetics. The apparent first-order rate constant is often referred to as the overall elimination rate constant (K_{el}) since it represents the sum of all rate constants due to metabolism (K_m) and excretion (K_{ex}) (Box 1.11).

The time required for the concentration of the drug to decrease by one half is the *biologic half-life* or *elimination half-life* ($t_{1/2}$). The half-life of a drug with apparent first-order elimination characteristics is independent of dose. Elimination half-life can be readily determined from a semilogarithmic plot of plasma concentration versus time after rapid IV injection by selecting a plasma concentration at any point along the straight line and calculating the time it takes for the concentration to fall by one half (Fig. 1.11).

Alternatively, the elimination half-life can be determined from the elimination rate constant (Box 1.12).

● **Distribution** Following an IV injection, a drug becomes mixed in the plasma water, is bound to plasma proteins and erythrocytes, and diffuses into erythrocytes and extravascular tissue to varying degrees. This distribution is usually rapid. Once the exchange of drug between blood and the various tissues reaches a dynamic equilibrium, a constant relationship exists between drug concentration in the plasma and the amount of drug in the body (X_b) (Box 1.13). V_d is the apparent volume of distribution.

When the distribution of the drug after IV injection is rapid and the plasma data form a semilogarithmic line, the drug is said to obey a *one-compartment model*. When the distribution is slow and the decline of drug concentration is multiexponential, a *multicompartment model* is proposed.

In the case of a one-compartment model (i.e., a drug with rapid distribution) the apparent volume of distribution (V_d) is determined from the dose (D) given IV and the extrapolated drug concentration in plasma (C_0).

Problem: What is the apparent volume of distribution (V_d) when 30 mg/kg of drug X given IV yields an extrapolated drug concentration at time zero in plasma (C_0) = 0.150 mg/ml (Box 1.14)?

When a drug obeys one-compartment kinetics, it appears to be distributed into one central compartment, which determines its elimination

Box 1.14

SOLUTION

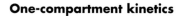

$$V_d = \frac{D_{IV}}{C_0}$$

$$V_d = \frac{30 \text{ mg/kg}}{0.15 \text{ mg/ml}} = 200 \text{ ml/kg or } 0.2 \text{ L/kg}$$

*Appears to distribute in extracellular water

kinetics. This does not mean that the drug concentrations in all tissues are equal, but rather that the concentration gradient between tissue and plasma is in rapid equilibrium. If the log concentration versus time of elimination for different tissues for a drug obeys one-compartment kinetics, a series of parallel lines will be obtained (Fig. 1.12).

For many drugs there is not a rapid distribution between the central (plasma) and the peripheral tissue compartments. An example of the log tissue concentration versus time graph after a bolus IV dose of thiopental is shown in Fig. 1.13. The elimination of such drugs is described by multicompartment kinetics.

● **Clearance** Clearance is used to describe the removal of a drug from a biologic system. Most simply, clearance of a drug is the rate of elimi-

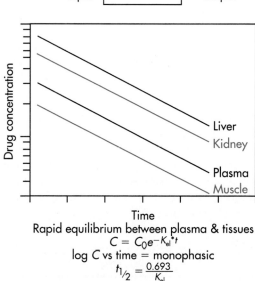

One-compartment kinetics

Fig. 1.12 Log concentration of drug versus time yields parallel lines between plasma and tissues for a one-compartment system.

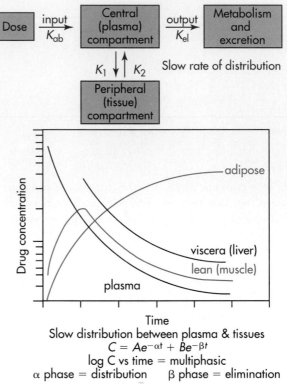

Multicompartment kinetics

Fig. 1.13 Log concentration of a drug versus time for plasma and tissues of a drug obeying multicompartment kinetics.

Box 1.15

CLEARANCE

Cl = rate of elimination/C
or
rate of elimination = Cl × C

CL = V_d × K_{el}

Cl = V_d × $\dfrac{0.693}{t_{1/2}}$

Box 1.16

RENAL CLEARANCE

$Cl_r = \dfrac{U \times C_{ur}}{C_p}$

nation by all routes relative to the concentration of the drug in the plasma. Clearance is also the apparent volume from which the drug is cleared per unit of time. Clearance can be defined by the relationships shown in Box 1.15.

— *Additivity of clearance* Plasma clearance (Cl_p) can be partitioned into components based on the various routes of elimination, e.g., $Cl_p = Cl_m + Cl_r$, where Cl_m and Cl_r are metabolic and renal clearances, respectively.

— *Renal clearance* The renal clearance of a drug is calculated by the formula shown in Box 1.16, where U is urine flow (ml/min), C_{ur} is concentration of drug in urine, and C_p is concentration of drug in plasma. For the renal clearance of an unbound drug, the concentration of unbound drug in the plasma is used rather than the total concentration.

Problem: What is the renal clearance of *unbound* Drug Z (Box 1.17)?

Box 1.17

SOLUTION

$Cl_r = \dfrac{90 \text{ ml/60 min} \times 10 \text{ mg/ml}}{0.25 \text{ mg/ml}} = 60 \text{ ml/min}$

Bioavailability

$$\text{Bioavailability} = \frac{\text{AUC}_{oral}}{\text{AUC}_{iv}} \times 100$$

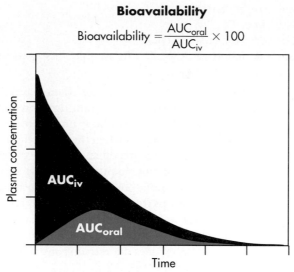

Fig. 1.14 The use of area under the curves (*AUC*) to calculate oral bioavailability.

Urine concentration = 10 mg/ml
Urine flow = 90 ml/hr
Drug Z is 75 % protein bound
Total plasma concentration = 1 mg/ml

Bioavailability Systemic bioavailability is the relative amount of administered drug that reaches the general circulation (i.e., venous blood). It is usually estimated by comparing the area under the blood, plasma, or serum concentration time curve after nonparenteral administration of a drug to that after an IV injection. The IV injection is considered to be 100% bioavailable (Fig. 1.14).

The bioavailability of a drug and the bioequivalence of two formulations of the same drug require the following identical characteristics:

Repetitive dosing

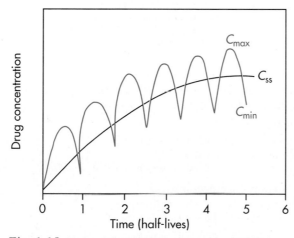

Fig. 1.15 Drug concentration versus time relationship for repeated administration of a drug. C_{ss}, concentration at steady state.

1. peak height concentration, C_{max}
2. peak time, T_{max}
3. area under the curve (AUC)

Factors That Influence Bioavailability

First-pass metabolism
Drug instability
Drug formulation

Factors that influence bioavailability include first-pass metabolism, drug instability, and drug formulation.

● **Repetitive dosing** Most drugs are administered on a chronic basis. Repeated administration of a fixed dose at constant time intervals gradually increases the concentration of drug in the body until a steady state is reached (Fig. 1.15). The steady state is reached when the rate of input of drug equals the rate of elimination. The average steady-state plasma concentration, the degree of accumulation, and the time required to achieve steady-state can be predicted from the pharmacokinetic characteristic of the drug. It is important to understand these relationships to achieve the desired target concentration (i.e., C_{ss}, or concentration at steady state). The dosing rate to achieve the target C_{ss} is equal to the clearance times the steady-state concentration. Although the plasma level of drug does not remain constant between doses, an average C_{ss} can be calculated (Box 1.18).

Box 1.19 highlights important points to consider with respect to the C_{ss}.

Box 1.18

CONCENTRATION AT STEADY STATE

$$C_{ss} = \frac{F \cdot D/\tau}{K_{el} \cdot V_d} = \frac{F \cdot D/\tau}{Cl} = \frac{1.44(F)(D/\tau) \cdot t\frac{1}{2}}{V_d}$$

F = availability fraction
D = dose
τ = dosage interval
Cl = clearance
V_d = apparent volume of distribution
$t\frac{1}{2}$ = half life
K_{el} = elimination rate constant

Box 1.19

STEADY-STATE CONCENTRATION

Plateau State

Attained after 4 to 5 half-lives
Time to plateau is independent of dose
Level of plateau is proportional to dose

Fluctuations

None with continuous IV infusion
Blunted by slow absorption
Proportional to dosage interval/half-life

Plateau Concentration

Proportional to dose/dose interval
Proportional to half-life
Inversely related to K_{el}
Inversely related to V_d
Proportional to F/Cl

- **Dosing rate** The effective dosing rate is the amount of drug (D) given divided by the time interval (τ) times the fraction availability (F). The actual dosing rate (i.e., the dose given to the patient) is D/τ and is defined by the relationships presented in Box 1.20.

  For many drugs the desired C_{ss} is known. Ideally, the drug concentration should always be in the therapeutic but not the toxic range. Because of individual variation, C_{ss} may differ from one patient to another. Thus dosage regimens must be adjusted for each patient to achieve the most desirable effects. Once a target C_{ss} is established for an individual patient, the dosing rate is as shown in Box 1.21.

- **Loading dose** Because it takes 4 to 5 half-lives to reach C_{ss}, it is necessary to give a loading dose (LD) for drugs with long half-lives. One approach to determine LD is to identify a target plasma concentration (C_p) for the first dose. This concentration should be about 1.44 times the C_{ss}. The LD can then be calculated (Box 1.22).

- **Intravenous infusion** The rate at which a drug must be infused (R_0) to obtain a desired plasma level is given by the equation shown in Box 1.23.

- **Effects of disease on pharmacokinetic processes** All pharmacokinetic processes can be affected by disease. Situations in which drug levels must be closely monitored and doses adjusted include impaired renal function, impaired hepatic function, gastrointestinal abnormalities, genetic differences, geriatric patients, and drugs with a low therapeutic index.

  Adjustment of dosage schedules for patients with impaired renal function can be made precisely for most drugs by the formula shown in Box 1.24, where G is the fraction of the usual maintenance dose given at the usual dosage interval, f is the fraction of the drug excreted, unchanged in the urine of patients with normal renal function, Cl_{cr} is normal creatinine clearance, and Cl'_{cr} is the creatinine clearance in a patient with impaired renal function.

  Adjustment of dosage schedules for patients with impaired liver function is more difficult because hepatic drug elimination does not correlate well with any of the routine hepatic function tests.

Section 1.3 Pharmacodynamics

- **Dose-response Relationships** A central question of drug therapy is the drug dose that produces a desired therapeutic action without harmful side effects. This is determined by the dose-response relations. Typically, log dose-response (LDR) curves are used for this purpose. For example, increasing doses of histamine causes a gradual contraction of the **guinea pig ileum** with low doses having virtually no effect. Responses are observed only beyond a threshold dose of about 20 ng. Higher doses of histamine (>50 µg) have no additional effect (Fig 1.16).

  - Properties of log dose-response curves
    1. LDR curves cover a wide range of doses.
    2. LDR curves are typically S-shaped, or sigmoidal with the central portion being almost a straight line, facilitating the analysis of the data.
    3. Frequently, the same effect is produced by different drugs acting with an identical, or at least similar, mechanism. For example, if drug A is twice as potent as drug B, twice as much B is needed to produce an identical response. This is true at all concentrations of B. Consequently, in a plot

Box 1.20

DOSING RATE
$\text{Dosing rate} = \dfrac{C_{ss} \cdot Cl}{F}$
$= \dfrac{C_{ss} \cdot K_{el} \cdot V_d}{F}$
$= \dfrac{0.693 \cdot C_{ss} \cdot V_d}{F \cdot t_{1/2}}$

Box 1.21

INDIVIDUAL DOSING RATE
$\text{Dosing rate} = \text{target } C_{ss} \cdot \dfrac{Cl}{F}$

Disease/Pharmacokinetic Adjustments

Impaired renal function
Impaired hepatic function
Patients with gastrointestinal abnormalities
Patients with genetic differences
Many geriatric patients
Drugs with a low therapeutic index

Box 1.22

LOADING DOSE
$\text{LD} = 1.44\, C_{ss} \cdot \dfrac{V_d}{F}$

Box 1.23

INTRAVENOUS INFUSION
$C_{ss} = \dfrac{R_0}{K_{el} \cdot V_d}$
$\text{LD} = V_d \cdot C_{ss}$

Box 1.24

RENAL DISEASE DOSE ADJUSTMENT
$G = 1 - f\left(1 - \dfrac{Cl'_{cr}}{Cl_{cr}}\right)$

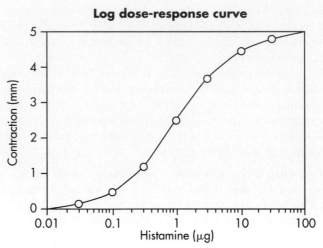

Fig. 1.16 Log dose-response curve for histamine-induced contraction of the guinea pig ileum.

contrasting a response with the corresponding dose, the curve representing drug B will always lie to the right of drug A (Fig. 1.17). In this situation the two curves in the LDR plot are parallel and easy to evaluate, unlike the two curves represented by a linear plot.

- **Relationship between LDR curves and receptor occupancy** According to one popular theory of drug action, drug molecules attach to receptors in the body to induce a biologic response. Thus the intensity of drug action is proportional to the number of receptors occupied or to the concentration of drug-receptor complexes (DR) (Box 1.25). This situation is analogous to enzymatic reactions in which an enzyme-substrate complex is in dynamic equilibrium forming a reaction product at a rate proportional to the concentration of the complex. It is not surprising that the mathematical descriptions of receptor binding and enzyme-substrate interactions are similar. The dependence of the response to a drug on the unbound concentration is characterized by an expression of a hyperbola, where $K = k_{-1}/k_1$ is the dissociation constant of the drug receptor complex. Brackets imply drug concentration. This expression is analogous to the relationship between the velocity of an enzyme-catalyzed reaction and the free substrate concentration.

Box 1.25

RESPONSE VERSUS RECEPTOR OCCUPANCY

$$\text{Response} = \alpha\ (DR)$$

$$D + R \underset{k_{-1}}{\overset{k_1}{\rightleftarrows}} DR$$

$$\text{Response} = \alpha\ \frac{(D)(R)}{K + (D)}$$

$$\frac{1}{\text{Resp}} = \frac{1}{\text{Resp}_{max}} + \frac{K}{\text{Resp}_{max}} \times \frac{1}{(D)}$$

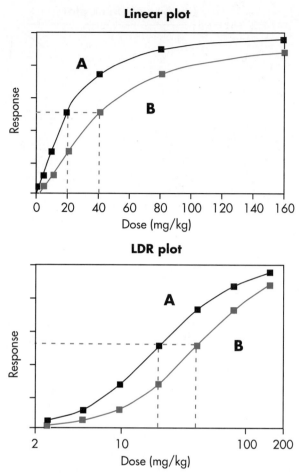

Linear plot

LDR plot

Fig. 1.17 Comparison of the linear and log dose-response curves. Drug A is twice as potent as Drug B.

The receptor-ligand interaction can be converted into a straight-line expression where Resp and $Resp_{max}$ refer to the response and its maximally attainable value, respectively (Fig. 1.18).

• **All-or-none effects** The histamine example describes a graded effect in which a slight increase in dose brings about a small increase in response in a given subject. In other situations, the number of subjects in a population responding to a given dose of the drug is assessed. Examples of such *quantal*, or *all-or-none*, responses include the presence or absence of convulsions, death, or anesthesia. Usually either the proportion, the percentage, or the actual number of subjects responding to a given dose of the drug is recorded.

Thus, for certain drug dosages, only a fraction of the subjects respond. This is usually due to biologic variations in the sensitivity of the subjects to the drug. Individuals range from very sensitive (hyperreactive individuals) to insensitive (hyporeactive individuals). Hyperreactive individuals respond to very low doses, whereas hyporeactive individuals require very large doses of drug.

• **Histograms and cumulative frequency plots** When the dosage is varied, the number (or fraction, or percentage) of subjects responding can be plot-

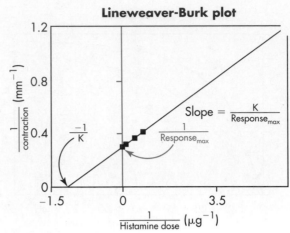

Lineweaver-Burk plot

Fig. 1.18 A double reciprocal plot of data presented in Fig. 1.16.

ted against the dose or log-dose. For example, in each of 60 dogs the rate of an intravenous epinephrine infusion is increased gradually until a 35% enhancement in heart rate is observed. At doses to 10 ng/kg/min the desired effect is attained in only 1 dog; between 10 and 13 ng/kg/min in 2 additional dogs; between 13 and 17 ng/kg/min in 6 more dogs; and so on. These data can be displayed in a *histogram* that illustrates the distribution of the sensitivity to heart rate increase in the various dogs. The histogram is bell-shaped, just as plots of any characteristic for a given population (normal distribution). The data can also be plotted as cumulative distributions (Fig. 1.19).

● **Median effective dose** It is possible to calculate doses to which 20%, 70%, 84%, or any other percentage of subjects respond. These *effective doses* are abbreviated ED_{20}, ED_{70}, ED_{84} and so on. Especially useful is the *medium effective dose*, or ED_{50}, the dose to which 50% of the subjects respond. When drugs have parallel LDR curves, their potencies can be compared through their ED_{50} values; the more potent the drug, the lower its ED_{50} value.

By definition, effective doses, specifically of the ED_{50}, relate to quantal responses. A looser, less rigorous definition, which is often used in the pharmacologic literature, extends the applicability to *graded* responses. In this case the ED_{50} represents the dose that yields 50% of the maximal response in a given subject.

Drug Receptors

● **Definition of receptor** A drug receptor is any biologic component that specifically interacts with a drug molecule with a resultant change in cellular activity. If the absorption or binding of a drug to a cellular component does not have any consequence, such as in the case of drugs binding to albumin or their sequestration in adipose tissue, the biologic sites are not receptors but rather are referred to as *binding sites* or *acceptor sites*. Thus there are binding sites associated with receptors coupled to biologic function as well as those associated with drug disposition.

● **Receptor-signal coupling mechanisms** Cells are surrounded by a plasma membrane composed of a lipid bilayer. Embedded in the lipid matrix are

A

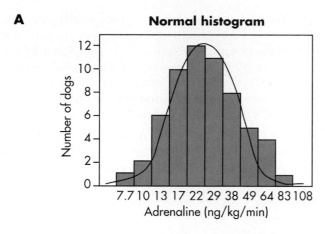

B

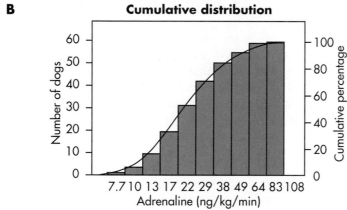

Fig. 1.19 Bar graphs illustrating the number of dogs responding to a 35% enhancement in heart rate versus increasing dose of adrenaline. **A,** A normal histogram profile. **B,** A cumulative distribution profile.

proteins that function in transport processes and intracellular signaling. The function of cell depends on changes in ion concentrations via transporters and ion channels and on biochemical signals that stimulate a cascade of phosphorylation reactions.

- **Intracellular receptors that regulate gene expressions** Several hormones are lipid soluble, cross the plasma membrane, and act on intracellular receptors. The ligand-receptor complex stimulates the transcription of genes in the nucleus by binding to specific DNA sequences. There are two important therapeutic consequences of hormones and drugs that act by this mechanism. All of these hormones exert their effects after a lag period of 30 minutes to several hours (time required for the synthesis of new proteins) and their effects persist for hours to even days after the hormone concentration has been reduced.

- **Ligand-gated channels** Many drugs act by mimicking or blocking the action of endogenous ligands that regulate the flow of ions through plasma membrane channels. These receptors transmit their signal across the membrane by increasing transmembrane ion conductance, altering the electrical potential of the cell.

Gene Expression

Corticosteroids
Mineralcorticoids
Sex steroids
Vitamin D
Thyroid hormone
P-450 inducers

Ligand-gated Channels

GABA → chloride
Nicotinic/ACh → sodium
Glutamate/AMPA → sodium
Glutamate/NMDA → calcium

— *Acetylcholine* binds to nicotinic receptors, which open sodium channels, producing a depolarization. This receptor is a pentamer composed of five polypeptide subunits. These polypeptides form a cylindrical structure 80 Å in diameter. When acetylcholine binds, a conformational change occurs that results in the transient opening of a central aqueous channel, allowing Na^+ ions to pass. The ligand-gated channel process is very fast (milliseconds).

— *Gamma-aminobutyric acid (GABA)* This binds to a GABA receptor that opens channels, resulting in an inward flow of chloride ion and hyperpolarization of the cell. The GABA receptor is composed of three recognition (binding) sites: (1) a GABA recognition site, (2) a benzodiazepine recognition site (benzodiazepines enhance GABA inhibition), and (3) a picrotoxinin recognition site. Agents that bind to the picrotoxinin site inhibit GABA receptor function and are generally convulsants.

● **Cyclic AMP as a second messenger** Numerous receptors act to either stimulate (R_s) or inhibit (R_i) adenylyl cyclase (Fig. 1.20). These receptors increase or decrease cyclic AMP (cyclic adenosine-3', 5'-monophosphate) formation. The polypeptide chain of these receptors is folded across the plasma membrane seven times, with the amino terminus in the extracellular space and the carboxy terminus in the cytoplasm. Such receptors bind to G proteins, which catalyze the formation of cAMP. Thus R_s binds to G_s, which stimulates cAMP production, whereas R_i binds to G_i, inhibiting the formation of cAMP. The coupling of a receptor to adenylyl cyclase through a G_s protein results in the conversion of ATP to cAMP. The cAMP serves as an intracellular regulatory molecule, or *second messenger*, for receptor-signal coupling for many neurotransmitters, hormones, autocoids, and drugs. The intracellular receptor for cAMP is protein kinase A (R_2C_2) which exists as a tetramer consisting of two regulatory (R) and catalytic (C) subunits. When cAMP binds to the inactive form of protein kinase A, there is a dissociation of the regulatory and catalytic units yielding two molecules of active catalytic subunits. The active catalytic subunits of protein kinase A catalyze the phosphorylation of a variety of enzymes such as lipase, phosphorylase kinase, and glycogen synthase, which are responsible for metabolic changes. These events are responsible for the metabolic effects of epinephrine on skeletal muscle, heart, liver, and adipose tissue. However, there are differences in the regulation of these reactions among tissues.

For example, isoproterenol increases cAMP levels by binding to the beta receptor (R_s), which couples to adenylyl cyclase through a G_s protein (a positive signal). In contrast, clonidine decreases cAMP levels by binding to the alpha-2 receptor (R_i), which influences adenylyl cyclase through a G_i protein (a negative signal). Caffeine increases cAMP levels by inhibiting phosphodiesterase (PDE), the enzyme responsible for the metabolic conversion of cAMP to 5 AMP, an inactive substance.

Calcium Channel Blockers
Diltiazem
Verapamil
Nifedipine

● **Potential sensitive calcium channels** Many cardiac drugs exert their effects through calcium channels. Cytoplasmic Ca^{++} regulates many intracellular functions. In some cases, it exerts its effects by binding to an intracellular Ca^{++}-dependent regulatory protein calmodulin (CaM).

● **Nitric oxide and carbon monoxide** Nitric oxide (NO) has been identified as a paracrine-type transmitter. When muscarinic receptors are activated on endothelial cells, there is an increase in intracellular Ca^{++}, which,

Cyclic AMP pathway

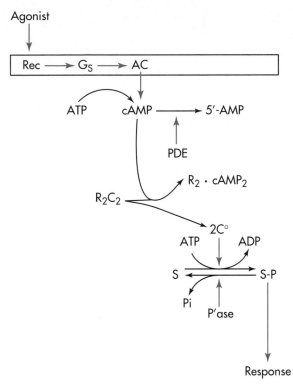

Fig. 1.20 The cyclic AMP second messenger pathway. See text for abbreviations.

through calmodulin, activates nitric oxide synthtase, which in turn converts arginine to citrulline and NO. NO is a diffusible substance that can be synthesized in one cell (e.g., endothelial cells) and then can exert its effect in another cell (e.g., epithelial cells), a *paracrine* effect. In the epithelial cell NO activates guanylyl cyclase to convert GTP to cGMP, which then activates protein kinase G, resulting in vasodilation. For this reason, NO was first referred to as endothelial derived relaxation factor (EDRF). More recently, NO has received considerable attention as an important substance in the central nervous system. Carbon monoxide (CO) may also be a paracrine transmitter in the brain. The enzyme heme oxidase converts heme to biliverdin and CO, which, like NO, activates guanylyl cyclase (Box 1.26).

● **The polyphosphoinositide signal** Hormones bind to receptors that couple with G proteins, which activate phospholipase C. Stimulation of phospholipase C results in the hydrolysis of a membrane phospholipid, phosphatidylinositol-4,5-bisphosphate (PtdInsP$_2$), resulting in the intracellular accumulation of inositol-1,4,5-triphosphate (Ins-P$_3$) and diacyglycerol DAG). The Ins-P$_3$ releases Ca^{++} from intracellular stores. Cytoplasmic Ca^{++} regulates some functions directly and others by binding to calmodulin. Also, Ca^{++} in the presence of DAG activates a protein kinase C (Fig. 1.21).

● **Ligand-regulated protein tyrosine kinases** This signaling pathway be-

Box 1.26

> **NO AND CO AS TRANSMITTERS**
>
> Activate guanylyl cyclase
> GTP → cGMP

Polyphosphoinositide signal

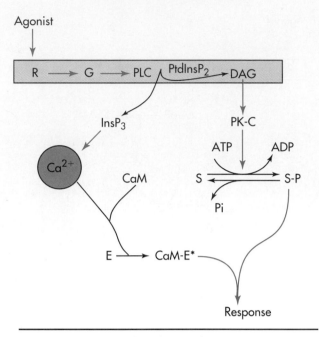

Fig. 1.21 The polyphosphoinositide signaling pathway. *PLC*, phospholipase C; *PK-C*, protein kinase C; *R*, receptor; *CaM*, calmodulin; *E*, calmodulin binding enzyme; *S*, substrates for protein kinase C. See text for other abbreviations.

Protein Tyrosine Kinase Signaling

Insulin
Epidermal growth factor
Platelet-derived growth factor
Nerve growth factor

G Proteins

G_s stimulates adenylyl cyclase
G_i inhibits adenylyl cyclase
G_p stimulates
   phospholipase C
G_o inhibits Ca^{++} channel
G_i opens K^+ channel

gins with a ligand-induced activation of a protein tyrosine kinase located in the cytoplasmic domain of the receptor protein. The autophosphorylation of the receptor causes a change that persists long after the ligand leaves the binding site. The next step is thought to be due to the phosphorylation of a tyrosine residue in a protein substrate.

● **G Proteins** There is a superfamily of diverse G proteins. The ligand receptor that couples to the G protein is thought to always be a polypeptide chain that crosses the membrane seven times with the amino terminus in the extracellular space and the carboxy terminus in the cytoplasm. When stimulated, the receptor activates the G protein located on the cytoplasmic face of the plasma membrane. The activated G protein allows the activity of an effector, usually an enzyme or ion channel. The G proteins are GTP-binding proteins. Receptor agonists promote the release of GDP from the G protein, allowing the attachment of GTP to the nucleotide binding site. When GTP is bound the G protein is capable of regulating the activity of an enzyme or ion channel. The signal is terminated by the hydrolysis of GTP to GDP by a component of the G protein itself. The slow hydrolysis of GTP allows active G protein to persist long after the ligand has dissociated from its receptor.

■ **Classical Terms Used to Describe Drug-receptor Interactions** Valuable information regarding the biologic responses to drugs following their interaction with receptors comes from dose-response studies where this relationship is studied either in isolated tissue preparations (in vitro) or in whole animals (in vivo). Some of the terminology used to describe these relations follows.

● **Affinity** Affinity is a measure of the propensity of a drug to bind with a given receptor. Thus a drug with an affinity (K_D) of 10^{-7} M has a greater affinity for the receptor than a drug with a K_D of 10^{-6} M.

● **Potency** A comparative expression relating to the dose required to produce a particular effect of given intensity relative to a standard reference. Thus a drug that exerts 50% of its maximal response (ED_{50}) at 10^{-7} M is more potent than one that has an ED_{50} of 10^{-6} M.

● **Efficacy** Efficacy is a biologic response resulting from the binding of a drug to its receptor. By definition, a receptor antagonist has no efficacy because it does not directly provoke a biologic response. However, an antagonist does have potency.

● **Intrinsic activity** Intrinsic activity is synonymous with efficacy.

● **Agonist** An agonist is a drug that stimulates a receptor, provoking a biologic response.

● **Antagonist** An antagonist is a drug whose interaction with a receptor blocks the effect of an agonist acting at the same site. Pure competitive antagonists have no intrinsic activity or efficacy.

● **Partial agonist** A partial agonist is a compound that provokes a maximal response somewhat less than a full agonist. Partial agonists act as antagonists in the presence of full agonists.

   Shown in Fig. 1.22 are semilogarithmic graphs of three full agonists with intrinsic activity (α) = 1.0 and K_A equal to 1, 10, and 100 respectively. K_A is the concentration that yields 50% of the maximal response. Under ideal conditions $K_A = K_D$, the dissociation constant for the agonist-receptor interaction. The drug represented by the curve furthest to the left

Properties of Competitive Inhibitors

• The effects of competitive inhibitors can be overcome by increasing the dose of the agonist (i.e, a reversible effect).

• A fixed dose of an antagonist will result in a *parallel* shift of the dose response curve for an agonist to the right.

• As the concentration of antagonist increases, E_{max} of agonist does not change.

• The intrinsic activity of a competitive antagonist = 0.0 (zero).

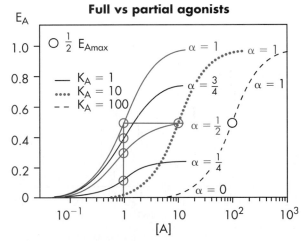

Fig. 1.22 Log dose response curve for drug A where drug A is a full or partial agonist. E_A, response; α, intrinsic activity; K_A, concentration of a drug that gives 50% maximum response.

Properties of Noncompetitive Inhibitors

Effect is **not** completely overcome by increasing the concentration of agonist.

A *fixed dose* of the antagonist will result in a *nonparallel,* downward shift to the right of the dose-response curve for the agonist.

The number of functional receptors decrease.

As the concentration of antagonist increases, E_{max} decreases because fewer functional receptors are available.

The intrinsic activity of a noncompetitive antagonist is actually a negative number because the number of active receptors actually decrease.

represents the most potent compound. This graph also depicts a series of partial agonists whose K_A all equal 1.0. As α decreases from 1 to 0, the response achieved at any concentration is less than maximal. When $\alpha = 0$, the compound is a competitive antagonist.

- **Competitive inhibitors** are compounds that reversibly compete for the same binding site as the agonist. An antagonist yields no dose-response curve itself because it has no intrinsic activity. Therefore its activity is assessed by studying its effects on the dose-response curve for an agonist (Fig. 1.23). In the example, the dose-response curve for agonist A is examined in the presence of increasing concentrations of the competitive antagonist B ($\beta = 0$). As the concentration of the antagonist is increased the dose-response curve for the agonist shifts to the right, although the maximal response to the agonist is unchanged. This indicates that it takes more of agonist A to provoke a maximal response in the presence of B because it has to compete with the antagonist for the binding site.

- **Noncompetitive inhibitors** are compounds that either irreversibly bind to the same site as an agonist or inhibit the agonist by binding to a secondary site on the receptor, which influences the binding property of the agonist site (allosteric interaction). Figure 1.24 depicts a dose-response curve for agonist A ($\alpha = 1$) in the presence of various concentrations of a noncompetitive antagonist B. In this case, as opposed to competitive antagonists, the noncompetitive agent reduces the maximal response to the agonist.

- **Partial agonists as inhibitors** All partial agonists can act as competitive inhibitors to full agonists (Fig. 1.25).

- **Physiologic Compensations and Altered Responses** When drugs are administered, the body compensates in several ways. Likewise, drug interactions, pathologic insults, and genetic differences alter drug responses. Thus several factors can modify the response to a drug.

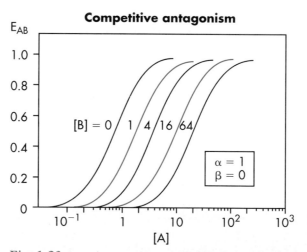

Fig. 1.23 Log dose-response curve for drug A in the presence of different concentrations of a competitive inhibitor. *B,* concentration of inhibitor; α, intrinsic activity of drug A; β, intrinsic activity of drug B; E_{AB}, response of drug A in the presence of drug B.

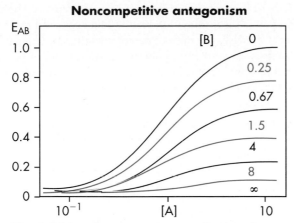

Fig. 1.24 Log dose-response curve for drug A in the presence of different concentrations of a non-competitive inhibitor (B). E_{AB}, response of drug A in the presence of drug B; B, concentration of drug B.

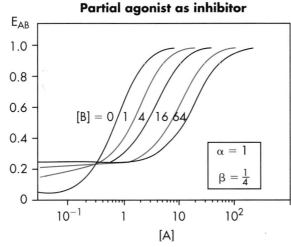

Fig. 1.25 Log dose-response curve for drug A in the presence of different concentrations of a partial agonist (B). E_{AB}, response of drug A in the presence of drug B; α, intrinsic activity of drug A; B, concentration of drug B.

● **Decreased activity** *tolerance*—the response to the drug diminishes with repeated administration.

— *In pharmacokinetic tolerance* the response is lessened because the drug induces the enzymes responsible for its own metabolism. This is also referred to as metabolic tolerance or drug disposition tolerance. For example, pentobarbital sleeping time is reduced in subjects pre-treated with barbiturates for several days. Moreover, the dose of warfarin (an oral anticoagulant) must be increased in patients taking barbiturates or phenytoin because these drugs induce the enzymes that metabolize the anticoagulant.

— *In pharmacodynamic tolerance,* tolerance develops at the cellular level. This is also referred to as cellular tolerance and may be due to changes in receptor number or function. For example, continuous exposure to β-adrenergic agonists, such as occurs in the treatment of asthma with isoproterenol, results in a decreased responsiveness to the drug. Likewise, the dose of narcotic analgesics (e.g., morphine) must be increased over time to obtain constant relief of pain because of the development of cellular tolerance. This type of tolerance is also observed with benzodiazepines (e.g., diazepam).

— *In tachyphylaxis* indirectly acting amines, such as tyramine or amphetamine, exert their effects by releasing monoamines. If several doses are given over a short time interval, the monoamine pool is depleted, reducing the response to successive doses. A rapidly developing tolerance such as that noted with tyramine, a hypertensive agent, is referred to as tachyphylaxis.

— *Physiologic tolerance* occurs when two agents that yield opposing physiologic effects are administered. For example, histamine causes vasodilation, and norepinephrine causes vasoconstriction. When administered together these agents tend to counteract each other.

— *Competitive tolerance* occurs when a receptor antagonist is administered with an agonist. For example, naloxone, an opioid receptor antagonist, blocks the effects of morphine. Likewise, atropine blocks the effects of acetylcholine at the muscarinic receptor, and propranolol blocks the effects of isoproterenol at the beta receptor.

● Mechanisms of tolerance

— *Desensitization* refers to a process that occurs rapidly, such as when continuous exposure to an agonist results in the conversion of a channel to an altered state that remains closed. Another type is when a receptor coupling element is phosphorylated to an inactive form.

— *Down-regulation* usually refers to the process of ligand-induced endocytosis and degradation of the receptor, thereby decreasing receptor number because the rate of degradation is enhanced without an increase in receptor synthesis. In general, agonists cause a down-regulation of receptors if administered at high doses for prolonged periods.

● Increased drug activity

— *Supersensitivity or hyperactivity* An enhanced response to a drug may be due to an increase in the number of its receptors. In the absence of ligand or in the prolonged presence of antagonist, ligand-induced receptor endocytosis and degradation is reduced, tipping the balance of receptor synthesis to degradation in favor of synthesis, increasing the number of receptors and therefore the response to a given dose of agonist.

— *Chemically induced* In some cases there is an increase in catecholamine sensitivity in patients administered certain general anesthetics, such as halothane. Catecholamine sensitivity may also be enhanced in subjects administered a β-adrenergic receptor antagonist (e.g., propranolol) for a prolonged period. In general, receptor antagonists tend to cause an increase in the number of receptors (up-regulation).

— *Surgically induced* A supersensitivity of postsynaptic receptors to agonists develops when the presynaptic nerve has been surgically destroyed or lesioned, resulting in a decrease in the amount of endogenous agonist and an increase in receptor number.

— *Deficiency in degrading enzymes* Such deficiencies are typically genetic in nature, with abnormal responses to drugs referred to in this case as *pharmacogenetic effects.*

  For example, there is an increased sensitivity to succinylcholine, a skeletal muscle relaxant, in patients with abnormal serum cholinesterase, and primaquine, an antimalarial, induces an acute hemolytic anemia in patients with glucose-6-phosphate dehydrogenase deficiency.

— *Competition for binding sites* Drugs may displace one another from plasma albumin binding sites, enhancing the response to one agent. Thus the dose of warfarin must be decreased in patients taking phenylbutazone, an antiinflammatory agent. If a drug is displaced from a plasma protein-binding site, the response to it is intensified and the duration of action is shortened.

— *Physiologic synergism* In this case, two drugs that produce the same or similar effects through different receptors or mechanisms are administered simultaneously, enhancing the response observed with either agent alone. For example, severe depression of the central nervous system is produced by diazepam (Valium) plus ethanol. Indeed, all central nervous system depressants act additively or synergistically with each other.

  Terminology used to describe these effects:
  Additive or summation: 5 + 5 = 10
  Synergism: 5 + 5 = 15
  Potentiation: 0 + 5 = 20

● Dependence

— *Physical dependence* Physical dependence is an altered or adaptive physiologic state produced by repeated administration of a drug. Physiologic disturbances (withdrawal, or abstinence syndrome) occur if the drug is not present. Termination of drug administration produces signs and symptoms that are often the opposite of those sought by the user. Alcohol, barbiturate, and narcotic withdrawal is a sign of physical dependence.

— *Psychic dependence* Psychic dependence is typified by compulsive drug-seeking behavior in which the individual uses the drug repetitively for personal satisfaction. Cigarette smoking and cocaine abuse are instances of psychic dependence.

— *Addiction* Addiction is a state of psychic or physical dependence.

Overextension of Response
Atropine-induced dry mouth
Diazepam-induced
  drowsiness
Pentobarbital-induced coma
Cocaine-induced convulsions

SECTION 1.4 ADVERSE EFFECTS (TOXICOLOGY)

Adverse effects of drugs may be due to a dose-dependent toxicity. Toxicity may also be assessed with dose-response curves. Other types of adverse responses to drugs are not predictably related to the dose. Examples are drug allergies and drug idiosyncrasies.

■ **Toxicity** The toxic effects of drugs are dose-related with all drugs being toxic if a sufficient dose is administered. Typically the toxicity of a drug is related to its pharmacologic activity. This relationship is usually expressed as the *therapeutic index* (Box 1.27, *A*) or the *margin of safety* (Box 1.27, *B*).

Box 1.27, A

THERAPEUTIC INDEX

$$TI = \frac{\text{Lethal dose for 50\% of population}}{\text{Effective dose for 50\% of population}}$$

$$TI = \frac{LD_{50}}{ED_{50}}$$

Box 1.27, B

MARGIN OF SAFETY

$$MS = \frac{\text{Lethal dose for 1\% of population}}{\text{Effective dose for 99\% of population}}$$

$$MS = \frac{LD_1}{ED_{99}}$$

To establish these values, studies are performed on laboratory animals to determine lethality. Results indicate the LD_{50}, the dose necessary to kill 50% of the animals. When these evaluations are made in humans, the end point is usually a toxic response (i.e., TD_{50}) (Fig. 1.26) Clinically, the concept of **benefit-to-risk ratio** is more valuable than the therapeutic index.

- **Overextension of the pharmacologic response** These may occur as mild, annoying side effects or severe adverse effects that can even be life-threatening.

- **Organ-directed toxicities** An organ-directed toxicity is associated with a particular organ or organ system.

  Some drugs are directly toxic to the fetus whereas others are teratogenic. The word teratogen is derived from the Greek work *teratos*, meaning monster. Thus a teratogen is an agent or factor that causes physical defects in the developing embryo. These effects are usually most pronounced during organogenesis, which in humans occurs from about day 20 of gestation to the end of the first trimester. The teratogenic potential of most drugs is unknown.

■ **Drug Allergies (Hypersensitivity)** A drug allergy is an abnormal response to a drug resulting from a previous sensitizing exposure that activates an immunologic mechanism. It differs from drug toxicity in a number of respects.

  - The altered reaction occurs in only a fraction of the population.
  - Its dose-response rate is unusual in that a minute amount of an otherwise safe drug may elicit a severe reaction.
  - The manifestations of the reaction are different from the usual pharmacologic and toxicologic effects of the drug.
  - There is a primary sensitization period before the individual experiences an allergic response.
  - Being small molecules, most drugs by themselves are not immunogenic.

Organ-Directed Toxicity

Aspirin-induced gastrointestinal toxicity
Epinephrine-induced arrhythmias
Propranolol-induced heart block
Aminoglycoside-induced renal toxicity
Acetaminophen-induced hepatotoxicity
Chloramphenicol-induced aplastic anemia

Fetal Toxicity

Sulfonamide-induced kernicterus
Chloramphenicol-induced *Gray baby* syndrome
Tetracycline-induced teeth discoloration and retardation of bone growth

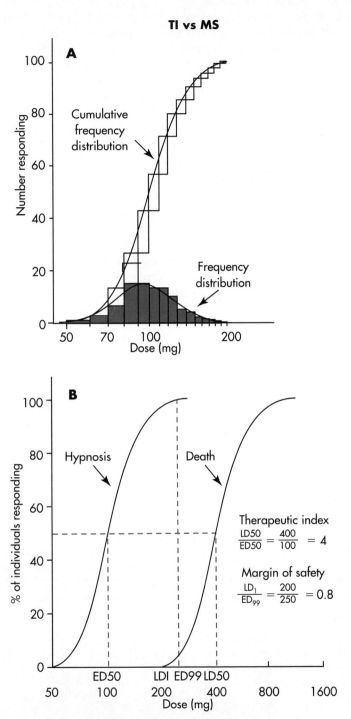

Fig. 1.26 **A,** Cumulative frequency distribution and frequency distribution curves versus drug dose. **B,** Cumulative frequency distribution of the therapeutic and lethal effects of a drug versus dose. *TI,* therapeutic index; *MS,* margin of safety.

Rather, they must bind covalently to a macromolecule or alter the structure of a macromolecule to produce antibodies.

Drug-induced hypersensitivity reactions have been reported for almost every drug. In most cases it is difficult to determine if a drug-induced adverse effect is mediated by an immunologic mechanism. Indeed, many drug reactions, such as those to biologicals containing horse serum and other foreign proteins (e.g., chymotrypsin, trypsin, streptokinase), penicillins, iodides, phenytoin, and sulfonamides, are truly allergic in nature. These drug reactions manifest as skin eruptions, edema, anaphylactoid reactions, fever, eosinophilia, anemia, immune complex disorders, and contact dermatitis. Thus drug-induced allergies can be mediated by any one of the four major types of hypersensitivity reactions (Table 1.9).

- **Type I** Allergic reactions to drugs produced by this mechanism include anaphylaxis, urticaria, and angioedema. This reaction is mediated by synthesis of the IgE antibody directed toward the allergen. The IgE molecules bind to blood basophils and tissue mast cells via F_c receptors for the antibody. When the offending drug is introduced into the body, it immediately binds to IgE bound to the sensitized cells, resulting in the release of mediators (e.g., histamine, leukotrienes, prostaglandins). These substances initiate skin and smooth muscle responses, cause tissue injury, and provoke the inflammatory response. Mediator-induced reactions can be lethal, especially when they produce bronchospasm, laryngospasm, or hypotension. Immediate treatment consists of an injection of epinephrine, 0.5 ml of 1 : 1000 solution, or 0.5 mg IV or IM. Corticosteroids are sometimes used in the treatment of severe allergic reactions. Penicillin-induced anaphylaxis is an example of a type I response. A type I-induced penicillin response may manifest as a mild urticaria, breathing problems, cardiovascular collapse, or death.

- **Type II** Some autoimmune syndromes can be induced by drugs. Damage is usually mediated by IgM or IgG binding to cells or tissue, resulting in the activation of complement. Fortunately, autoimmune reactions to drugs usually subside within months after drug withdrawal. Immunosuppressive therapy is required only in unusually severe cases.

Human Teratogens

Thalidomide
Antifolates (ex.methotrexate)
Phenytoin
Warfarin

Type II Reactions

Penicillin-induced hemolytic anemia
Methyldopa-induced autoimmune hemolytic anemia
Quinidine-induced thrombocytopenic purpura
Sulfonamide-induced granulocytopenia
Hydralazine or procainamide-induced systemic lupus erythematosus

Table 1.9   *Types of Drug-Induced Hypersensitivities*

TYPE	TARGET ORGAN	CLINICAL MANIFESTATIONS	MECHANISM
I **Anaphylactic** (immediate)	Gastrointestinal tract Skin Lung Vasculature	Gastrointestinal allergy Urticaria Asthma Anaphylactic shock	IgE
II **Cytotoxic** (autoimmune)	Circulating Blood Cells	Leukopenia Thrombocytopenia Hemolytic anemia Granulocytopenia	IgM, IgG
III **Arthus** (immune complex)	Blood vessels Skin Joints Kidney	Serum sickness Vasculitis Arthritis Glomerular nephritis	Ag-Ab complexes
IV **Cell-mediated** (delayed)	Skin Lungs Central nervous system	Contact dermatitis Tuberculosis Allergic encephalitis	Sensitized T-cells

- **Type III** This reaction is mediated by immune complexes. Serum sickness to drugs is more common than are immediate anaphylactic responses. The clinical symptoms of serum sickness include urticarial skin eruptions, arthralgia or arthritis, lymphadenopathy, and fever. These reactions usually last 6 to 12 days and subside once the offending agent is eliminated. Corticosteroids are useful in treating severe cases of serum sickness. Several drugs, such as sulfonamides, penicillins, thiouracil, anticonvulsants, and iodides can induce immune vasculitis. Erythema multiforme is a relatively mild vasculitic skin disorder that may be secondary to drug hypersensitivity. Stevens-Johnson syndrome, such as that induced by sulfonamides, is a more severe form of immune vasculitis. Symptoms of this reaction, which may be fatal, include erythema multiforme, arthritis, nephritis, central nervous system abnormalities, and myocarditis.

- **Type IV** Cell-mediated or delayed hypersensitivity often occurs when drugs are applied topically. This reaction is mediated by sensitized T-cells. Many drugs induce a contact dermatitis by this mechanism. Poison ivy is an example of delayed hypersensitivity.

■ **Drug Idiosyncrasies** A drug idiosyncrasy is an abnormal response to a drug that is not immunologically mediated. It is likely that all drug idiosyncrasies are genetically determined abnormalities of enzymes and receptors. Therefore these abnormal responses are often referred to as *pharmacogenetic disorders*. Examples include the following:

- **Apnea caused by succinylcholine in patients with abnormal serum cholinesterase** Succinylcholine acts postsynaptically at the neuromuscular junction of skeletal muscle to block the action of acetylcholine. The ensuing paralysis and relaxation of all voluntary muscles is of value in certain kinds of surgery. Normal individuals are paralyzed for about 5 minutes after an IV injection of 30 mg of succinylcholine. Occasionally patients who receive this dose during surgery remain paralyzed for 4 to 8 hours. This extreme sensitivity to succinylcholine is caused by an abnormal serum cholinesterase that is incapable of destroying the drug. Normally this enzyme reduces the amount of drug that reaches the neuromuscular junction after an IV injection and rapidly inactivates the drug as it is released from the postjunctional site and diffuses back into the bloodstream. About 1 of every 4000 persons is homozygous for the abnormal cholinesterase. Heterozygotes are intermediate in their ability to destroy succinylcholine, but they are close enough to normal not to be a clinical problem.

- **Fast and slow acetylation of isoniazid** Genetic studies in humans have identified individuals as either "fast" or "slow" acetylators. Slow acetylators have low hepatic N-acetyltransferase activity and are homozygous for an autosomal recessive gene. There is a bimodal distribution of fast and slow acetylators in the general population. Slow acetylators are more prone to isoniazid-induced vitamin B6 deficiency, which may produce anemia and various neuropathies. It has been suggested that fast acetylators are more susceptible to isoniazid-induced hepatotoxicity by the formation of a reactive intermediate leading to hepatotoxicity (Fig. 1.27). However, recent information points to the complexity of isoniazid-induced hepatotoxicity and suggests that the age of the patient is more important than the rate of acetylation. Isoniazid should be used with extreme caution in patients above 35 years of age.

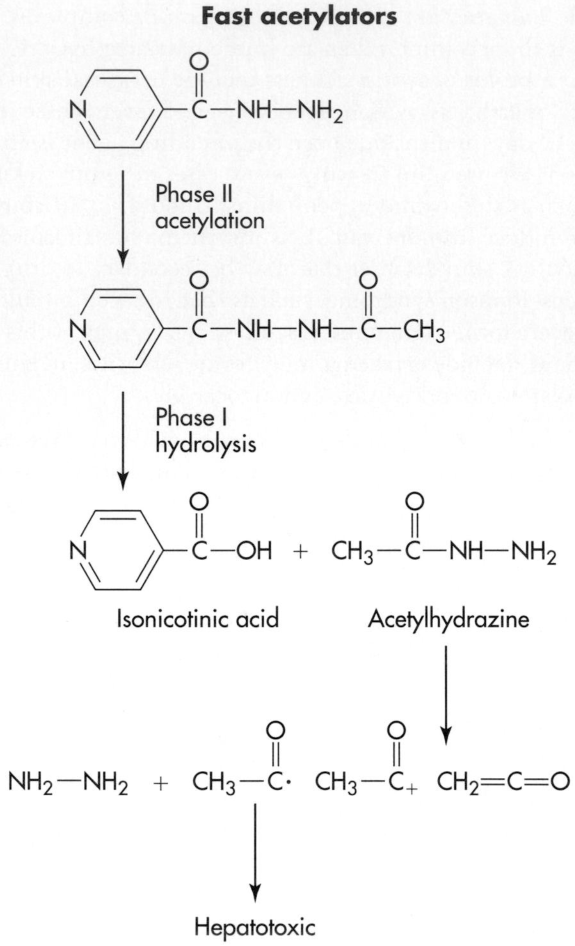

Fast acetylators

Fig. 1.27 The biotransformation pathways of isoniazid illustrating the formation of reactive intermediates.

Hemolytic Anemia in G-6-PDH Deficiency

Primaquine
Phenacetin
Antipyrine
Furadantin
Probenecid
Sulfonamides
Aspirin

● **Hemolytic anemia elicited by primaquine in patients whose red blood cells are deficient in glucose-6-phosphate dehydrogenase** About 10% of African-American males develop acute hemolytic anemia when administered normal doses of primaquine. This sensitivity is also observed in some darker-skinned Caucasians including Sardinians, Sephardic Jews, Greeks, and Iranians. In normal erythrocytes there are several processes that protect cells against injury by oxidative drugs such as the metabolic derivatives of primaquine. Primaquine-sensitive erythrocytes are incapable of regenerating NADPH because of their deficiency of glucose-6-phosphate dehydrogenase. Therefore all of the reductive processes within the cell that depend on NADPH are impaired. The erythrocytes of these individuals are much more susceptible to oxidative lysis and methemoglobin formation. Because primaquine sensitivity is inherited by a gene carried on the X chromosome, the hemolysis is often of intermediate severity in heterozygous females. Many drugs other than primaquine may also induce hemolytic anemia in sensitive individuals.

● **Barbiturate-induced prophyria in patients with abnormal heme**

biosynthesis Acute attacks of porphyria may be induced by barbiturates. Porphyria is a condition characterized by excretion of porphyrins, which turn the urine dark red on standing. In acute attacks there are various neurologic disturbances, including psychosis and peripheral neuritis. Abdominal pain is common. The genetic abnormality is in the pathway of heme biosynthesis. It appears that barbituratic acid mimics part of the heme structure, thereby occupying a portion of the heme site on the protein that regulates production of ALA synthetase. Heme is a repressor, inhibiting production of ALA synthetase, thereby reducing porphyrin production. If barbituraic acid is a less effective repressor, more ALA synthetase is produced. Because the step mediated by ALA synthetase is rate limiting for heme biosynthesis, an increased activity of this enzyme increases the rate of porphyrin biosynthesis.

SECTION 1.5 PHARMACOTHERAPEUTICS

This section covers clinical considerations that must be taken into account to administer drugs properly. Pharmacotherapeutics is based on the principles of pharmacokinetics, pharmacodynamics, and adverse effects.

Pharmacotherapeutics is Based on Principles of

Pharmacokinetics
Pharmacodynamics
Adverse effects

The rational selection of an appropriate therapeutic regimen is based on the following:

- An accurate diagnosis
- Thorough knowledge of the pathophysiology of the disease
- Knowledge of the pharmacokinetics of the drug and its metabolites in normal and diseased patients
- The ability to transfer this knowledge to effective bedside action
- A plan to make specific measurements that will reveal efficacy and toxicity and determine the course of continued therapy

This is a time-consuming process that may seem unrealistic for application in every case. For the beginning student in pharmacology a considerable investment of time is required. However, if the principles are understood, and if the results of their application are carefully assessed, objectively catalogued, and integrated with knowledge obtained in other basic and clinical sciences, the process becomes nearly automatic. Each time a prescription is written the benefits and risks of the therapy for the individual patient must be assessed. Every drug presents a risk; it may or may not benefit the patient.

Many failures in drug therapy are based on the fact that the wrong drug was used or that the drug selected was not administered using the dosage schedules that yield maximum efficacy. Other failures result when the drug therapy was not indicated in the first place. Drugs cannot substitute for thorough history taking, physical examination, diagnostic study, and non-drug management of the condition. It is just as important to know when not to use a drug as it is to know when to use it.

■ **The Placebo Response** Most patients perceive any therapeutic intervention by caring, interested, and enthusiastic health care professionals as a positive measure. The manifestation of this effect is the *placebo response* and may involve objective physiologic and biochemical changes, as well as changes in subjective complaints associated with the disease. The placebo response is quantified by giving an inert material (placebo or "dummy" medication) with the same physical appearance and properties as the active dosage form to a control group. The incidence of a placebo response is usually fairly constant, between 20% and 40% in most clinical trials. Placebo "toxicity" also occurs, usually involving subjective effects such as stomach upset, insomnia, and sedation. As expected, the placebo response greatly complicates the evaluation of efficacy and toxicity in clinical trials by *single-blind* or *double-blind* techniques. The single-blind design involves the use of a placebo administered to the same subjects in a crossover design if possible or to a separate control group. This procedure does not protect against observer bias because the clinical scientist knows which patients are receiving test agent and which are administered a placebo (single-blind). In the double-blind design, neither the patient not the clinical scientist knows who is receiving the test agent. A third party holds the code identifying each medication. The code is not broken until all the clinical data are collected. This protects against investigator and subject bias in the collections and evaluation of data.

■ **Drug Interactions**   The response to a drug may be altered by the concurrent administration of other drugs. As the number of drugs given to a patient increases, there is greater than an additive increase in the potential number of significantly important drug-drug interactions. There are several ways in which drugs may interact. Most may be classified as pharmacokinetic (absorption, distribution, metabolism, excretion), pharmacodynamic, or combined toxicity.

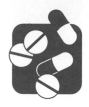

●   **Pharmacokinetic mechanisms**   The gastrointestinal absorption of drugs may be affected by the concurrent use of other agents. An effort must be made to distinguish between effects on rate and extent of absorption. A reduction in the rate of absorption may not be clinically important, whereas a reduction in the extent of absorption may result in subtherapeutic serum levels of the drug. Agents with a large surface area to which other drugs may be adsorbed may affect the extent of absorption (e.g., cholestyramine, a resin used to bind bile acid, adsorbs may drugs). Antacids also absorb or chelate drugs (e.g., tetracyclines). Anticholinergics (e.g., atropine) decrease gastrointestinal motility, slowing absorption. This may increase bioavailability of drugs that are poorly lipid soluble or may reduce bioavailability of drugs degraded in the gut (e.g., levodopa). Alteration in gastrointestinal pH may alter the absorption of drugs. For example, antacids may delay the absorption of some weak organic acids.

Drug interactions can also occur by processes associated with drug distribution. The most commonly cited example involves displacement from plasma protein-binding sites. The importance of this has probably been overemphasized, but some examples are of significant clinical importance, such as that observed with oral anticoagulants (e.g., warfarin), oral hypoglycemic agents (e.g., tolbutamide), and methotrexate, an antimetabolite. Drugs can also displace other drugs from tissue-binding sites. This may partially account for the elevation of serum digoxin levels by quinidine therapy.

The biotransformation of drugs may be increased or decreased by concurrent therapy. Hepatic microsomal enzymes are induced by many drugs. Likewise, drugs may inhibit hepatic microsomal drug-metabolizing enzymes, enhancing and prolonging the response to other agents.

The renal excretion of active drug can also be affected by concurrent therapies. The effect of urinary pH on the urinary elimination of weak organic acids or bases has already been described. The active renal tubular secretion of drugs may be blocked by some agents (e.g., probenecid inhibition of penicillin secretion).

Inducers

Barbiturates
Phenytoin
Rifampin
Carbamazepine
Primidone

Inhibitors

Ketoconazole
Erythromycin
Isoniazid
Disulfiram
Cimetidine
Chloramphenicol
Metronidazole
Phenylbutazone

●   **Pharmacodynamic mechanisms**   When drugs with similar pharmacologic effects (e.g., Valium and ethanol) are administered concurrently, an additive or synergistic effect may be observed. The two drugs may or may not act on the same receptor to produce synergistic effects. Conversely, drugs with opposing pharmacologic effects (e.g., propranolol and iso-proternenol; naloxone and morphine) may reduce the response to one or both drugs.

- ● **Combined toxicity** The use of two or more drugs, each of which has toxic effects on a given organ, greatly enhances the likelihood of organ damage. For example, the administration of two nephrotoxic drugs (e.g., amino-glycoside and cephalosporin) produces kidney damage even when the dose of either alone may have been insufficient to produce this toxicity.

- ■ **Aging and Pharmacokinetics** Some of the important effects of aging on phar-macokinetics are summarized in Tables 1.10 through 1.13.

- ■ **Federal Regulations** Once a potential drug is judged safe for human studies, a Notice of Claimed Investigational Exemption for a New Drug (IND) is filed with the Food and Drug Administration (FDA). The IND includes information

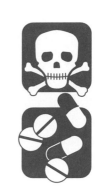

Table 1.10 *How Aging Affects Drug Absorption*

PHYSIOLOGIC CHANGES	DRUGS AFFECTED
Decreased number of absorptive cells	May decrease absorption of substances requiring active transport (mainly nutrients)
Decrease in some active transport processes	Lower levels of sugars, amino acids, Ca^{++}, Fe^{++}, and thiamine
Decrease in gastric acidity and increased (10×) incidence of achlorhydria	May decrease dissolution and acid degradation of some drugs
Decrease in volume of intestinal fluids, gastric emptying, gastrointestinal motility, and intestinal blood flow	Variable effects on rate and extent

Table 1.11 *How Aging Affects Drug Distribution*

PHYSIOLOGIC CHANGES	DRUGS AFFECTED
Decreased total body water	Decreased V_d of water-soluble drugs (e.g., ethanol)
Decreased lean body mass, decreased parenchymal cells, and decreased perfusion to tissues (with decreased cardiac output, decreased hepatic and renal blood flow, and decreased tissue perfusion)	Decreased V_d and decreased clearance
Increased fat-to-muscle ratio	Increased V_d of highly lipid-soluble drugs (e.g., diazepam)
Decreased plasma albumin concentration	Increased availability to tissues of highly bound drugs may increase response and may increase clearance (e.g., phenytoin, warfarin)

Table 1.12 *How Aging Affects Metabolism*

Physiologic Changes	Drugs Affected
Possibly reduced oxidative enzyme activity	Reduced oxidative metabolism of drugs*
Decreased hepatic blood flow (1%/yr for >25 yr) (40% from 25 to 75 yr)	Reduced metabolism of drugs with high hepatic extraction ratios (e.g., morphine, propranolol, meperidine, and lidocaine)†
Decreased liver mass and volume (1%/yr for >40 yr)	Decreased metabolism
Decreased enzyme activity (?)	Decreased metabolism (e.g., phenytoin)

*Phase II-type metabolism (e.g., acetylation, glucuronidation and sulfation) not affected.
†Drugs with low hepatic extraction ratios (e.g., antipyrine warfarin, tolbutamide, and phenylbutazone) not affected.

Table 1.13 *How Aging Affects Renal Excretion of Drugs*

Physiologic Changes	Drugs Affected
Decreased body weight	All drugs eliminated primarily by glomerular filtration or tubular secretion have decreased elimination rate and should be dosed according to creatinine clearance (e.g., aminoglycosides, penicillin, dihydrostreptomycin, kanamycin, colistin, ethambutol, tetracyclines, digoxin, procainamide, lithium, practolol, phenobarbital, and methotrexate)
Decreased parenchymal cells	
Decreased renal blood flow	
Decreased active tubular secretion	

on the composition and source of the compound, manufacturing information, data from animal studies, clinical plans and protocols, and names and credentials of physicians who will conduct the trials.

■ **Human Testing** Clinical trials are divided into four phases:

● **Phase I** (clinical pharmacology) is the first time the agent is administered to humans. This step can be taken only after adequate laboratory animal testing to ensure minimal risk. Although formerly all Phase I testing was done in healthy volunteers, patient volunteers are being used more frequently. Morally, it is thought a person should be able to benefit from the risk of taking a new chemical substance; pharmacologically, it has been found that unexpected benefits are more likely to manifest themselves in the sick than in the well.

— *Informed consent* is required from volunteers for all phases of drug testing. This entails informing the subject as honestly, clearly, and completely as possible of the risks and potential benefits associated with participation in the trial. This information must be in writing for Phases I and II. Peer review (Committee on Human Experimentation) also helps protect the interests of the volunteers.

The first dose (sometimes the first several doses) may be a placebo in a Phase I study. Because the patient's anxiety may produce psychic or physiologic changes, the placebo helps keep the clinical investigator from confusing these responses with pharmacologic actions of the drug.

The first dose administered is the minimal dose found to produce an effect in the most sensitive test animal. This is usually a nonpharmacologic dose. The dose is then gradually increased until side effects or toxicity is encountered. If it is concluded that the compounds may have clinical potential, the company begins ADME tests (absorption, distribution, metabolism, excretion) if they have not been included in the Phase I study. Phase I testing is never double-blind and usually involves 1 to 20 patients. Typically, Phase I examines only the safety of the medication and is used to establish the doses to be employed when attempting to determine efficacy in Phase II and III.

- **Phase II** involves attempts to determine the clinical effectiveness of the test agent. These tests may be single-blind or double-blind and may involve hundreds of patients depending on the condition being treated.

- **Phase III** is an extensive and comprehensive test of efficacy and toxicity and is undertaken only if the data from Phase II are positive. Phases I and II are usually conducted by clinical scientists, but Phase III may include physicians in private practice.

    After Phase III the company files a New Drug Application (NDA) with the FDA. Records of all patients treated with the drug, as well as all other data, must be included in this application. If the NDA is approved, the FDA licenses the drug and it may be dispensed with a prescription.

    Before the drug is marketed, its label must be formulated. The package insert is the official label for the drug and provides specific indications for which it has been licensed. For example, propranolol was originally licensed only for arrhythmias and could be advertised only for this condition, although it was also widely employed in the treatment of angina pectoris. Although a doctor may use a drug for any purpose, there is significant liability for difficulties encountered when administering a drug for a nonindicated condition.

    Fewer than 10,000 subjects are usually tested before Phase IV, which is postmarketing surveillance.

- **Phase IV** follows licensing, and it is here that adverse effects and toxicities become most evident. For example, the incidence of aplastic anemia in chloramphenicol therapy is only 1/40,000. Therefore the drug must be followed after licensing, especially more potent agents. As an example, companies selling L-Dopa are required to obtain autopsies of those undergoing long-term treatment with the drug. These long-term studies also help determine whether a drug is of any value in arresting the course of a chronic illness.

MULTIPLE CHOICE REVIEW QUESTIONS

1. Refer to Figure 1.28. Drug C:

    a. is a competitive antagonist.
    b. is a partial agonist.
    c. is a noncompetitive antagonist.
    d. potentiates the effects of Drug A.
    e. potentiates the effects of Drug B.

2. A 50 kg female receives a drug by IV administration. The dosage is 15 mg and the extrapolated time 0 plasma concentration is 0.003 mg/ml. What is the volume of distribution, and what is the primary compartment apparently containing the drug?

    a. 0.1 L/kg: mostly plasma water
    b. 10 L/kg: tissue concentration, like chloroquine
    c. 0.07 L/kg: mostly plasma water
    d. 0.07 L/kg: mostly total body water
    e. 0.01 L/kg: total body water

3. A 40-year-old female (50 kg) is prescribed propranolol (50 mg in the mornings) to treat hypertension. What would be the total body clearance for propranolol if the volume of distribution is 4 L/kg, oral bioavailability (F) is 0.25, and its half-life is 4 hours?

    a. 0.69 ml/min
    b. 69 ml/min
    c. 120 ml/min
    d. 600 ml/min
    e. 1200 ml/min

4. A 43-year-old male weighs 60 kg with normal hepatic function. About 80% of a drug he is taking is excreted unchanged in the urine. This drug has a half-life of 18 hours and has a volume of distribution of 10 L. As a result of recent-onset renal dysfunction, his previously normal steady-state serum creatinine value of 0.8 mg/dl has increased to 2.4 mg/dl. It was decided to change his maintenance dosage, which had been 100 mg. The new maintenance dosage should be:

    a. 100 mg.
    b. 45 mg.
    c. 75 mg.
    d. 10 mg.
    e. 5 mg.

5. The volume of distribution of tolbutamide is about 0.1 L/kg. The half-life is about 6 hours. The patient is a 50-year-old male weighing 70 kg. The total body clearance for tolbutamide is about:

    a. 1 ml/min.
    b. 13 ml/min.
    c. 26 ml/min.
    d. 80 ml/min.
    e. 100 ml/min.

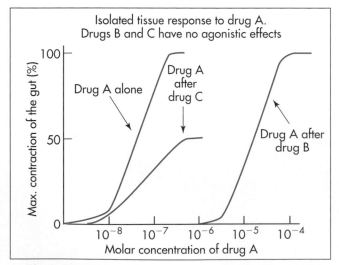

Fig. 1.28 Dose response curves for drug A alone or after addition of drug B or drug C to the organ bath.

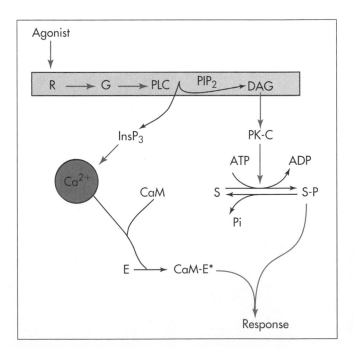

Fig. 1.29 Diagrammatic representation of the polyphosphoinosidide signaling pathway.

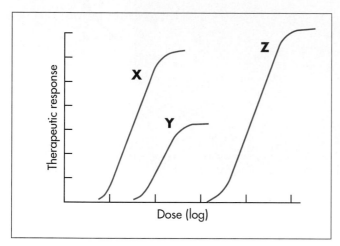

Fig. 1.30 Dose response curves for agonists X, Y, and Z.

6. Refer to Figure 1.29. Which agonist exerts its effects via this signaling pathway?

    a. Acetylcholine acting on a muscarinic receptor
    b. Acetylcholine acting on a nicotinic receptor
    c. Isoproterenol acting on a beta-1 receptor
    d. Diazepam acting on a benzodiazepine receptor
    e. Diazepam acting on an insulin receptor

7. Refer to Figure 1.30. Which drug has the greatest efficacy?

    a. X
    b. Z
    c. Y
    d. All the same

8. A placebo is:

    a. a highly toxic drug.
    b. mediated via an immunological response.
    c. a person showing an unusual reaction to a drug.
    d. an inert or dummy medication.
    e. a cellular compartment where drug transformation occurs.

9. Two pharmaceutically equivalent drug products differ only in their rates of absorption. This difference will affect:

    a. C_{max} (peak height concentration).
    b. T_{max} (peak time).
    c. both.
    d. neither.

10. The time required to reach a steady-state plasma concentration with a drug that is eliminated by first order kinetics depends on:

    a. drug dosage.
    b. the elimination rate constant of the drug.
    c. the magnitude of the drug's plasma concentration necessary for therapeutic efficacy.
    d. bioavailability.
    e. all of the above.

Chapter 2

The Autonomic Nervous System

SECTION 2.1 INTRODUCTION

■ **Overview** The nervous system can be divided functionally into two subdivisions: the autonomic nervous system (ANS) and the somatic nervous system. The activity of the ANS is generally not under direct conscious control and is concerned primarily with regulating visceral functions necessary for life (e.g., cardiac output, regional blood flows, digestion, elimination). The somatic nervous system is largely concerned with conscious control of function such as locomotion, breathing, and posture. ANS pharmacology is concerned with the study of drugs that directly affect the ANS or influence autonomic receptors on effector organs (e.g., cardiac muscle, vascular smooth muscle, endothelial cells, and glands) controlled by the ANS. To understand the pharmacology of the ANS, an understanding of the anatomy, biochemistry, and physiology of the ANS is essential.

The ANS is divided anatomically into two subdivisions: the parasympathetic nervous system (PNS) and the sympathetic nervous system (SNS). Both have afferent and efferent limbs. The afferent neurons carry information toward the central nervous system (CNS), whereas the efferents transmit information from the CNS to effector organs (Fig. 2.1). The two-neuron efferent pathways are of primary importance to pharmacology. In both the PNS and the SNS, the preganglionic cell originates within the CNS (the brain or the spinal cord) and terminates in ganglia on postganglionic nerves, which in turn project to the effectors. The only exception to this is the adrenal medulla (sometimes considered a modified postganglionic neuron), which is directly innervated by preganglionic nerve fibers. Most organs are innervated by both the PNS and SNS, which mediate opposing actions. For example, the PNS slows the heart rate, whereas the SNS accelerates the heart rate.

There are several important anatomic distinctions between the PNS and the SNS.

● **Parasympathetic nervous system** The PNS is also known as the *craniosacral division* of the autonomic nervous system. Thus the preganglionic nerves of the PNS leave the CNS through the cranial nerves (particularly III, VII, IX, X, and XI) and the second, third, and fourth sacral segments of the spinal cord. In general, parasympathetic preganglionic fibers are long and terminate in ganglia located near or within the innervated organ or tissue. The ratio of preganglionic to postganglionic fibers in the PNS is generally 1:1 or 1:2, providing for a discrete, limited response. An exception is Auerbach's plexus, also known as the myenteric nerve plexus, located between the outer longitudinal and middle circular muscle layers of the

It is important to remember that the terms *parasympathetic* and *sympathetic* are anatomic (i.e., based on site of origin) and do not depend on the neurotransmitter released or the physiologic response to nerve activation.

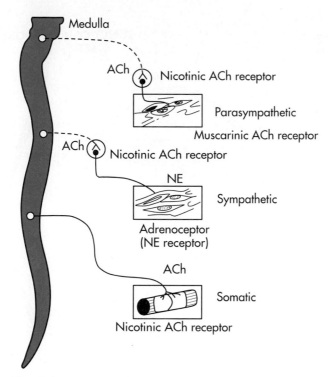

Fig. 2.1 Schematic diagram comparing anatomic and neurochemical features of the parasympathetic, sympathetic, and somatic nerves. *ACh,* Acetylcholine; *NE,* norepinephrine.

gastrointestinal tract. In this case the ratio of preganglionic to postganglionic fibers may be as high as 1:8000. The parasympathetic ganglia are located near or within the effector organ, so the postganglionic fibers are relatively short.

● **Sympathetic nervous system** The SNS is also known as the thoracolumbar subdivision of the ANS. Preganglionic sympathetic nerve fibers originate in the intermediolateral columns of the spinal cord from the eighth cervical to the second or third lumbar segments. The short preganglionic neurons pass out of the spinal cord in the anterior nerve roots and synapse with the postganglionic fibers in 22 pairs, one on either side of the spinal cord, or sympathetic ganglia. These ganglia are connected in chains, the paravertebral ganglionic chains, to each other and to the spinal nerves by rami communicantes. A single preganglionic fiber will frequently terminate on many postganglionic fibers, with ratios of 1:20 or more being common. Moreover, a postganglionic fiber may receive input from many preganglionic fibers. Because of this anatomic distribution, activation of the SNS often causes a diffuse, generalized response. After exiting the ganglia, the long sympathetic postganglionic nerve fibers traverse from near the spinal cord to the effector organ.

The *adrenal medulla* is innervated by preganglionic sympathetic nerve fibers. The release of the contents of the chromaffin cells into the bloodstream is controlled in a manner similar to postganglionic sympathetic nerves.

In general, postganglionic parasympathetic nerves release acetylcholine (ACh) to activate muscarinic receptors on effector organs, whereas post-

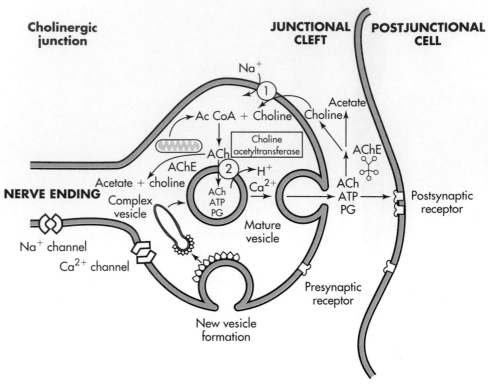

Fig. 2.2 Schematic illustration of a generalized cholinergic junction. *PG*, Prostaglandin; *ACh*, acetylcholine; *Ac CoA*, acetyl coenzyme A; *AChE*, acetylcholine esterase.

ganglionic sympathetic nerves release norepinephrine (NE), which activates adrenoceptors on the effector organs. Some important exceptions to this rule will be discussed later.

 ■ **Neurochemistry**   Neurons of the ANS communicate by releasing chemicals into the synaptic cleft to induce an excitatory or inhibitory response on the postsynaptic cell. The postganglionic neurons also release neurotransmitters to act on the effector organs, heart, blood vessels, smooth muscle, etc. Neurons of the ANS are classified according to their primary neurotransmitter: cholinergic fibers synthesize and release acetylcholine, while noradrenergic or adrenergic fibers synthesize and release norepinephrine.

● Acetylcholine

— *Acetylcholine synthesis*   Acetylcholine (ACh) is synthesized and stored in synaptic vesicles in cholinergic nerve terminals (Fig. 2.2). The synaptic vesicles contain high concentrations of ACh and peptides, particularly vasoactive intestinal peptide (VIP), which act as neuromodulators.

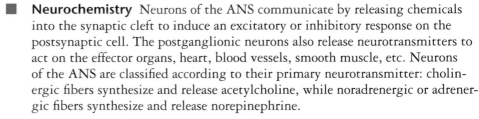

This enzymatic reaction occurs in the cytoplasm of presynaptic cholinergic nerve terminals. Choline is transported from extracellular fluid into the neuron by an active transport process. Acetyl coenzyme A is synthesized in the mitochondria of the cholinergic fiber.

— *Storage of ACh* Newly synthesized ACh is stored in synaptic vesicles, also known as storage granules, in the nerve terminal.

— *Release of ACh* When an action potential reaches the nerve terminal, calcium channels are opened. When sufficient Ca^{2+} enters the neuron the synaptic vesicle fuses with the nerve terminal membranes, releasing its contents into the synaptic cleft.

— *Activation of ACh receptors* ACh molecules released from the presynaptic nerve terminal into the synaptic cleft activate cholinoceptors on presynaptic neurons, postsynaptic neurons, or effector cells. There are several pharmacologically and molecularly distinct subtypes of ACh receptors, but all are activated by ACh.

— *Inactivation of ACh* Normally, inactivation of ACh is rapid, with the transmitter being enzymatically cleaved to choline and acetate by the enzyme acetylcholinesterase (AChE).

$$ACh \xrightarrow[\text{Esterase}]{\text{Acetylcholine}} Choline + Acetate$$

Found in the synaptic cleft associated with the receptors in the postsynaptic cell membrane, AChE is also present in tissues lacking innervation, such as red blood cells. Pseudocholinesterase, or butyrylcholinesterase, has less specificity for ACh than AChE but has pharmacologic importance. This enzyme is found in the blood, liver, glia, and other tissues.

● Catecholamines

— *Catecholamine synthesis* The catecholamines dopamine (DA), NE, and epinephrine (EPI) are synthesized in a multienzymatic process (Fig. 2.3). The amino acid tyrosine is transported by a Na^+-dependent carrier mechanism into the noradrenergic terminal, where it is transformed by tyrosine hydroxylase, the rate-limiting step in catecholamine synthesis, to dihydroxyphenylalanine (DOPA). DOPA is rapidly decarboxylated by DOPA decarboxylase (more correctly known as aromatic 1-amino acid decarboxylase) to DA in the cytoplasm. The DA is transported into synaptic vesicles by a carrier mechanism. In the synaptic vesicle the enzyme dopamine-β-hydroxylase (DβH) converts DA to NE. In the adrenal medulla and some CNS neurons, the enzyme phenylethanolamine-*N*-methyltransferase (PNMT) converts NE to EPI. Within the NE-containing synaptic vesicle is also found adenosine triphosphate ATP and peptides such as neuropeptide Y and enkaphalin. The role of the cotransmitter substances such as ATP and the neuropeptides in synaptic transmission is not yet clear.

Catecholamines
Norepinephrine (NE)
Epinephrine (EPI)
Dopamine (DA)

— *Storage of catecholamines* Most of the newly synthesized NE is stored in synaptic vesicles. There is a portion, however, present in the cytoplasm that is not in vesicles but is protected from enzymatic degradation. This nonvesicular NE is not released by action potentials but may be liberated by indirect-acting sympathomimetic amines such as tyramine.

— *Release of catecholamines* Similar to ACh, the noradrenergic vesicle releases its contents, including DβH, ATP, and peptide cotransmitters into the synaptic cleft after activation of the neuron.

— *Activation of catecholamine receptors* Released NE diffuses into

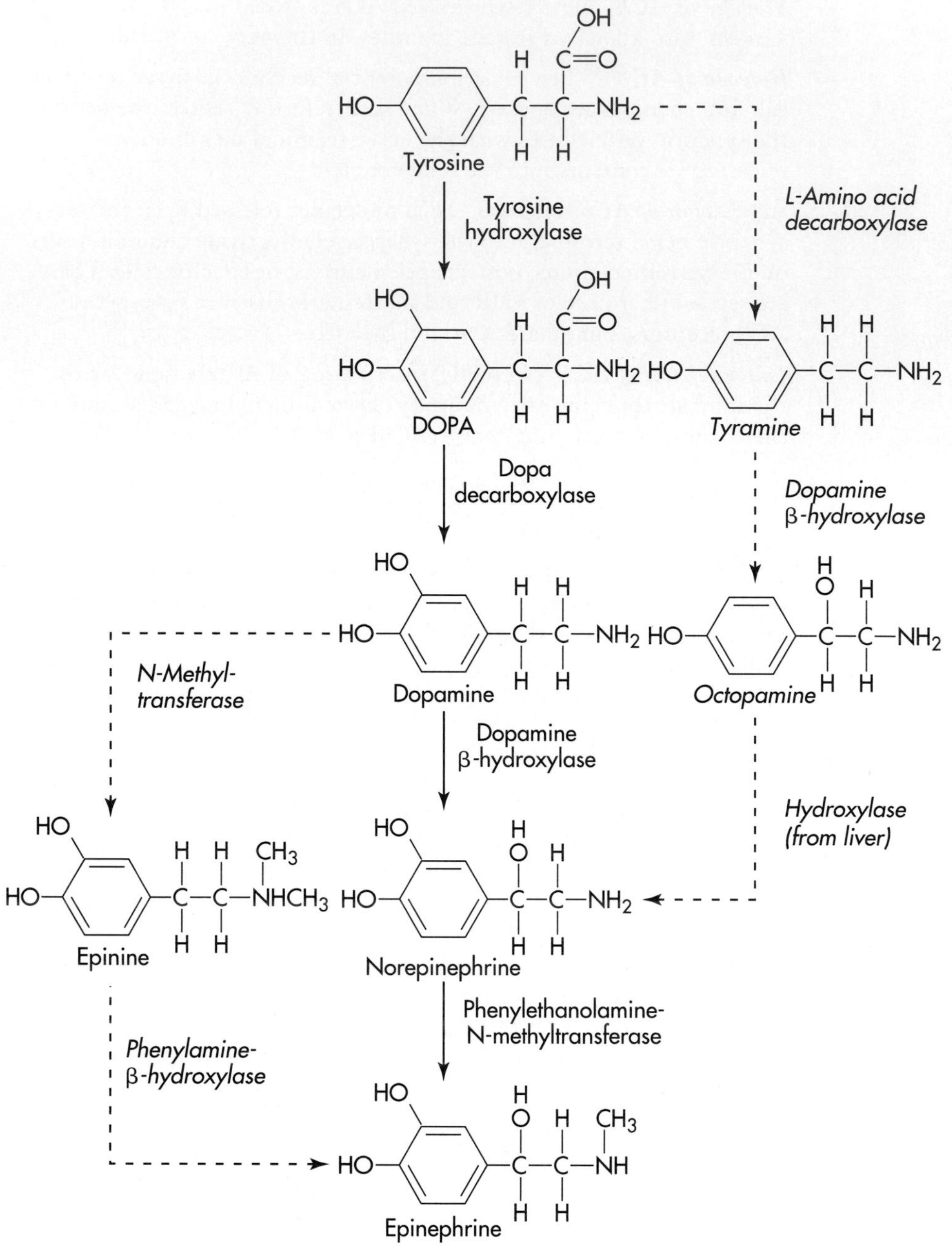

Fig. 2.3 Biosynthesis of catecholamines. The alternative pathways shown by the dashed arrows have not been found to be of physiologic significance in humans. However, tyramine and octopamine may accumulate in patients with monoamine oxidase inhibitors. *DOPA,* Dihydroxyphenylalanine.

the synaptic cleft where it can act on presynaptic or postsynaptic receptors. These adrenoceptors are subdivided into several categories (α_1, α_2, β_1, β_2) based on their molecular characteristics and affinity for various pharmacologic agents.

— **Inactivation of catecholamines** The major route of inactivation for catecholamines is active reuptake into the presynaptic nerve ter-

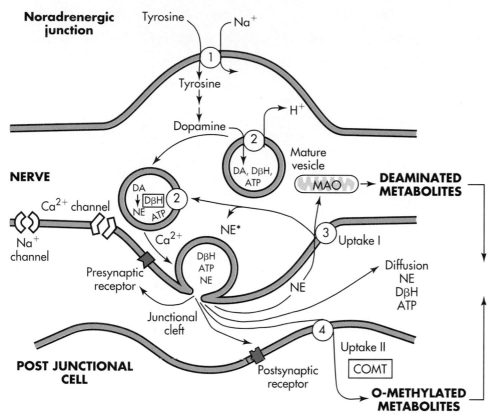

Fig. 2.4 Schematic diagram of the neuroeffector junction of the peripheral sympathetic nervous system. *DA,* dopamine; *DβH,* dopamine-β-hydroxylase; *MAO,* monoamine oxidase; *COMT,* catechol-*O*-methyltransferase; *NE,* norepinephrine; *ATP,* adenosine triphosphate.

minal (uptake I), removing the neurotransmitter from the synaptic cleft (Fig. 2.4). Subtle differences among the carriers for DA, NE, and EPI allow these substances to be selectively manipulated by various pharmacologic agents. Uptake I is inhibited by cocaine and tricyclic antidepressants. After reuptake into the presynaptic neuron the catecholamines are stored in synaptic vesicles to be released once again or are enzymatically inactivated by monoamine oxidase (MAO), a mitochondrial enzyme (Fig. 2.5). This enzyme is found in neurons, blood, the liver, and the lungs.

Another uptake mechanism (uptake II), located in glial and smooth muscle cells, also participates in the inactivation of catecholamines. Uptake II is not as important a process as uptake I. After accumulation into the postganglionic cell by uptake II, catecholamines are metabolized by catechol-*O*-methyltransferase (COMT). Uptake II is blocked by steroids, phenoxybenzamine, and metanephrine.

Deaminated metabolites formed by MAO diffuse from the presynaptic neuron, after which they are *O*-methylated by COMT. The *O*-methylated products formed by COMT diffuse from the glia or postganglionic cell and are deaminated by MAO. The inactive metabolites are excreted in the urine and serve as an estimate of catecholamine turnover. The major metabolites are homovanillic acid

Uptake I Inhibitors

Cocaine
Tricyclic antidepressants

Uptake II Inhibitors

Steroids
Phenoxybenzamine
Metanephrine

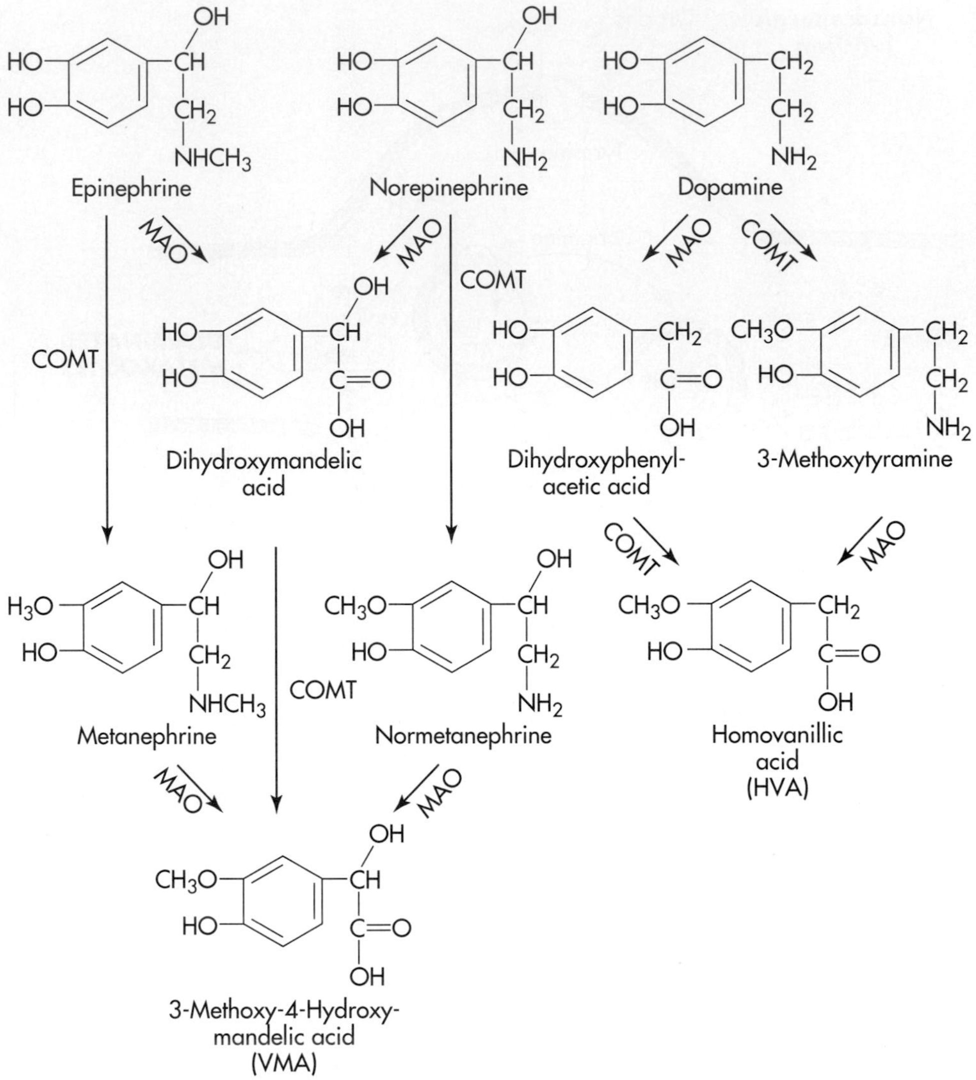

Fig. 2.5 Metabolism of catecholamines by catechol-*O*-methyltransferase (*COMT*) and monoamine oxidase (*MAO*).

(HVA) for DA and vanillyl mandelic acid (VMA) for NE and EPI.

- **Overview** In the ANS, all preganglionic fibers are cholinergic, as well as the postganglionic parasympathetic neurons. In contrast, most postganglionic sympathetic fibers are noradrenergic. Exceptions include postganglionic sympathetic nerves innervating most sweat glands and a small number of blood vessels in skeletal muscle. There is also evidence that some postganglionic sympathetic fibers innervating the kidney release DA.

■ **Neurotransmitter Receptors** Released neurotransmitters enter the synaptic cleft or bloodstream and interact with specific, membrane-bound receptors. The various receptor subtypes and their locations are summarized in Table 2.1.

- **Cholinoceptors** Endogenous ACh, when liberated from nerve terminals, acts on cholinoceptors to produce a response. Although ACh activates all

Table 2.1 *Autonomic Receptor Types*

NAME	TYPICAL LOCATIONS
Cholinoceptors	
Muscarinic (M_1)	Central nervous system neurons, sympathetic postganglionic neurons, some presynaptic sites
Muscarinic (M_2)	Myocardium, endothelium lining of vascular smooth muscle, some presynaptic sites
Nicotinic	All autonomic ganglia, skeletal muscle neuromuscular end plate, spinal cord, central nervous system
Adrenoceptors	
Alpha$_1$ (α_1)	Postsynaptic effector cells, especially smooth muscles
Alpha$_2$ (α_2)	Presynaptic adrenergic nerve terminals, platelets, lipocytes, smooth muscle
Beta$_1$ (β_1)	Postsynaptic effector cells, especially heart, lipocytes, brain, presynaptic noradrenergic nerve terminals
Beta$_2$ (β_2)	Postsynaptic effector cells, especially smooth muscle, brain
Dopamine	Brain and postsynaptic effectors, especially vascular smooth muscle of the splanchnic and renal vascular beds, presynaptic receptors on nerve terminals, especially in the heart, vessels, and gastrointestinal system

cholinoceptors, these receptors can be subdivided on the basis of their affinity for various xenobiotics. The two major subtypes of ACh receptor are muscarinic and nicotinic. *Muscarinic receptors* are activated by muscarine, a plant alkaloid isolated from certain poisonous mushrooms and are blocked by **atropine**. Muscarinic receptors are subdivided further into M_1 and M_2 receptors located on endothelial cells lining vascular smooth muscle. Although not innervated, these receptors respond to muscarinic agonists by releasing endothelium derived relaxing factor (EDRF) to cause vasodilation and lower arterial blood pressure. Other locations of M_1 and M_2 receptors are listed in Table 2.1.

ACh Receptors
Muscarinic
Nicotinic

    Nicotinic receptors are selectively activated by nicotine, a plant alkaloid. All preganglionic autonomic nerve fibers release ACh to stimulate ganglionic nicotinic receptors located on the postganglionic nerve cell (or chromaffin cell in the adrenal medulla). Ganglionic nicotinic ACh receptors are blocked by **hexamethonium.**

    Nicotine also mimics the actions of ACh at neuromuscular nicotinic receptors located on motor endplates of striated muscle innervated by somatic cholinergic nerve fibers. In contrast to the ganglionic nicotinic receptors, nicotinic ACh receptors at the neuromuscular junction are blocked by **d-tubocurarine** but not by hexamethonium or atropine.

● **Adrenoceptors** Adrenergic receptors, or adrenoceptors, respond to NE, EPI, and DA. Adrenoceptors are subdivided into α_1, α_2, β_1, β_2, and dopamine receptors based on agonist and antagonist selectivity. Adrenergic neuronal activity is regulated in part by negative feedback control at the presynaptic level. Although some α_2-adrenoceptors are located postsynaptically, most are found on the presynaptic adrenergic nerve terminal. Activation of presynaptic α_2-adrenoceptors by NE or pharmacologic agents

Table 2.2   *Some Prototypic Autonomic Drugs*

DRUGS	PROCESS
Reserpine	Promotes transmitter depletion
Carbachol	Promotes transmitter release
Tyramine	Promotes transmitter release
Tricyclic antidepressants	Inhibit transmitter reuptake
Amphetamine	Promotes transmitter release
Botulinus toxin	Inhibits transmitter release
Norepinephrine	Receptor agonist
Prazosin	Receptor antagonist
Isoproterenol	Receptor agonist
Propranolol	Receptor antagonist
Nicotine	Receptor agonist
Hexamethonium	Receptor antagonist
Bethanechol	Receptor agonist
Atropine	Receptor antagonist
Neostigmine	Inhibits transmitter degradation
Pargyline; tranylcypromine	Inhibit transmitter degradation

decreases the release of NE from the nerve terminal. Thus selective activation of α_2-receptors by drugs such as **clonidine** or **guanabenz** reduces sympathetic activity by decreasing the release of endogenous NE, although the presynaptic receptor is not their major site of action as discussed later. Likewise, activation of α_2-adrenoceptors located on parasympathetic nerve terminals decreases ACh release. Evidence suggests that activation of presynaptic β_1-adrenoceptors facilitates NE release. Presynaptic receptors that regulate the release of their own transmitters are known as *autoreceptors*. Hormones and peptides can also regulate transmitter release presynaptically. An example is the facilitation of NE release by the circulating octapeptide angiotensin II. The general location of adrenoceptors is summarized in Table 2.1.

Because of the organization of the ANS, there are many sites at which drugs can influence its activity. Table 2.2 lists some drugs and the effects they have on the ANS.

● **Physiology**   Most visceral organs are dually innervated. Usually the PNS and SNS have opposing effects, with one division predominating over the other. The predominant tone for most organ systems at rest is via the PNS. An exception to this is blood vessels, which are exclusively under sympathetic tone. The main activities associated with the PNS are as follows:

- Decrease in heart rate and blood pressure
- Relaxation of smooth muscle
- Eating and digestion
- Defecation
- Eye — the lens is accommodated for close work; the pupil is constricted for close work

The main activities associated with the SNS are as follows:

- Fear, flight, fight

Parasympathomimetic—
   mimics PNS response
Parasympatholytic—blocks
   PNS response
Sympathomimetic—mimics
   SNS response
Sympatholytic—blocks SNS
   response

- Increases in blood pressure and heart rate
- Maximum energy utilization
- Anxiety, nervousness
- Eye — lens is not accommodated for far vision; the pupil is dilated for far vision

Table 2.3 describes the physiologic effects of the PNS and SNS on visceral organs. This information is crucial to understanding the clinical response to a variety of therapeutic agents.

When considering the effects of ANS drugs on blood pressure and heart rate, both direct effects and reflex responses must be considered. Recall that an increase in mean arterial pressure causes a reflex slowing of the heart. When the NE is infused intravenously (IV), for example, it produces a powerful vasoconstriction and an increase in mean arterial pressure. Although NE released from cardiac sympathetic nerves increases heart rate, during IV infusion NE causes a reflex bradycardia by increasing the parasympathetic tone to the heart. In the absence of baroreflexes or if autonomic ganglia are pharmacologically blocked, IV NE will increase both mean arterial pressure and heart rate. This illustrates the importance of understanding the integration of cardiovascular function to predict the cardiovascular responses to drugs affecting the ANS.

Pharmacology Some generalizations can be made to help learn the responses to various drugs. It must be remembered, however, that these are generalizations and therefore do not hold true for all drugs and all circumstances. Thus activation of α-adrenoceptors usually produces excitatory responses such as contraction of smooth muscle, whereas activation of β_1-adrenoceptors increases renin release from the kidney and increases heart rate and contractility. In general, β_2-adrenoceptors mediate inhibitory responses such as relaxation of smooth muscle.

The adrenal medulla does not receive dual innervation, being influenced exclusively by preganglionic sympathetic fibers. Upon activation, ACh is released from these preganglionic sympathetic cholinergic fibers to act on ganglionic-type nicotinic ACh receptors located on adrenal chromaffin cells. The stimulated chromaffin cells release NE and EPI into the circulation. Because these catecholamines act at distant sites, they serve as hormones for α-adrenoceptors and β-adrenoceptors. The effects of circulating catecholamines are particularly important in cardiovascular homeostasis.

Circulating catecholamines, neurally released NE, and pharmacologic agents act primarily on β_1-adrenoceptors to increase heart rate (positive chronotropy) and increase the force of contraction (positive inotropy). There is also evidence of β_2-adrenoceptors in heart tissue. The heart has dual innervation from the ANS. Parasympathetic fibers originate from the vagus nerve and release ACh to act on cardiac muscarinic receptors to decrease heart rate (negative chronotropy) and decrease force of contraction (negative inotropy).

Arterial blood pressure is predominantly under sympathetic noradrenergic tone. Although exogenous ACh causes vasodilation, there is little evidence that activation of vascular muscarinic receptors occurs normally. An exception is the coronary circulation, which is enhanced by PNS-induced vasodilation. Even the sympathetic cholinergic fibers of the skeletal muscle vasculature is of questionable physiologic importance. The direct effect of adrenergic agonists on blood vessels is vasoconstriction, mediated by α_1-adrenoceptors, or vasodilation by way of β_2-adrenoceptors. Whether a

The importance of autonomic pharmacology is greater than that of the drugs themselves because it is the foundation for understanding other areas such as cardiovascular pharmacology and the pharmacology of the central nervous system. In addition, autonomic nerves or their effector organs are the sites of action responsible for adverse effects of many drugs whose primary site of action is elsewhere.

Heart
NE
  Positive chronotropy
  Positive ionotropy
ACh
  Negative chronotropy
  Negative ionotropy

Table 2.3 *Direct Effects of Autonomic Nerve Activity on Some Organ Systems*

ORGAN	SYMPATHETIC RESPONSE		PARASYMPATHETIC RESPONSE	
	ACTION[a]	RECEPTOR[b]	ACTION[a]	RECEPTOR[b]
Eye				
Iris				
Radial muscle	Contracts (mydriasis)	α_1	—	—
Circular muscle	—	—	Contracts	M
Ciliary muscle	Relaxes for far vision	β_2	Contracts	M
Heart				
Sinoatrial node	Accelerates	$\beta_1 > \beta_2$	Decelerates	M
Ectopic pacemakers	Accelerates	β_1	—	—
Contractility	Increases	$\beta_1 > \alpha_1$	Decreases (atria)	M
Arterioles				
Coronary	Dilation	β_2	Dilation	M
	Constriction	$\alpha_1 > \alpha_2$	—	—
Skin and mucosa	Constriction	$\alpha_1 > \alpha_2$	Dilation	M[c]
Skeletal muscle	[Constriction]	$\alpha_1 > \alpha_2$	Dilation	M[c]
	Dilation	β_2	—	—
		M[d]	—	—
Splanchnic	Constriction	$\alpha_1 > \alpha_2$	Dilation	M[c]
Renal and mesenteric	Dilation	Dopamine, β_2	—	—
	Constriction	$\alpha_1 > \alpha_2$	—	—
Veins				
Systemic	Dilation	β_2	—	—
	Constriction	$\alpha_1 > \alpha_2$	—	—
Bronchiolar Muscle	Relaxes	β_2	Contracts	M
Gastrointestinal Tract				
Smooth muscle				
Walls	Relaxes	α_2[e], β_2	Contracts	M
Sphincters	Contracts	α_1	Relaxes	M
Secretion	Inhibits	α_2	Increases	M
Genitourinary Smooth Muscle				
Bladder wall	Relaxes	β_2	Contracts	M
Sphincter	Contracts	α_1	Relaxes	M
Uterus, pregnant	Relaxes	β_2	—	—
	Contracts	α_1	—	—
Penis, seminal vesicles	Ejaculation	α_2	Erection	M
Skin				
Pilomotor smooth muscle	Contracts	α_1	—	—
Sweat glands				
Thermoregulatory	Increases	M	—	—
Apocrine (stress)	Increases	α_1	—	—
Muscle Functions				
Liver	Gluconeogenesis	α, β_2[f]	—	—
Liver	Glycogenolysis	α_1, β_2	—	—
Fat cells	Lipolysis	β_3	—	—
Kidney	Renin release	β_1, α_1[g]	—	—
	Na$^+$ reabsorption	α_1		

[a]Less important actions are in brackets.

[b]Specific receptor type: α = alpha, β = beta, M = muscarinic.

[c]The endothelium of most blood vessels releases endothelium-derived relaxing factor, which causes marked vasodilation in response to muscarinic stimuli. However, unlike the receptors innervated by sympathetic cholinergic fibers in skeletal muscle blood vessels, these muscarinic receptors are not innervated and respond only to *circulating* muscarinic agonists.

[d]Vascular smooth muscle has sympathetic cholinergic dilator fibers.

[e]Probably through presynaptic inhibition of parasympathetic activity.

[f]Depends on species.

[g]α_1 inhibits; β_1 stimulates.

drug produces vasodilation or vasoconstriction depends on its relative affinity for α_1-adrenoceptors and β_2-adrenoceptors and for the number of receptor subtypes in a given vascular bed. Inasmuch as the sympathetic response is "fight or flight," it controls the redistribution of blood from the skin, gastrointestinal tract, glands, and kidney to the heart and skeletal muscle. Thus there is a predominance of α_1-adrenoceptors within the vasculature perfusing those organs that do not need high blood flow under stress, whereas the blood vessels of the heart and skeletal muscle have primarily β_2-adrenoceptors to allow for stress-induced, sympathetically mediated vasodilation.

A fall in blood pressure caused by physiologic changes or drugs is detected by baroreceptors in the carotid sinus and aortic arch. This information is transmitted to the brain stem by afferent fibers to increase central sympathetic outflow. This results in sympathetic stimulation of heart rate, or reflex tachycardia, which helps return blood pressure to normal. On the other hand, an increase in blood pressure results in an increase in parasympathetic outflow by way of the baroreceptors and a slowing of the heart (reflex bradycardia). Because of these reflexes and the redistribution of blood flow, it is sometimes difficult to alter blood pressure in a predictable and precise manner.

Sweat glands are innervated only by sympathetic nerves. In this case most of the postganglionic fibers are cholinergic rather than adrenergic. The released ACh stimulates muscarinic receptors on the gland. This innervation is responsible for generalized sweating, often referred to as cholinergic sweating. Certain regional sweat glands, like those of the armpits, soles of the feet, and palms of the hand, are innervated by the SNS, which contains the characteristic adrenergic postganglionic fibers. Here the released NE acts on α-adrenoceptors, which mediate this localized response (sometimes referred to as adrenergic sweating).

In the pancreas, activation of α_2-adrenoceptors decreases insulin release from the β cells, whereas stimulation of β_2-adrenoceptors increases insulin release. The response to neurally derived NE during sympathetic activation is inhibition of insulin release mediated by α_2-adrenoceptors, whereas β_2-adrenergic stimulation of insulin release is induced only by drugs and not by the SNS.

Sweat Glands/Sympathetic Nerves

Cholinergic sweating (ACh)
Adrenergic sweating (NE)

Section 2.2 Cholinoceptor Agonists

■ **Overview** Drugs that mimic ACh are known as cholinomimetics or cholinergic agonists. Their classification is based on receptor selectivity and mechanism of action (Fig. 2.6).

■ **Muscarinic Receptor Agonists** Muscarinic receptor agonists (parasympathomimetics) produce effects that are generally equivalent to activation of postganglionic parasympathetic nerves. The direct-acting receptor agonists are classified further according to their chemical structure: choline esters (acetylcholine, carbachol, bethanechol, methacholine) and alkaloids (muscarine, pilocarpine). Muscarinic receptors are coupled to G proteins. Receptor stimulation initiates several biochemical events within the plasma membrane, including inhibition of adenylyl cyclase, stimulation of phosphoinositide hydrolysis, and activation of K^+ channels. These biochemical events lead to changes in intracellular Ca^{2+} concentrations, cyclic adenosine monophosphate (cAMP) levels, and protein phosphorylation, all of which influence various cellular and organ systems.

● **Cardiovascular** When muscarinic agonists are administered at doses

Responses produced by cholinomimetics are generally predictable based on knowledge of responses to parasympathetic nerve stimulation and the physiology of autonomic ganglia and the skeletal muscle motor end plate.

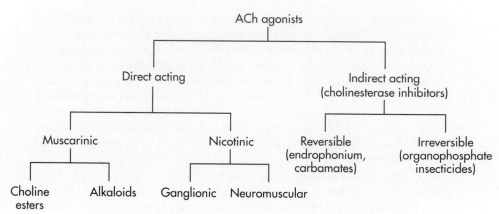

Fig. 2.6 A flow diagram of acetylcholine (*ACh*) agonists.

Direct Acting Receptor Agonists

Choline esters
  Acetylcholine
  Carbachol
  Bethanecol
  Methacholine
Alkaloids
  Muscarine
  Pilocarpine

too small to produce direct cardiac effects, they activate noninnervated muscarinic ACh receptors located on the endothelial lining of vascular smooth muscle. This causes the release of EDRF to produce vasodilation, hypotension, and reflex tachycardia. Larger doses of a muscarinic agonist cause hypotension and act directly on cardiac muscarinic receptors mimicking vagal stimulation. Thus bradycardia is produced by decreasing the rate of diastolic depolarization of the sinoatrial (SA) node, decreasing conduction, prolonging the refractory period of the atrioventricular (AV) node, decreasing myocardial contractions, and shortening the atrial refractory period. The decrease in atrial refractory period can lead to atrial flutter or fibrillation.

- **Eye** Parasympathomimetics cause contraction of the sphincter muscle (miosis) resulting in decreased intraocular pressure and contraction of the ciliary muscle (accommodation). Both effects facilitate outflow of aqueous humor into the canal of Schlemm draining the anterior chamber and reducing intraocular pressure.

- **Respiratory** Muscarinic agonists contract the smooth muscle of the bronchial tree and increase secretions from the glands of the tracheobronchial mucosa. This may have serious consequences in asthmatics.

- **Gastrointestinal** Stimulation of the PNS, or administration of muscarinic agonists, increases peristaltic activity throughout the intestine, relaxes most sphincters, and increases hydrochloric acid (HCl) secretion in the gastrointestinal tract. Salivary glands are also stimulated by muscarinic agonists, as are the pancreas and to a lesser extent the glands in the small intestine.

- **Genitourinary** Muscarinic agonists induce contraction of the detrusor muscle and relaxation of the trigone and sphincter muscles of the bladder, promoting urination.

- **Glands** In general, muscarinic agonists increase secretory activity, especially from sweat, lacrimal, and nasopharyngeal glands. Recall that most sweat glands are innervated by cholinergic sympathetic neurons.

- **Peripheral nervous system/neuromuscular junction** Cholinomimetics influence these systems through nicotinic, not muscarinic, receptors. Because muscarinic agonists are highly selective, they have little effect on nicotinic receptors. Thus parasympathomimetics do not normally influence these systems.

- **Central nervous system** Of the muscarinic agonists previously listed, all but pilocarpine are quaternary amines and therefore do not enter the CNS.

- **Basic pharmacology**

  — *Choline esters* Acetylcholine is inactivated by both ACh esterase and pseudocholinesterase. Because ACh is metabolized so readily, it is of limited clinical use as a therapeutic agent. **Methacholine** is more useful because it is more slowly metabolized by AChE than ACh and is resistant to hydrolysis by pseudocholinesterase. Carbachol and bethanechol are resistant to both esterases and therefore have much longer half-lives than other choline esters.

    Selective muscarinic agonists produce their effects by binding directly to the muscarinic ACh receptor. **Carbachol** is unique in that it also increases the release of endogenous ACh. Because of this indirect action, nicotinic effects are frequently encountered with its use.

    Most esters have low lipid solubility, are poorly absorbed, and have difficulty penetrating the CNS. **Bethanechol** is administered orally or parenterally for its systemic effects, whereas carbachol, ACh, and pilocarpine are used topically in ophthalmology.

Choline Esters
Acetylcholine
Bethanechol
Carbachol
Methacholine

- **Pharmacotherapeutics**

  • Because of its rapid hydrolysis, **ACh** has limited clinical usefulness, although a 1% topical solution is used to produce miosis in cataract extractions and other surgical procedures on the anterior segment of the eye.

  • **Methacholine** is used primarily as a diagnostic agent. If a patient is suspected of having poisoning from atropine or atropine-like compounds, subcutaneous methacholine administration will *not* produce the characteristic signs of flush, sweating, lacrimation, and so forth. It is also used to test pancreatic enzyme function because methacholine increases plasma amylase levels.

  • **Carbachol** is completely resistant to hydrolysis by cholinesterases. It has some indirect ACh-releasing effects that can produce adverse effects associated with nicotinic receptor activation. When administered directly into the eye for the treatment of noncongestive, wide-angle glaucoma, the nicotinic effects are avoided. This is the primary use of carbachol.

  • **Bethanechol** is not metabolized by cholinesterases and has a selective action on muscarinic receptors of the gastrointestinal tract and urinary bladder. Bethanechol is administered orally and subcutaneously (SQ) and is useful in certain cases of postoperative abdominal distention, gastric atony, and retention when organic obstruction is not present. The cardiovascular effects of bethanechol and carbachol are less common than those elicited by ACh and methacholine; they consist of a transient hypotension and reflex tachycardia.

- **Adverse effects** Adverse effects associated with muscarinic agonists are predictable and are generally due to overstimulation of the organs receiving parasympathetic innervation. Adverse effects include nausea, vomiting, diarrhea, salivation, cutaneous vasodilation, and bronchial constriction. These responses are competitively blocked by atropine and other muscarinic receptor antagonists. Muscarinic agonists should not be administered IV or intramuscularly (IM) because they tend to lose their selectivity for muscarinic receptors when given these ways, increasing the incidence and severity of adverse effects.

    Major contraindications to the use of choline esters include asthma, car-

Adverse Effects
Vomiting
Diarrhea
Salivation
Cutaneous vasodilation
Bronchial constriction

diac insufficiency, and peptic ulcer. Hyperthyroidism is also a contraindication because these patients may develop atrial fibrillation when administered a cholinomimetic.

Overdose is treated with atropine sulfate. Epinephrine, a physiologic antagonist for muscarinic agonists, may be useful in overcoming severe cardiovascular or bronchoconstrictor responses.

Alkaloids
Muscarine
Pilocarpine

■ Alkaloids

- ● Basic pharmacology

  - **Muscarine** is an alkaloid isolated from the mushroom *Amanita muscaria.* It is of no therapeutic use but is frequently responsible for mushroom poisoning.

  - **Pilocarpine** is a muscarinic agonist used in the initial treatment of open-angle glaucoma. Reduction of intraocular pressure is rapid and lasts 4 to 8 hours. Adverse systemic effects are nonexistent because the drug is applied directly into the eye.

■ Nicotinic Agonists

- ● Basic pharmacology

  - **Nicotine,** a volatile alkaloid, has no therapeutic use but is important as a prototype for understanding responses to activation of nicotinic ACh receptors. It is found not only in tobacco smoke but also in insecticides and therefore is of toxicologic importance. After dermal absorption, injection, or inhalation, nicotine acts at both parasympathetic and sympathetic ganglia to stimulate *all* postganglionic autonomic nerves to release their transmitters. Furthermore, nicotinic agonists stimulate the adrenal medulla to release EPI and NE into the circulation and act at the neuromuscular junction to contract skeletal muscles. At low doses nicotinic agonists produce muscle fasciculation, tachycardia, hypertension, an increase in respiratory rate from stimulation of chemoreceptors in the carotid and aortic bodies, a decrease in cutaneous blood flow, which decreases skin temperature, an increase in vasopressin (ADH) secretion, and an increase in blood sugar. Toxic doses cause pronounced hypertension with slow pulse rate, diarrhea, urination, vomiting, and flaccid paralysis, because at high doses nicotine behaves like a depolarizing muscle relaxant. Convulsions often occur, with death from failure of the respiratory muscles.

  - Although nicotinic agonists have been synthesized and isolated as natural products (DMPP, lobeline), they have no therapeutic value.

■ Acetylcholinesterase Inhibitors

- ● **Overview** Cholinesterase inhibitors are indirect-acting cholinomimetics. They produce their effects by inhibiting AChE and pseudocholinesterase, thereby decreasing the metabolism of ACh and increasing its concentration in the synaptic cleft. Because cholinesterase inhibitors act by enhancing the response to ACh, these agents have virtually no selectivity for cholinergic receptor subtypes. The most important use of cholinesterase inhibitors is as insecticides, some are used in nerve gas, and a few have therapeutic applications. Although the pharmacodynamic properties of these agents are similar, there are differences in their chemistry and pharmacokinetics.

- ● **Basic pharmacology** There are two major classes of AChE inhibitors: carbamates, which are reversible, and organophosphates, which form stable complexes with the esterase and are irreversible.

  — *Reversible cholinesterase inhibitors* Reversible AChE inhibitors

Table 2.4	*Duration of Action of Some Cholinesterase Inhibitors*
AChE INHIBITOR	**APPROXIMATE DURATION OF ACTION**
Edrophonium	2-10 min
Neostigmine	0.5-2 hr
Physostigmine	0.5-2 hr
Pyridostigmine	3-6 hr
Demecarium	4-6 hr
Ambenonium	4-8 hr
Echothiophate	100 hr

include physostigmine, neostigmine, pyridostigmine, demecarium, ambenonium, and edrophonium.

Edrophonium is a competitive inhibitor of ACh at the AChE reactive site. Its duration of action (2 to 10 minutes) is short, and because it is a quaternary ammonium compound, it does not cross the blood-brain barrier. Edrophonium is administered IV to distinguish between myasthenia gravis, where it produces a transient improvement, and a cholinergic crisis, which it will make transiently worse. Edrophonium has also been used for treatment of supraventricular tacharrhythmias, particularly paroxysmal supraventricular tachycardia. Table 2.4 lists the duration of action of some cholinesterase inhibitors.

Longer-acting carbamates include **neostigmine, pyridostigmine,** and **ambenonium.** Because all are quaternary ammonium compounds, they have difficulty crossing the blood-brain barrier, although ambenonium induces adverse CNS effects. All act primarily by binding to the active site of AChE, with the resulting carbamylated enzyme reactivated within ½ to 6 hours. These agents are useful in treating myasthenia gravis because they have some direct nicotinic action on skeletal muscle. Although they are quaternary ammonium compounds and therefore poorly absorbed, they are administered orally.

Physostigmine, a tertiary amine, is lipid soluble, and penetrates the CNS. It is used mainly as an eye drop to increase ACh, which will reduce intraocular pressure in patients with glaucoma. Because physostigmine crosses the blood-brain barrier it is used in the treatment of atropine poisoning.

Another quaternary ammonium compound used in the treatment of glaucoma is **demecarium.** This cholinesterase inhibitor has a longer duration of action than physostigmine.

Pralidoxime (2-PAM) is not a useful antidote for carbamate toxicity.

— *Irreversible cholinesterase inhibitors* Although these compounds, all of which are organophosphates, are most important from a toxicologic perspective, echothiophate and isoflurophate (DFP) are used in the treatment of glaucoma. Other organophosphates are nerve gases (soman, sarin, tabun) or insecticides (parathion and its active metabolite paraoxon, malathion and its active metabolite, malaoxon). Organophosphate cholinesterase inhibitors produce phosphonylation or

Carbamates (reversible)
Neostigmine
Physostigmine
Edrophonium

Organophosphates (irreversible)
Echothiophate
Isoflurophate
Soman
Parathion
Malathion

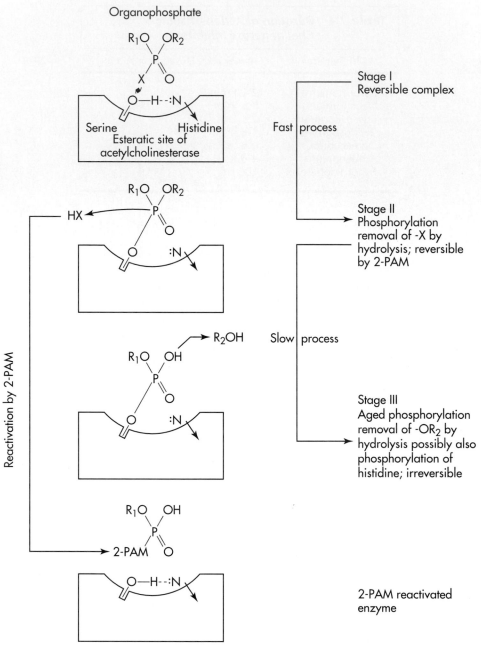

Fig. 2.7 The steps of acetylcholinesterase inhibition by organophosphorus compounds and enzyme reactivation with pralidoxime (*2-PAM*).

phosphorylation of the esteratic site of AChE (Fig. 2.7). Because this forms a covalent bond, once the reaction is complete it cannot be reversed. The reaction takes place in three stages:

1. The first step is the formation of a reversible complex in which the inhibitor competes with ACh for the binding site on AChE. At this stage there are rarely symptoms of organophosphate intoxication.

2. Next the irreversible inhibitor phosphorylates a serine residue in the esteratic site of the enzyme. At this stage the AChE can be reactivated by 2-PAM.

3. The third stage is known as aging and is characterized by the loss of an alkyl group or migration of the phosphoryl group to another amino acid residue. At this point the AChE is irreversibly inactivated and restoration of cholinesterase activity is dependent on synthesis of a new enzyme.

● **Pharmacotherapeutics**

• A therapeutic use of **physostigmine** takes advantage of its ability to penetrate the CNS. Physostigmine is used to reverse the CNS effects of anticholinergic drugs. Physostigmine may be administered IM, IV, or topically to treat acute congestive glaucoma and chronic simple glaucoma.

• **Neostigmine** can be administered SQ or IM in the prevention and treatment of postoperative distention and urinary retention after mechanical obstruction has been excluded. It is also used orally to ameliorate the symptoms of myasthenia gravis and to reverse the effects of nondepolarizing neuromuscular blockers such as tubocurarine, gallamine, and pancuronium. In this case neostigmine is administered by slow IV infusion in patients pretreated with atropine to minimize muscarinic responses.

• **Pyridostigmine,** similar to neostigmine, is administered orally for the treatment of myasthenia gravis or by slow IV infusion to reverse the effects of nondepolarizing muscle relaxants. All of the same precautions for neostigmine apply to pyridostigmine.

• **Demecarium** is a potent AChE inhibitor and must be used with caution. Demecarium is administered only topically in the conjunctival sac after iridectomy or in wide-angle glaucoma when short-acting mitotics are ineffective.

• **Edrophonium,** a short-acting cholinesterase inhibitor, is used IV to reverse the effects of nondepolarizing muscle relaxants and IV or IM in the diagnosis of myasthenia gravis. IV administration of edrophonium improves the muscle strength of a myasthenic within 30 to 60 seconds. If the muscle weakness is a result of cholinergic crisis (e.g., overdose of neostigmine), decreased muscle strength and other adverse cholinergic symptoms will become severe when edrophonium is administered. The effects of IV edrophonium dissipate within 10 minutes.

Only two of the irreversible cholinesterase inhibitors are used clinically: echothiophate and isoflurophate.

• **Echothiophate** is used in chronic, wide-angle (simple) glaucoma. It is contraindicated in congestive glaucoma.

• **Isoflurophate** (DFP; Diisopropylfluorophosphate) is used in wide-angle glaucoma when short-acting mitotics are ineffective, in conditions where aqueous outflow is obstructed, and after iridectomy. Both echothiophate and isoflurophate are applied topically to the conjunctival sac to minimize systemic effects.

• Echothiphate and isoflurophate are administered directly into the eyes to treat glaucoma. Because they are irreversible AChE inhibitors their duration of action is prolonged, which is beneficial. Even when applied topically, these drugs may enter the systemic circulation and therefore must be used cautiously to prevent systemic adverse effects.

• Because the nerve gases soman, sarin, and tabun are lipid soluble they rapidly penetrate intact skin and mucous membranes, enter the circulation, and rapidly inhibit AChE throughout the body. Because the "aging process" is extremely rapid with these compounds, 2-PAM is effective

Table 2.5 *Adverse Effects of AChE Inhibitors*

Muscarinic Manifestations	Nicotinic Manifestations	CNS Manifestations
Bronchoconstriction	Muscular fasciculations	Restlessness
Increased bronchial secretions	Paralysis (eventually)	Insomnia
Sweating		Tremors
Salivation		Confusion
Lacrimation		Ataxia
Bradycardia		Convulsions
Hypotension		Respiratory depression
Miosis		Circulatory collapse
Blurring of vision		
Uncontrolled urination		
Uncontrolled diarrhea		

CNS, Central nervous system.

in reactivating the enzyme only within the first few minutes of exposure. High doses of 2-PAM may cause neuromuscular blockade and slight inhibition of AChE. These actions of 2-PAM are nonexistent or minimal at the usual doses.

• Insecticide organophosphates are designed to be selectively toxic to insects. For example, **parathion** must be converted to **paraoxon** to inhibit AChE. This process occurs rapidly in insects but very slowly in humans. **Malathion** is converted to **malaoxon,** the active inhibitor of AChE. Malaoxon is rapidly converted to an inactive metabolite in humans, but not in insects. Toxicity can result from exposure to a high dose of malaoxon or repeated exposure to smaller quantities.

● **Adverse effects** Organophosphate toxicity is directly related to overstimulation of ACh receptors, including those in the ganglia, intestine, neuromuscular junction, and CNS. Adverse effects on the CNS are less severe with quaternary ammonium compounds. The most common manifestations of toxicity associated with cholinesterase inhibition are summarized in Table 2.5.

In addition, organophosphates cause polyneuritis, neuronal degeneration, and demyelination, which are unrelated to their action on AChE. Death from acute intoxication is due to respiratory failure and cardiovascular collapse. Respiratory problems include laryngospasm, bronchoconstriction, increased tracheobronchial and salivary secretions, and paralysis of the respiratory muscles and the control centers in the brain. Besides maintaining vital signs, treatment includes pralidoximine. Pralidoximine (2-PAM) is contraindicated in poisoning with carbamates.

Section 2.3 Cholinoceptor Antagonists

■ **Overview** In the periphery, ACh activates three molecularly and pharmacologically distinct receptors: muscarinic and nicotinic sites located on ganglia and at the neuromuscular junction. Xenobiotics have been identified that block these receptors with a great deal of selectivity. For example, at therapeutic doses, **atropine** inhibits actions of ACh at muscarinic sites, such as in the heart, but not at autonomic ganglia or the neuromuscular junction.

■ **Antimuscarinic Agents** Drugs in this category selectively compete with ACh in binding to muscarinic receptors at parasympathetic postganglionic sites, at cholinergic sympathetic postganglionic sites (sweating), and at muscarinic receptor sites in the CNS. This class is sometimes termed *parasympatholytics*. Until recently it was believed that there was only one type of muscarinic receptor. Gene cloning and expression have revealed at least four distinct muscarinic receptors. Two of these, M_1 and M_2, can be differentiated pharmacologically.

The M_1 receptor, which has high affinity for the receptor antagonist **pirenzepine**, is found in high concentrations in the cerebral cortex, hippocampus, autonomic ganglia, and gastric parietal cells. Stimulation of M_1 activates a G protein coupled to phospholipase C, activation of which increases intracellular Ca^{2+}. Accordingly, M_1 receptors mediate Ca^{2+}-dependent activations such as contraction of smooth muscle and secretion. The M_1 stimulation of phopholipase C also results in the activation of protein kinase C through production of di-acylglycerol.

The M_2 receptor has low affinity for pirenzepine and is found in the myocardium, secretory glands, and smooth muscle. The M_2 and M_4 receptors interact with G proteins and inhibit adenylyl cyclase activity, activate K^+ channels, and modulate the activity of some Ca^{2+} channels. Activation of cardiac M_2 receptors and the subsequent effects on adenylyl cyclase and K^+ conductances are responsible for the negative chronotropic and inotropic effects of muscarinic agonists. Evidence suggests that M_2 receptors located in the heart and the secretory glands are not identical, pointing to the possibility of developing drugs that selectively activate or inhibit these sites.

● **Basic pharmacology** All muscarinic receptor antagonists are competitive inhibitors of ACh. At therapeutic doses these antagonists have high selectivity for muscarinic receptors, being essentially devoid of any effects on ganglionic or neuromuscular cholinergic receptors.

In general, **atropine,** the prototypical muscarinic receptor antagonist, produces effects opposite to those observed after stimulation of the PNS.

— *Exocrine glands* Perhaps the most prominent effect noted with these agents is dry mouth. **Atropine** is potent in decreasing salivary secretions, producing xerotomia and difficulty in swallowing. Although not life threatening, these effects may be discomforting enough to effect patient compliance. Atropine decreases gastric secretions, but not sufficiently to increase gastric pH. The effectiveness of parasympatholytics in the treatment of peptic ulcer is related to their effects on the gastrointestinal motility not in decreasing HCl secretion. Bronchial secretions and sweating are suppressed with atropine. The former is of use in general anesthesia, and the latter can have a fatal consequence as hyperthermia can ensue with overdose.

— *Smooth muscle* Although atropine does not affect normal gastrointestinal motility, it abolishes excessive tone and motility. Thus parasympatholytics are antispasmodic but not constipating.

Atropine is moderately effective in relieving biliary colic without altering the formation of bile.

Atropine also causes relaxation of the smooth muscle of the ureters and the bladder wall. These effects can lead to urinary retention, a potentially serious problem in elderly men with prostatic hypertrophy.

— *Cardiovascular system* Large doses of atropine produce tachycardia (40 to 50 beats per minute) caused by inhibition of the vagal tone on

Muscarinic Antagonists
Atropine
Scopolamine
Ipratropium
Pirenzepine (M_1 selective)

Pralidoxime (2-PAM) is a *reactivator* of acetylcholinesterase in the periphery, *not* a competitive muscarinic antagonist.

It is important to note that not all parasympathetic neuroeffector junctions are equally sensitive to blockade. The order of sensitivity is salivary, bronchial, and sweat glands > iris, ciliary muscle and vagal effects > urinary bladder and gastrointestinal muscles > gastric secretion (> means "is more sensitive than"). Thus low doses depress salivary, bronchial, and sweat secretion whereas much larger doses are required to inhibit gastric secretions.

the SA nodal pacemaker. Because there is essentially no cholinergic innervation of blood vessels and no ACh is found in the circulation, atropine has no direct effect on vascular tone. Toxic doses of atropine dilate cutaneous vessels, producing what is known as the "atropine flush."

— *Eye* The two primary effects of atropine and other antimuscarinics on the eye are mydriasis and cycloplegia. Both occur after systemic administration of atropine, but they are more prominent after topical application. In those with a narrow chamber angle in the eye, atropine may precipitate glaucoma and blindness because drainage of the aqueous humor through the canal of Schlemm is inhibited. Local application of atropine to the eye may cause noticeable changes for as long as 1 week. Accordingly, atropine must be used cautiously as a mydriatic.

— *Central nervous system* Clinical doses of atropine may cause a mild vagal excitation, transiently decreasing heart rate. **Scopolamine** produces sedation in low doses and is used prophylactically to prevent motion sickness through its action on the vestibular system. Scopolamine is not effective against other types of nausea or vomiting. Other muscarinic antagonists (**trihexyphenidyl** and **benzotropine**) are used to reduce tremor and rigidity in Parkinson's disease.

Toxic doses of atropine cause disorientation with the subject becoming restless, quarrelsome, and irritable. This state of excitation may be followed by delirium and hallucinations. Normally there is no residual CNS damage, but occasionally the intoxication proceeds to coma, respiratory failure, and death. Although fatalities are rare, poisoning is common because many over-the-counter medications contain antimuscarinic agents. Treatment of overdose includes gastric lavage, administration of **physostigmine,** and possibly **diazepam** if excitation or convulsions are present.

● **Pharmacotherapeutics** Although there are many antimuscarinics available for clinical use, only pirenzepine differentiates between muscarinic sites. An M_1-selective antagonist, pirenzepine preferentially inhibits gastrointestinal secretions. Although many other parasympatholytics have been used for this purpose, their value is questionable and their use is declining with the development of newer agents.

Scopolamine has more CNS effects than any other antimuscarinic. It is used as a preanesthetic medication to produce drowsiness and amnesia and to inhibit secretions. It is also used routinely for motion sickness.

Atropine is used primarily as a preanesthetic medication, although it is also used to treat overdoses of muscarinic agonists and AChE inhibitors, as well as in some cases of mushroom poisoning if muscarine is involved.

Antimuscarinics are commonly used in ophthalmology. Although they can precipitate glaucoma in susceptible patients, they are used when prolonged pupillary dilation is necessary and for their cyclopolegic effect to permit the measurement of refractive error without interference by the accommodative ability of the eye. Because locally applied atropine or scopolamine has an extremely long duration of action, shorter-acting antimuscarinics such as homatropine, cyclopentolate and tropicamide are preferred for eye examinations.

There are many atropine-like drugs. A major difference among them is related to their chemical structures. In general, quaternary amines are less selective for muscarinic sites, with high doses causing ganglionic blockade.

Used for Eye Examinations
Homatropine
Cyclopentolate
Tropocainamide

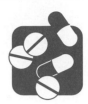

● **Pharmacokinetics** Atropine and **scopolamine** are plant alkaloids. Many congeners have been synthesized, including tertiary ammonium analogs. Furthermore, some antihistamines, antipsychotics, and antidepressants have similar structures and significant antimuscarinic effects. Atropine analogs have been formulated as quaternary ammonium compounds to reduce their effects on the CNS (Box 2.1).

Box 2.1

REPRESENTATIVE ANTIMUSCARINIC DRUGS	
Tertiary Amines	**Quaternary Amines**
Atropine	Propantheline
Scopolamine	Methscopolamine
	Glycopyrrolate

Most of the naturally occurring alkaloids and tertiary antimuscarinics are well absorbed orally, cross the conjunctival membrane, and are distributed through the body, including the CNS. Scopolamine is prepared in a special vehicle to allow transdermal absorption. A patch containing **scopolamine** is placed behind the ear to prevent motion sickness without significant adverse effects. The quaternary ammonium compounds are poorly absorbed (10% to 30%) after oral administration and do not enter the CNS.

Atropine has a half-life of 2 hours and about 80% is excreted in the urine. Approximately one third of an administered dose is excreted unchanged, and the rest as glucuronidated metabolites. Although the parasympatholytic effect is relatively short, effects on the iris and ciliary muscle last for 48 to 72 hours.

● **Adverse effects** The adverse effects of parasympatholytics are an extension of their pharmacologic actions. The most common signs of overdose are xerotomia, hot, dry, flushed skin, dilated pupils, tachycardia, blurred vision, and CNS disturbances. Convulsions, coma, and death can occur with toxic doses.

Blockade of muscarinic receptors precipitates acute glaucoma, so parasympatholytics are contraindicated in this condition. These drugs may worsen gastric ulcers by decreasing gastric emptying, and they should be used with caution in elderly men because of effects on the bladder.

■ **Nicotinic Antagonists**

● **Overview** Nicotinic antagonists are defined by their ability to block the effects of ACh on the nicotinic receptors located in the autonomic ganglia and at the neuromuscular junction.

● **Basic pharmacology** Acetylcholine is the primary neurotransmitter released by all preganglionic autonomic neurons. It activates nicotinic ACh receptors located on postganglionic sympathetic neurons, on postganglionic parasympathetic neurons, and on adrenal chromaffin cells in the adrenal medulla. Ganglionic blockers inhibit the actions of ACh at all three sites. At high doses, nicotine, a nicotinic receptor agonist, can also inhibit these receptors by depolarization blockade.

Ganglionic Antagonists
Hexamethonium
Trimethaphan
Mecamylamine

The effects of ganglionic blockade depend on the predominant tone for each organ. Table 2.6 summarizes the physiologic effects of ganglionic blockade.

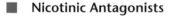

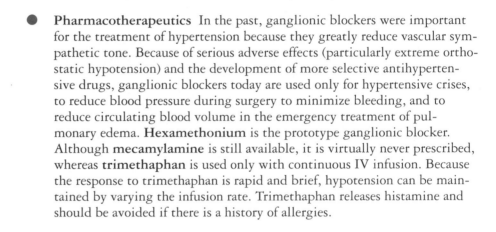

Table 2.6 *Physiologic Effects of Ganglionic Blockade*

SITE	PREDOMINANT TONE	EFFECT OF GANGLIONIC BLOCKADE
Arterioles	Sympathetic (adrenergic)	Vasodilatation; increased peripheral flow; hypotension
Veins	Sympathetic (adrenergic)	Dilation; pooling of blood; decreased venous return, decreased output
Heart	Parasympathetic (cholinergic)	Tachycardia
Iris	Parasympathetic (cholinergic)	Mydriasis
Ciliary muscle	Parasympathetic (cholinergic)	Cycloplegia
Gastrointestinal tract	Parasympathetic (cholinergic)	Reduced tone and motility; constipation
Urinary bladder	Parasympathetic (cholinergic)	Urinary retention
Salivary glands	Parasympathetic (cholinergic)	Xerostomia (dry mouth)

Experimentally or clinically, in the presence of ganglionic blockade only *direct* effects of parasympathomimetics, sympathomimetics, and other vasoactive compounds will be observed; *there will be no reflex control of any autonomically innervated organ.*

● **Pharmacotherapeutics** In the past, ganglionic blockers were important for the treatment of hypertension because they greatly reduce vascular sympathetic tone. Because of serious adverse effects (particularly extreme orthostatic hypotension) and the development of more selective antihypertensive drugs, ganglionic blockers today are used only for hypertensive crises, to reduce blood pressure during surgery to minimize bleeding, and to reduce circulating blood volume in the emergency treatment of pulmonary edema. **Hexamethonium** is the prototype ganglionic blocker. Although **mecamylamine** is still available, it is virtually never prescribed, whereas **trimethaphan** is used only with continuous IV infusion. Because the response to trimethaphan is rapid and brief, hypotension can be maintained by varying the infusion rate. Trimethaphan releases histamine and should be avoided if there is a history of allergies.

SECTION 2.4 ADRENOCEPTOR AGONISTS

■ Adrenoceptor Classification

● **Overview** Receptors for sympathomimetic agents are membrane bound and are divided into two major classes: α-adrenoceptors and β-adrenoceptors. Both α-adrenoceptors and β-adrenoceptors are subcategorized into α_1-, α_2-, β_1-, and β_2-adrenoceptors based on their affinities for various agonists and antagonists. Recent studies suggest an even greater diversity of adrenoceptor subtypes (e.g., α_{1A}, α_{1B}, α_{2A}, α_{2B}, β_3), but the physiologic and pharmacologic significance of these receptors is as yet unclear. The anatomic distribution and function of the various adrenoceptor subtypes are summarized in Table 2.7.

In general, activation of α_1-adrenoceptors causes contraction of smooth muscle. The major exception is nonsphincter muscle of the intestine, which is relaxed.

   ● Activation of α_1-adrenoceptors is frequently associated with an increase in cytosolic calcium. The molecular mechanisms leading to this include an increase in calcium influx through receptor-operated calcium channels and stimulation in phospholipase C resulting in the degradation of phosphoinositides, which promotes the release of calcium from intracellular stores.

   ● Activation of α_2-adrenoceptors is of pharmacologic importance primarily because it decreases NE release from central and peripheral neurons. In the CNS, activation of postsynaptic α_2-adrenoceptors decreases sympathetic outflow and increases parasympathetic tone. In the periphery, α_2-

---

Table 2.7   *Distribution and Function of Adrenoceptors*

Type	Tissue	Actions
Alpha$_1$ (α_1)	Most vascular smooth muscle (innervated)	Contraction
	Pupillary dilator muscle	Contraction (*dilates pupil*)
	Pilomotor smooth muscle	Erects hair
	Kidney	Increases Na$^+$ reabsorption; inhibits renin release
	Heart	Increases force of contraction
Alpha$_2$ (α_2)	Postsynaptic central nervous system neurons	Decrease sympathetic and increase parasympathetic outflow
	Platelets	Aggregation
	Presynaptic adrenergic and cholinergic nerve terminals	Inhibition of transmitter release
	Some vascular smooth muscle (noninnervated)	Contraction
	Pancreas (beta cells)	Inhibition of insulin release
Beta$_1$ (β_1)	Heart	Increases force and rate of contraction
	Kidney (JG cells)	Stimulates renin release
	Postganglionic sympathetic nerve terminals	Increase norepinephrine release
Beta$_2$ (β_2)	Respiratory, uterine, and vascular smooth muscle	Promotes smooth muscle relaxation
	Skeletal muscle	Promotes potassium uptake; increases contractility
	Human liver	Activates glycogenolysis
	Pancreas	Increases insulin secretion

---

adrenoceptors are primarily located presynaptically on some sympathetic and parasympathetic nerve terminals. Activation of these receptors decreases neurotransmitter release.

- Although certain α_2-adrenoceptor agonists inhibit adenylyl cyclase, the physiologic significance of this is as yet unknown.

- β_1-Adrenoceptors are located primarily in heart tissue, but are also found on fat cells, currently thought to be β_3-adrenoceptors, and on juxtaglomerular cells in the kidney. Activation of β_1-adrenoceptors greatly increases heart rate and force of contraction: both NE and EPI activate β_1-receptors.

- β_2-adrenoceptors occur primarily in certain vascular beds and other smooth muscle cells where they promote relaxation. Epinephrine is a potent agonist at β_2-adrenoceptors, whereas NE is nearly devoid of activity at those sites. The synthetic catecholamine isoproterenol is a potent β-adrenoceptor agonist at both β_1 and β_2 sites.

- In the heart, β_2-adrenoceptors make up approximately 30% of the total β-adrenoceptor population. These receptors may not be functional under normal conditions, but they have pharmacologic significance in the failing heart.

- Activation of β_1-receptors and β_2-receptors results in activation of adenylyl cyclase through the stimulatory G protein, increasing cAMP production.

An important example of this presynaptic inhibition is in the gastrointestinal tract, where sympathetic activation relaxes the smooth muscle tone of the walls not directly, but by the release of NE to act on α_2-adrenoceptors found on parasympathetic nerve terminals to inhibit ACh release.

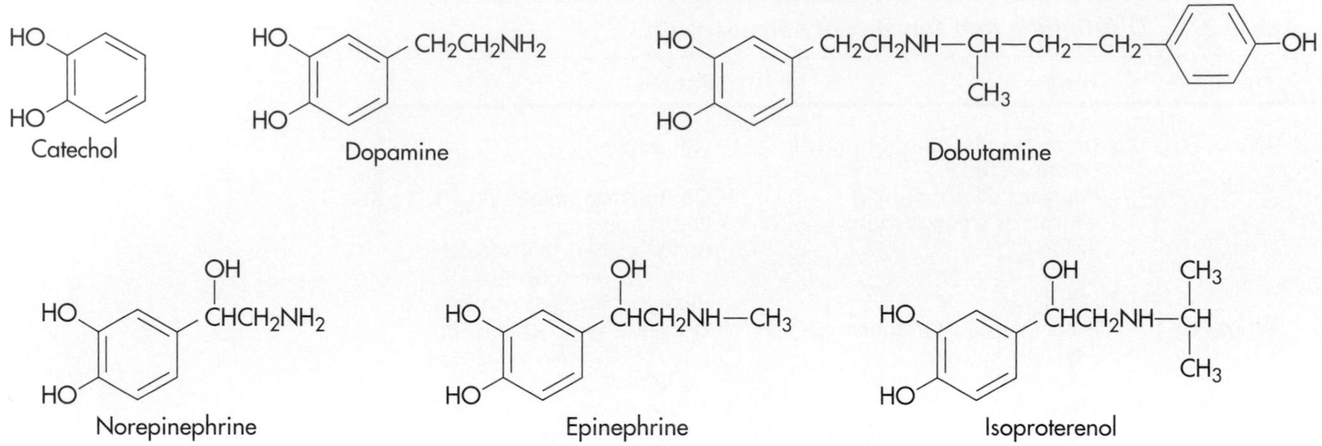

Catechol

Dopamine

Dobutamine

Norepinephrine

Epinephrine

Isoproterenol

Fig. 2.8 Formula structures of catechol and catecholamines.

- The dopamine receptor is distinct from the α-adrenoceptors and β-adrenoceptors and is subclassified into D_1 and D_2 sites. Dopamine receptors are not activated by NE or EPI, although at high doses dopamine can stimulate α_1-adrenoceptors and β_1-adrenoceptors. The D_1 receptor is coupled to a G protein, accumulating adenylyl cyclase in vascular beds and producing vasodilation. The D_2 receptors are located in the CNS and anterior pituitary. Activation of these sites inhibits the formation of cAMP.

- Many factors alter responses to adrenoceptor activation. Numerous hormones, drugs, and disease states modify the number or function of the membrane-bound receptor. These receptors are subject to up-regulation and down-regulation depending on the state of innervation. If a cell or tissue is exposed to a receptor agonist for a prolonged period of time, receptor down-regulation occurs with the tissue becoming less responsive because of a decrease in the number of receptors. If a cell or tissue is exposed to a receptor antagonist for a period of time or is deprived of agonist because of denervation, supersensitivity occurs because of an increase in the number of receptors. These changes may limit the therapeutic potential of some drugs and must be considered when discontinuing long-term therapy with a receptor agonist or antagonist.

■ Adrenoceptor Agonists

- **Overview** Stimulation of sympathetic nerves causes a release of NE from the nerve terminal and a release of EPI and NE from the adrenal medulla. The EPI and NE act at adrenoceptors. Drugs that mimic the actions of NE or EPI are known as *sympathomimetics* and display a wide range of effects.

■ Catecholamines

- **Overview** The basic structure of the catecholamines is the catechol nucleus (Fig. 2.8). The three endogenous catecholamines of physiologic importance are NE, EPI, and dopamine. **NE** is found in peripheral sympathetic neurons, the brain, and the adrenal medulla. **EPI** is located primarily in chromaffin cells in the adrenal medulla and in the brain. **Dopamine** is highly concentrated in certain regions of the brain and is also found in sympathetic ganglia and some renal nerves. Dopamine receptors (but not dopamine neurons) are located in the renal and mesenteric blood vessels and thus are of pharmacologic importance.

Table 2.8 *Relative Potencies of Epinephrine, Norepinephrine, and Isoproterenol*

Adrenoceptor Receptor Subtype	Relative Potency
α_1	EPI ≥ NE >>> Iso
α_2	EPI ≥ NE >>> Iso
β_1	Iso > EPI = NE
β_2	Iso > EPI >> NE

EPI, epinephrine; *NE,* norepinephrine; *ISO,* isoproterenol.

● **Basic pharmacology** The relative potencies of EPI, NE, and isoproterenol are summarized in Table 2.8.

EPI is equally potent at α_1-adrenoceptors and α_2-adrenoceptors as is NE, although the latter is generally less potent than EPI at the two sites.

The catecholamines mediate a variety of responses.

  • When administered IV, NE displays primarily an α_1-adrenoceptor profile. Although endogenously released NE increases heart rate through β_1-adrenoceptors, exogenously administered NE generally produces a decrease in heart rate by increasing blood pressure and activating the baroreceptor reflex. However, along with the reflex decrease in heart rate, NE produces a β_1-mediated positive inotropy.

  • EPI stimulates responses mediated by both α-adrenoceptors and β-adrenoceptors. The effect of EPI depends on the relative number of receptors in the affected tissue, the dose, and the rate of infusion. In skeletal muscle, for example, low doses of EPI produce a vasodilation because of activation of β_2-adrenoceptors, for which EPI has a high affinity, whereas high doses cause vasoconstriction because there are more α_1-adrenoceptors than β_2-adrenoceptors in skeletal muscle vessels. Because isoproterenol acts exclusively on β-adrenoceptors, it produces responses consistent with β_1- and β_2-adrenoceptor activation, such as hypotension and tachycardia. At low doses dopamine stimulates only D_1-receptors, causing vasodilation. At higher doses dopamine increases heart rate by acting at β_1-adrenoceptor sites and causes vasoconstriction through stimulation of α_1-adrenoceptors.

The pharmacologic effects generally observed after catecholamine infusion are summarized in Table 2.9.

The α-adrenoceptor-mediated relaxation of intestinal smooth muscle is probably of greater pharmacologic significance than β-adrenoceptor-induced relaxation. α-Adrenoceptor agonists, especially those acting at α_2-adrenoceptor sites, decrease gastrointestinal muscle activity indirectly by decreasing ACh release through presynaptic receptors.

● **Pharmacotherapeutics** The catecholamines are *never* administered orally because of rapid metabolism by MAO in the lining of the intestine and the first-pass effect. Although isoproterenol is not a good substrate for MAO, it is rapidly metabolized by COMT in the liver. Dopamine, NE, and dobutamine are generally administered by slow IV infusion; EPI is given IV, SQ, or directly into the heart during cardiac arrest; and isoproterenol is given by sublingual tablets or inhalation. The duration of action for all

Epinephrine is the most potent endogenous stimulator of α_1-receptors, followed by norepinephrine and only weakly by dopamine. Isoproterenol, a synthetic catecholamine, has no efficacy at any α-adrenoceptor.

Table 2.9   *Effects of Norepinephrine, Epinephrine, Isoproterenol, or Dopamine Infusion*

	NOREPINEPHRINE α-EFFECT	EPINEPHRINE α1β EFFECT	ISOPROTERENOL B-EFFECT	DOPAMINE
1. Cardiovascular System				
Heart rate (β_1)	Decrease (reflex)	Increase (direct)	Increase (direct and reflex)	Slight increase (through β_1)
Cardiac output	Decrease	Increase	Increase	Variable
Force of contraction (β_1)	Little effect	Increase (direct)	Increase (direct)	—
Systolic pressure	Increase	Increase	Slight increase	Slight increase
Mean arterial blood pressure	Increase	Slight increase	Decrease	Slight increase
Diastolic pressure	Increase	Decrease	Decrease	—
Pulse pressure	No effect	Increase	Increase	—
Skin vasculature (α_1)	Constrict	Constrict	—	Constrict (high dose)
Skeletal muscle vasculature				
β_2	—	Dilate (low doses)	Dilate	—
α_1	Constrict	Constrict (high doses)	—	Constrict (high doses)
D_1	—	—	—	Dilate (low doses)
Visceral vasculature	Constrict	Variable	Dilate	Dilate
Coronary vasculature	Dilate (?)	Dilate	Dilate	Dilate
Renal vasculature	Constrict	Constrict	Dilate	Dilate
Total peripheral resistance	Increase	Variable	Decrease	Slight increase (high doses)
2. Nonvascular Smooth Muscle				
Bronchi	Little effect	Relax	Relax	—
Intestinal	Little effect	Relax	Relax	—
Bladder (detrussor)	Little effect	Relax	Relax	—
Sphincter (of bladder)	Little effect	Constrict	Relax	—
Uterus (pregnant)	Stimulate	Usually inhibit	Inhibit	—
3. Eye				
Aqueous humor production	Unchanged	Decrease	Decrease	—
Outflow	Increase	Unchanged or slight increase	Unchanged	—
Radial muscle	Contract (mydriasis)	Weak contraction	Unchanged	—
4. Intermediary Metabolism				
Liver				
Glycogenolysis	Slight increase	Large increase	Slight increase	—
Gluconeogenesis	Slight increase	Increase	Slight increase	
Pancreatic Hormones				
Insulin	Decrease	Decrease	Increase (β_2)	—
Glucagon	Increase	Increase	Increase	
Adipose Tissue				
Glycerol	Increase	Increase	Large increase	—
NEFA	Increase	Increase	Large increase	
Skeletal Muscle				
Lactate release	Slight increase	Increase	Large increase	—

catecholamines is extremely short because of rapid metabolism. The catecholamines have only limited selectivity for the various adrenoceptors (Table 2.10).

• **EPI (adrenaline)** is a potent vasoconstrictor, producing direct positive inotropic and chronotropic effects in the heart. It dilates several

Table 2.10 *Receptor Selectivity of Catecholamine*	
CATECHOLAMINE	RECEPTOR
Epinephrine	α_1, α_2, β_1, β_2
Norepinephrine	α_1, α_2, β_1
Isoproterenol	β_1, β_2
Dopamine	D_1 (α_1 and β_1 at high doses)
Dobutamine	β_1 (α_1)

vascular beds to produce a decrease in total peripheral resistance and diastolic pressure. It is sometimes applied locally to reduce bleeding in facial, oropharyngeal, and nasopharyngeal surgery (an α_1-adrenoceptor-mediated action) mixed with local anesthetics to prolong the duration of nerve block and to reduce the likelihood of the anesthetic entering the systemic circulation. EPI is injected intracardially in the temporary emergency management of complete heart block and cardiac arrest, and in the emergency treatment of anaphylactic shock and acute hypersensitivity reactions, and it is applied topically for glaucoma.

• **NE** (levarterenol, noradrenaline) differs from EPI primarily because it lacks potency on β_2-adrenoceptors. That is, NE activates α_1-, α_2-, and β_1-adrenoceptors, increasing peripheral resistance, systolic blood pressure, and diastolic blood pressure. As a drug, the vascular effects of NE activate vagal reflexes, decreasing heart rate even though a positive inotropic effect is maintained. NE is occasionally used in hypotensive crises to preserve cerebral and coronary blood flow while fluids or blood are being administered. Because shock-induced hypotension is generally associated with reflex sympathetic activation, NE is normally of no benefit. In shock, tissue perfusion, not blood pressure, must be optimized.

• **Isoproterenol** is a potent and selective β-adrenoceptor agonist, but it does not discriminate between the β_1- and β_2-sites. Isoproterenol is a potent vasodilator through its action at β_2-adrenoceptors; it produces a reflex increase in heart rate. Because isoproterenol is also a potent β_1-adrenoceptor agonist it provokes positive inotropic and chronotropic effects through a direct effect on the heart as well. Thus isoproterenol greatly increases cardiac output while decreasing diastolic, systolic, and mean arterial pressure. Isoproterenol is used in the temporary emergency treatment of complete heart block and cardiac arrest. An aerosol formulation is used for bronchodilation in the treatment of asthma. Adverse cardiac effects (e.g., tachycardia and arrhythmias) can occur when high doses of isoproterenol are inhaled.

• The effects of **dopamine** are dose dependent, with selectivity for D_1-receptor activation at low doses and EPI-like activity at higher doses. In cardiogenic shock, a positive inotropic agent such as dopamine increases cardiac output with low to moderate doses. At these same doses dopamine produces minimal peripheral vasoconstriction and increases renal blood flow, preserving renal function.

• **Dobutamine** is a β_1-adrenoceptor-selective synthetic catecholamine that displays some α_1-adrenoceptor activity. Dobutamine is used in cardiogenic shock and congestive heart failure.

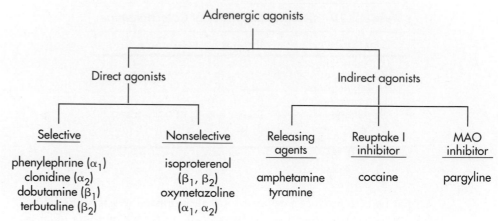

Fig. 2.9 A flow diagram of adrenergic agonists.

● **Adverse effects** The most serious adverse response to all catecholamines is an increased cardiac excitability and arrhythmias, which can lead to fatal ventricular fibrillation. Patients anesthetized with any of the halogenated hydrocarbon anesthetics or cyclopropane are particularly susceptible to catecholamine-induced arrhythmias.

The most common adverse effect of EPI and NE is elevated blood pressure, which can produce headache, cerebral hemorrhage, pulmonary edema, and anxiety.

Isoproterenol administration is associated with tachycardia, hypotension, palpitations, and arrhythmias. Overdoses of isoproterenol can be fatal.

Dopamine can cause nausea and vomiting by an action on dopamine receptors in the chemoreceptor trigger zone. Other adverse effects include tachycardia, anginal pain, arrhythmias, headache, and hypertension. All of these symptoms disappear rapidly when the infusion is stopped. Prolonged infusion of dopamine can produce gangrene in fingers and toes because of ischemic necrosis. This can be prevented with **phentolamine,** an α-adrenoceptor antagonist.

The dose of any catecholamine should be reduced and used with caution in patients taking an MAO inhibitor, a tricyclic antidepressant, or cocaine and in patients with a history of arrhythmias, coronary artery disease, hypertension, or hyperthyroidism.

■ **Sympathomimetic Drugs**

● **Overview** In addition to the endogenous and synthetic catecholamines, many other drugs stimulate adrenoceptors. Collectively these are referred to as *sympathomimetics.* Direct-acting sympathomimetics were developed to act selectively on one of the adrenoceptor subtypes. Indirect-acting adrenoceptor agonists are nonselective because their pharmacologic responses are mediated by altering the release, metabolism, or uptake of endogenous catecholamines. The responses to indirect-acting agents generally are reduced or eliminated after denervation or depletion of the catecholamine stores.

Sympathomimetics (Fig. 2.9) are frequently more useful than the catecholamines themselves because of their pharmacokinetic features, such as oral availability, CNS activity, and resistance to metabolism, or because of their receptor selectivity (Table 2.11).

Use catecholamines cautiously with MAO inhibitors, tricyclic antidepressants, and cocaine.

Table 2.11	*Receptor Selectivity of Some Direct Adrenoceptor Agonists*
ADRENOCEPTOR	**DRUG**
α-Adrenoceptors	
$\alpha_1 \approx \alpha_2$	Xylometazoline
	Oxymetazoline
α_1 selective	Phenylephrine
	Methoxamine
	Naphazoline
α_2 selective	Clonidine
	Methyldopa
	Guanfacine
	Guanabenz
β-Adrenoceptors	
$\beta_1 \approx \beta_2$	Isoproterenol
$\beta_1 > \beta_2$	Dobutamine (plus α_1)
$\beta_2 > \beta_1$	Terbutaline
	Metaproterenol
	Isoethanine
	Albuterol
	Ritodrine
	Pirbuterol
	Bitoterol

- **α_1-Adrenoceptor agonists**
  - *Basic pharmacology* **Phenylephrine** is the prototype α_1-adreno-ceptor agonist. It has great selectivity for α_1-adrenoceptors with little effect at other adrenoceptor subtypes. Phenylephrine differs from NE only by the removal of one hydroxyl group from the phenol nucleus. Therefore, phenylephrine is not a catechol, is not inactivated by COMT, and has a substantially longer duration of action (20 minutes after IV infusion) than the catecholamines. When administered systemically, phenylephrine induces vasoconstriction and increases arterial pressure and reflex bradycardia. The reflex bradycardia is used clinically to terminate paroxysmal and atrial tachycardia. More commonly, phenylephrine is used topically as a nasal decongestant and to produce mydriasis before ophthalmic examinations.

    Methoxamine and **naphazoline** are also direct-acting selective α_1-adrenoceptor agonists. Methoxamine is used to maintain blood pressure during anesthesia because it produces fewer arrhythmias than other sympathomimetics when used in conjunction with general anesthetics and to terminate supraventricular tachycardia. Naphazoline is used in ophthalmology as a mydriatic.

α_1-Selective Adrenoceptors
Phenylephrine
Methoxamine

- **α_2-Adrenoceptor agonists**
  - *Basic pharmacology* Clonidine, methyldopa, guanfacine, and guanabenz act selectively on α_2-adrenoceptors. α_2-Adrenoceptors are located in non-innervated regions of vascular smooth muscle and promote vasoconstriction. α_2-Adrenoceptors of pharmacologic impor-

α_2-Selective Adrenoceptors
Clonidine
Methyldopa
Guanabenz
Guanfacine

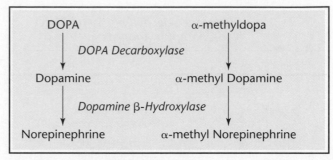

Fig. 2.10 Metabolism of *DOPA* and α-methyldopa.

tance are located in the CNS and decrease sympathetic outflow. The reduction in sympathetic nerve activity produced by α_2-adrenoceptor agonists decrease both blood pressure and heart rate. When clonidine is administered IV, vascular α_2-adrenoceptors are activated to produce a transient hypertension prior to a prolonged centrally-mediated hypotension and bradycardia.

Methyldopa is the precursor of the α_2-adrenoceptor agonist α-methyl NE (Fig. 2.10). After administration, methyldopa enters noradrenergic neurons, where it is converted by DOPA decarboxylase and dopamine β-hydroxylase to the active agent.

Unlike NE, α-methyl NE is more potent on α_2-adrenoceptor sites than on α_1-adrenoceptor sites. With chronic administration of methyldopa, endogenous NE is replaced by α-methyl NE in the peripheral nervous system (PNS) and CNS, where it is released and acts like an endogenous neurotransmitter.

Nonselective α-Agonists

Oxymetazoline
Xylometazoline

● **Nonselective α-agonists**

— *Basic pharmacology* Many sympathomimetics are used as topical nasal decongestants because they constrict blood vessels of the nasal mucosa. The α-adrenoceptor agonists most frequently used are nonselective, activating α_1-adrenoceptor and α_2-adrenoceptor sites. Of the two, the action at α_1-adrenoceptors are of greater clinical importance. Two such agents are **xylometazoline** and **oxymetazoline.** At high doses oxymetazoline can produce hypotension, presumably by a clonidine-like action at central α_2-adrenoceptor sites.

β_1-Selective Agonists

Dobutamine (slight α_1)

● **β_1-Adrenoceptor agonists**

— *Basic pharmacology* **Dobutamine** is a synthetic catecholamine that is a selective agonist for β_1-adrenoceptors. It produces a marked increase in the force of contraction with little effect on heart rate or total peripheral resistance. This combination of effects is thought to be due to its agonistic effects on α_1-adrenoceptor sites.

β_2-Agonists

Terbutaline
Ritodrine
Bitoterol

● **β_2-Adrenoceptor agonists**

— *Basic pharmacology* β_2-adrenoceptor agonists are important in the treatment of asthma because they induce bronchodilation. Members of this class include terbutaline, metaproterenol, isoethanine, pirbuterol, bitoterol, and albuterol.

   • **Bitoterol** is a prodrug that is hydrolyzed by esterases in the lung and other tissues to its active form, colterol. Because esterases are present in higher concentrations in the lung than in other tissues, this metabolic transformation improves the specificity of the drug.

• **Ritodrine** is a β_2-adrenoceptor agonist used as a uterine relaxant during premature labor.

• In severe heart failure there is a down regulation of cardiac β_1-adrenoceptors, decreasing the efficacy of dobutamine, a β_1-adrenoceptor agonist, to increase the force of contraction. Inasmuch as cardiac β_2-adrenoceptors remain functional in heart failure and mediate a positive inotropic response, β_2-adrenoceptors may be used as positive inotropic agents in this condition.

Indirect-acting sympathomimetics

● **Overview** The effects of endogenous NE and EPI can be augmented by stimulating their release, blocking their reuptake into the presynaptic terminal, or by inhibiting MAO. In general, drugs that act in these ways lack the specificity of direct-acting agonists, more closely resembling the responses to generalized sympathetic activation.

● **Norepinephrine-Releasing Agents**

— *Basic pharmacology* In general, NE-releasing agents are transported via uptake I into noradrenergic neurons where they displace NE from storage sites releasing it into the synaptic cleft. Drugs that block uptake I, such as cocaine, imipramine, and other tricyclic antidepressants, block the action of some releasing agents because they must be actively transported into the neuron. Some releasing agents, such as metaraminol, ephedrine, and pseudoephedrine, not only release NE but also directly stimulate adrenoceptors. Because releasing agents rely on endogenous stores of NE to produce their effects, tachyphylaxis is observed. That is, with repeated administration of the releasing agent, the intraneuronal pool of NE becomes depleted. This is most frequently observed with ephedrine and tyramine.

The amphetamines are releasing agents used primarily for their CNS effects. The peripheral cardiovascular responses to amphetamines, including cardiac arrhythmias, hypertension, and anginal pain, are unavoidable adverse effects.

• Because **amphetamine** lacks a catechol nucleus and possesses a methyl substituted α-carbon, it is not a substrate for either COMT or MAO. It is lipophilic and is used primarily because it releases NE, dopamine, and serotonin from CNS neurons. It does not require uptake I to enter neurons or adrenal chromaffin cells so its actions are not eliminated by uptake I inhibitors.

• Although similar in action to amphetamine, methamphetamine has even more CNS effects. Phenmetrazine, methylphenidate, and pemoline are all variants of amphetamine with similar pharmacologic effects and abuse potential.

• **Ephedrine** and **pseudoephedrine** are mixed receptor agonists. Their sympathomimetic effects are caused primarily by release of NE from postganglionic sympathetic neurons, but these agents also directly stimulate α_1-, β_1-, and β_2-adrenoceptors. Tachyphylaxis occurs to the peripheral sympathomimetic effects but not to the CNS effects of those agonists. Ephedrine and pseudoephedrine are orally effective and have relatively long duration of action. They may increase arterial blood pressure, dilate coronary vessels, increase heart rate, dilate bronchioles, and increase the tone of skeletal muscle. These

NE-Releasing Agents
Amphetamine
Methamphetamine
Ephedrine
Tyramine

Direct and Indirect Affects
Metaraminol
Ephedrine
Pseudoephedrine

Amphetamine-like Compounds
Phenmetrazine
Methylphenidate
Pemoline

drugs are used primarily in asthma, as nasal decongestants, and occasionally as pressor agents. Ephedrine has also been used in the treatment of myasthenia gravis.

• **Metaraminol** is a mixed agonist used almost exclusively for the treatment of hypotension. Although it releases catecholamines, its overall effects are similar to those of NE; however, it is less potent and longer acting. Metaraminol increases blood pressure, reflexly decreases heart rate, and slightly decreases cardiac output (although it increases the force of contraction). If the reflex bradycardia is prevented by atropine, a marked increase in cardiac output is observed.

• **Tyramine** acts only on peripheral neurons to release NE from noradrenergic terminals. It is metabolized by MAO and produces a spectrum of action similar to NE. Tyramine is not used clinically but is found in high concentrations in fermented foods and beverages such as cheese, beer, and wine. Because tyramine is inactivated by MAO, patients being treated with MAO inhibitors are particularly susceptible to hypertensive crises after ingesting foods containing tyramine. The effects of tyramine are blocked by uptake I inhibitors, NE depletion, and repeated administration (tachyphylaxis).

● **Uptake I Inhibitors**

— *Overview* The major route of inactivation of NE is by reuptake into the presynaptic neuron by uptake I. Many drugs act to inhibit this transport process. None of these agents are used therapeutically for their peripheral effects. When uptake I is inhibited, the concentration of NE in the synaptic cleft is elevated, resulting in stimulation of adrenoceptors.

— *Basic pharmacology* The uptake I inhibitors also prevent the uptake of any drug or endogenous substance transported by the catecholamine uptake system into neurons. The response to ephedrine is diminished and the response to tyramine is abolished by uptake I inhibitors. Drugs that block uptake I include cocaine, tricyclic antidepressants, and certain antipsychotics.

Uptake I Inhibitors
Cocaine
Trycyclic antidepressants
Some antipsychotics

● **Monoamine Oxidase Inhibitors**

— *Overview* Inhibitors of MAO prevent the intracellular deamination and inactivation of NE in nerve terminals and extraneuronal tissue. At one time these drugs were used as antihypertensive agents because they promote the formation of octopamine, a weak adrenoceptor agonist, which replaces NE in sympathetic neurons, thereby decreasing vasoconstriction. Today, MAO inhibitors are used primarily to treat depression and Parkinson's disease. Severe hypertensive crises have developed in patients receiving MAO inhibitors after ingesting foods rich in tyramine. Adverse effects can result from administering a catecholamine during surgery to a patient treated with an MAO inhibitor and when combining an indirect-acting sympathomimetic with an MAO inhibitor.

— *Basic pharmacology* There are two forms of MAO: MAO-A and MAO-B. MAO-A is more effective in degrading NE and serotonin, and MAO-B is less selective for individual monoamines. Older MAO inhibitors, such as **pargyline** and **tranylcypromine**, inhibit MAO-A and MAO-B equally. There are newer agents that selectively block MAO-A, such as **clorgyline,** and MAO-B, such as **(-)deprenyl.**

Table 2.12 *Receptor Selectivity of Some* *α-Adrenoceptor Antagonists*	
RECEPTOR SELECTIVITY	DRUG
$\alpha_1 \approx \alpha_2$	Phentolamine Tolazoline Phenoxybenzamine*
α_1 selective	Prazosin Terazosin Doxazosin Labetalol†
α_2 selective	Yohimbine

*Irreversible covalent binding; noncompetitive antagonist.
†Also blocks β_1-adrenoceptors and β_2-adrenoceptors.

SECTION 2.5 ADRENOCEPTOR ANTAGONISTS AND OTHER SYMPATHOLYTIC AGENTS

■ **Overview** The characteristic physiologic responses to sympathetic excitation are blocked in a variety of ways. Some drugs competitively antagonize the effects of NE and EPI at α-adrenoceptors and β-adrenoceptors, some deplete NE from sympathetic nerves, and some act on the CNS to inhibit sympathetic nerve activity. All of these drugs are classified as sympatholytics.

■ **α-Adrenoceptor Antagonists** (Table 2.12) In general, α-adrenoceptor antagonists have limited clinical utility. Arteriolar and venous tone are tonically maintained by the sympathetic nervous system with NE acting on α_1-adrenoceptors. Thus blockade of α_1-adrenoceptors lowers peripheral vascular resistance and blood pressure, causing reflex tachycardia, a reflex increase in renin release, and can precipitate orthostatic hypotension. The tachycardic and renin responses are greater with agents that block both α_1-adrenoceptors and α_2-adrenoceptors. Selective α_1-antagonists, such as prazosin, have less of an effect on heart rate and renin release than nonselective antagonists because they do not block the pre-synaptic inhibitory α_2-adrenoceptors. Although cardiac output is usually unchanged after administration of an α_1-adrenoceptor antagonist, cardiac output increases during long-term treatment with these agents. Blockade of presynaptic α_2-adrenoceptors increases NE release from adrenergic neurons to act on β-adrenoceptors, increasing heart rate and renin release. Other effects produced by α-adrenoceptor antagonists include miosis, decreased adrenergic sweating, nasal stuffiness, decreased resistance to urinary outflow, increased insulin release, and impaired ejaculation. All of these adverse effects can be predicted on the basis of physiology. Individual α-blockers have other adverse effects unrelated to their ability to block α-adrenoceptors.

● **Basic pharmacology**

• **Phentolamine** is a competitive, reversible, nonselective α-adrenoceptor antagonist. It also blocks serotonin receptors and is an agonist at muscarinic and histamine receptors. Phentolamine is poorly absorbed from the gastrointestinal tract and has a short duration of action. Phentolamine administration results in a marked tachycardia that is in part reflex because of the hypotension caused by this agent and, in part, caused by increased NE release in response to blockade of presynaptic α_2-adrenoceptors on the cardiac sympathetic nerves. Adverse effects include severe tachycardia, arrhythmias, angina, diarrhea, and excessive gastric acid secretion.

- **Tolazoline** is similar to phentolamine but is less potent and more readily absorbed after oral administration.

- **Phenoxybenzamine** binds covalently to α-adrenoceptors, causing irreversible blockade. The duration of action is 14 to 48 hours after a single dose. It displays almost no selectivity in vivo. Other pharmacologic actions of phenoxybenzamine include inhibition of uptakes I and II and blockade of histamine, acetylcholine, and serotonin receptors. Although phenoxybenzamine produces only a slight reduction in blood pressure in supine individuals, it causes significant hypotension when sympathetic tone or circulating catecholamines are high, such as on standing with blood volume depletion or with pheochromocytoma. Phenoxybenzamine increases cardiac output. Adverse effects include postural hypotension, tachycardia, nasal stuffiness, impaired ejaculation, sedation, and nausea.

- **Prazosin** is a selective, competitive antagonist at α_1-adrenoceptors, with little affinity for α_2-adrenoceptor sites. Thus prazosin causes less tachycardia, positive inotropy, and renin release than nonselective α-adrenoceptor antagonists or direct vasodilators. Chronic administration of selective α_1-adrenoceptor antagonists has little effect on heart rate and renin secretion. This class of drugs can be used for the treatment of hypertension.

- **Terazosin** and **doxazosin** are analogs of prazosin, possessing similar properties but with longer half-lives.

- A unique α-adrenoceptor antagonist is **yohimbine.** Yohimbine is the only selective α_2-adrenoceptor antagonist on the market. It may have usefulness in autonomic insufficiency because it stimulates NE release by blocking presynaptic α_2-adrenoceptors. It has also been reported to improve symptoms in patients with painful diabetic neuropathies and may enhance sexual function.

- **Labetalol** is an α_1-adrenoceptor antagonist with β-adrenoceptor blocking activity.

Many drugs used in the treatment of schizophrenia block α-adrenoceptors. Although these drugs are not used clinically for this purpose, the α-adrenoceptor antagonism may contribute to such adverse effects as orthostatic hypotension.

Pharmacotherapeutics

- The α-adrenoceptor antagonists are theoretically useful in hypertensive crises, although other drugs, especially diuretics, are more commonly used for this condition.

- The primary use of **phenoxybenzamine** and **phentolamine** is in the management of pheochromocytoma. This condition is characterized by hypertension, tachycardia, arrhythmias, and high levels of circulating catecholamines and urinary catecholamine metabolites. Phentolamine has been used in the diagnosis of pheochromocytoma because patients with the tumor will display a much greater fall in blood pressure than normal, although measurements of catecholamines in plasma and urinary excretion is a more reliable and safer approach. During removal of the tumor release

Table 2.13   *Characteristics of Some β-Adrenoceptor Antagonists*

	SELECTIVITY	PARTIAL AGONIST ACTIVITY	LOCAL ANESTHETIC ACTIVITY	ELIMINATION HALF-LIFE
Acebutolol	$\beta_1 > \beta_2$	Yes	Yes	3-4 hr
Atenolol	$\beta_1 > \beta_2$	No	No	6-9 hr
Metoprolol	$\beta_1 > \beta_2$	No	Yes	3-4 hr
Esmolol	$\beta_1 > \beta_2$	No	No	10 min
Propranolol	None	No	Yes	3.5-6 hr
Labetalol	None	No	Yes	5 hr
Nadolol	None	No	No	14-24 hr
Pindolol	None	Yes	Yes	3-4 hr
Timolol	None	No	Yes	4-5 hr

of stored catecholamines cannot always be prevented. The resulting hypertension can be controlled with phentolamine.

- **Phentolamine** is used to prevent local vasoconstriction produced by sympathomimetics by infiltration into the ischemic tissue.

- **Phenoxybenzamine** is useful in the preoperative management of pheochromocytoma and in chronic treatment of inoperable or metastatic pheochromocytoma.

- **Prazosin, terazosin,** and **doxazosin** are effective in the chronic management of mild to moderate hypertension. These drugs can produce profound orthostatic hypotension with syncope, especially after the first dose is administered. This adverse effect generally disappears with repeated administration.

- Selective α_1-adrenoceptor antagonists such as prazosin and terazosin are useful in patients with inoperable obstructive prostatic hyperplasia. Because the α_1-adrenoceptor subtype that mediates contraction of prostatic smooth muscles is molecularly distinct from that regulating vascular smooth muscle tone, selective α_1-adrenoceptor antagonists may be developed to relieve the symptoms of bladder outlet obstruction associated with symptomatic benign prostatic hyperplasia without affecting blood pressure.

- In general, α-adrenoceptor antagonists do not adversely affect serum lipids and may actually increase the high-density lipoprotein total cholesterol ratio.

Treatment of Hypertension

Prazosin
Terazosin
Doxazosin

Treatment of Obstructive Prostatic Hyperplasia

Prazosin
Terazosin
Doxazosin

■ β-Adrenoceptor Antagonists

- **Overview** β-adrenoceptor antagonists are some of the most commonly used drugs, particularly in hypertension. They are all competitive antagonists of catecholamines. β-Adrenoceptor blockers, such as **acebutolol** and **pindolol,** have partial agonist activity, and some have greater affinity for one or the other of the β-adrenoceptor subtypes. Others display local anesthetic-like membrane-stabilizing effects. The local anesthetic effect does not appear to be clinically important except when these drugs are used as eye drops. Table 2.13 lists the characteristics of some β-adrenoceptor antagonists.

- **Pharmacokinetics** β-adrenoceptor antagonists are well absorbed after oral administration. The prototypic β-adrenoceptor antagonist **propranolol** undergoes extensive first-pass metabolism. There is great individual varia-

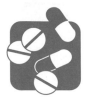

tion in the plasma concentration of propranolol after oral administration. Bioavailability is limited to varying degrees, except for **pindolol,** which is 90% absorbed.

In general, β-adrenoceptor antagonists have a large volume of distribution. Propranolol is lipophilic and readily crosses the blood-brain barrier. The clinical use of propranolol in treating migraine and other neurologic disorders may be related to its CNS effects.

The half-lives are generally several hours. An exception is **esmolol,** which has a half-life of approximately 10 minutes (Table 2.13).

Pharmacodynamics Most of the effects of β-adrenoceptor antagonists are directly related to blockade of catecholamines at these receptors. Thus these drugs lower blood pressure in patients with hypertension, produce negative inotropic and chronotropic effects on the heart, decrease AV conduction, block β_2-adrenoceptor-mediated vasodilation (increasing total peripheral resistance), and decrease renin release. The cardiac effects result in decreased oxygen consumption of the heart. Hence, β-adrenoceptor antagonists are useful in treating angina.

• Nonselective β-adrenoceptor antagonists counteract the bronchodilation produced by circulations EPI and increase airway resistance, particularly in asthmatics. Even the β_1-adrenoceptor-selective drugs produce some bronchoconstriction. Thus this class should generally be avoided in patients with asthma.

• Several β-adrenoceptor blockers, such as timolol, betaxolol, and levobunolol, are used in the treatment of open-angle glaucoma to reduce intraocular pressure, presumably by decreasing aqueous humor production.

• Because β-adrenoceptor antagonists inhibit sympathetic stimulation of glycolysis they should be used with caution in insulin-dependent diabetics.

• Frequently associated with β-adrenoceptor antagonist therapy are increases in plasma levels of triglycerides and decreases in high-density lipoproteins, neither of which is desirable.

• Pindolol, penbutolol, carteolol, and acebutolol have partial agonist activity, also known as intrinsic sympathomimetic activity. This may explain why these drugs cause less bradycardia than propranolol.

• The local anesthetic effect of some β-adrenoceptor antagonists results from their ability to block sodium channels in neurons and in heart and skeletal muscle. It is unlikely that this is of clinical consequence, except when used as eye drops, because the normal drug concentration is probably insufficient to block the channels.

— *Specific β-adrenoceptor antagonists (Table 2.14)*

• **Propranolol** is the prototypic agent in this class. It undergoes extensive first-pass metabolism and is nonselective (β_1, β_2).

• **Nadolol** is distinctive for its long duration of action.

• **Timolol** is used primarily in glaucoma because it greatly decreases intraocular pressure.

• **Labetalol** is not only a potent, nonselective β-adrenoceptor antagonist, it is also a competitive, selective α_1-adrenoceptor antagonist. The hypotensive response to labetalol is accompanied by less tachycardia than is typically associated with α-adrenoceptor antagonists.

• **Metoprolol, atenolol, esmolol,** and **acebutolol** are all relatively

Treatment of Open-Angle Glaucoma

Timolol
Betaxolol
Levobunolol

Partial Agonist Activity

Pindolol
Penbutolol
Carteolol
Acebutolol

B_1 Selective

Metoprolol
Atenolol
Esmolol
Acebutolol

Table 2.14	*Receptor Selectivity of Some β-Adrenoceptor Antagonists*
RECEPTOR SELECTIVITY	**DRUG**
$\beta_1 \approx \beta_2$	Propranolol Timolol Nadolol Levobunolol Pindolol* Penbutolol* Carteolol* Labetalol†
$\beta_1 > \beta_2$	Metoprolol Acebutolol* Atenolol Betaxolol Esmolol
$\beta_2 > \beta_1$	Butoxamine

*Also have intrinsic sympathomimetic activity.
†Also a selective α_1-adrenoceptor antagonist.

selective β_1-adrenoceptor antagonists. These drugs are generally safer than nonselective agents in patients with history of bronchospasm, although they should be used with great caution in such patients. β_1-adrenoceptor-selective drugs are preferable for use in diabetics because they are less likely to delay recovery from hypoglycemia or cause severe hypertension when hypoglycemia leads to an increase in circulating EPI levels. They are also useful in patients with peripheral vascular disease.

• **Esmolol** is noteworthy for its short duration. It is typically administered IV with its actions terminated almost immediately after discontinuation of the infusion. During surgery, infusion of esmolol blocks the reflex tachycardia and renin response elicited by vasodilators. Therefore, in the presence of emolol, lower doses of vasodilators produce the same degree of hypotension without the severe tachycardia as normally encountered with these agents.

• **Butoxamine** is a selective β_2-adrenoceptor antagonist. Currently there is no clinical indication for its use. With the recent interest in cardiac β_2-receptors, clinical investigations are ongoing to determine whether such agents have therapeutic value.

• **Pindolol, penbutolol, carteolol** (nonselective β-adrenoceptor antagonists) and **acebutolol** (a β_1-adrenoceptor selective antagonist) possess intrinsic sympathomimetic activity. Accordingly, they lower blood pressure with less of a decrease in cardiac output or heart rate at rest. The clinical significance of this effect is not yet clear.

● **Pharmacotherapeutics** β-Adrenoceptor antagonists are one of the most important classes of drugs for the treatment of hypertension. They are also useful in reducing the frequency of anginal episodes, in ischemic heart disease and in the treatment of supraventricular and ventricular arrhythmias. In certain circumstances they are useful in treating congestive heart failure, in the treatment of glaucoma, in reducing the symptomology associated with hyperthyroidism, and in some neurologic disorders.

● **Adverse effects** The major adverse effects of these drugs are extensions of their pharmacologic properties. Even selective β_1-adrenoceptor antagonists should be used with extreme caution in asthmatics and in patients with severe peripheral vascular disease or vasospastic disorders.

The β-adrenoceptor antagonists are used to decrease myocardial contractility and excitability which is beneficial in treating hypertension and arrhythmias. However, if a patient has partial AV block, or some underlying heart disease, such as a previous myocardial infarction or congestive heart failure, β-adrenoceptor antagonists should be used sparingly, if at all.

A serious problem can occur with abrupt withdrawal of a β-adrenoceptor blocker after chronic use. Under this circumstance, β-adrenoceptor antagonists cause up regulation, or supersensitivity of β-adrenoceptors. With abrupt withdrawal there may be a large number of unoccupied receptors which, upon normal stimulation, may produce extensive cardiac stimulation and hypertension. The dose of β-adrenoceptor blockers should be gradually reduced rather than abruptly discontinued.

Nonselective β-adrenoceptor antagonists generally increase serum triglycerides or decrease high-density lipoprotein cholesterol. These adverse effects are less with selective β_1-adrenoceptor antagonists.

■ **Adrenergic Neuron-Blocking Drugs**

● **Overview** Drugs in this category are sympatholytic by preventing the normal physiologic release of NE from the sympathetic neuron. These agents are used in hypertension, normally when all other therapies fail.

■ **Specific Agents**

NE-Releasing Agents
Guanethidine
Guanadrel
Reserpine
Bretylium

• Guanethidine acts to reduce sympathetic tone by two mechanisms: inhibition of NE release and displacement and gradual depletion of NE from the storage granules. To be effective, guanethidine must enter the adrenergic neuron by uptake I. Accordingly, its effects are blocked by cocaine and other inhibitors of this transport process. Upon entry into the neuron, guanethidine initially displaces NE. Thus if it is administered by rapid IV infusion it can produce hypertension. In the early phase of treatment, the decrease in blood pressure produced by guanethidine is associated with reduced cardiac output because of bradycardia and relaxation of capacitance vessels with no significant change in total peripheral resistance. With chronic treatment, cardiac output may return to normal and a substantial decrease in peripheral resistance is observed. A period of 1 to 2 weeks of continuous treatment is required to reduce blood pressure.

The major adverse responses to guanethidine are orthostatic hypotension from elimination of reflex control of the sympathetic nervous system, diarrhea, and failure of ejaculation. There are no CNS effects because guanethidine does not cross the blood-brain barrier.

• Guanadrel is similar to guanethidine, but has a shorter duration of action.

• Reserpine is an alkaloid that was used as an antihypertensive drug but is rarely employed today because of its adverse effects. Reserpine blocks the transport of biogenic amines into neuronal storage vesicles. Because of this, reserpine depletes peripheral and central stores of NE, dopamine, and serotonin, as well as adrenal EPI. The effect of reserpine on synaptic vesicles is irreversible with a single dose effectively depleting the amines until the neurons resynthesize active vesicles. Although reserpine decreases blood pressure, its primary site of action, central or peripheral, is not known.

Adverse effects of reserpine include sedation, a Parkinson-like syndrome caused by depletion of dopamine, psychic depression, nightmares, diarrhea, and increased gastric acid secretions. Thus it should not be used in patients with peptic ulcers. Because of its effects on CNS function it should not be used in patients with a history of depression.

  • Bretylium is similar to guanethidine in that it blocks the neural release of NE. It is used as an antiarrhythmic agent because of its direct actions on the heart. Like guanethidine, rapid IV infusions of bretylium may release sufficient NE to precipitate ventricular arrhythmias.

■ **Central-Acting Sympatholytic Drugs** Included in this group are the selective α_2-adrenoceptor agonists clonidine, methyldopa, guanabenz, and guanfacine. These drugs stimulate postsynaptic α_2-adrenoceptors in the CNS and thereby decrease outflow to all sympathetically innervated organs.

Central-Acting

Clonidine
Methyldopa
Guanabenz
Guanfacine

MULTIPLE CHOICE REVIEW QUESTIONS

1. After an acute myocardial infarction, a 55-year-old male exhibits sinus bradycardia with a ventricular rate of 42 beats per minute. He is significantly hypotensive. After atropine administration, his ventricular rate increased to 80, but his pupils became fixed and dilated, although he remained alert. Why was atropine administered and why might the pupils have changed appearance?

    a. Atropine's sympathomimetic effects increased heart rate directly, whereas its ganglionic effects changed pupil size.
    b. Atropine use results in a release of histamine, further reducing blood pressure but eliciting a stronger reflex response, thus increasing heart rate. Increased pupil size was an incidental effect of histamine.
    c. Atropine was administered because its antimuscarinic effect would inhibit vagal influences at the SA node. The same anticholinergic effect could, especially at higher concentrations, induce pupillary dilation.
    d. Atropine was administered to inhibit vascular smooth muscle relaxation and counteract the hypotension induced by increased circulating acetylcholine. Atropine caused the pupillary dilation.

2. Isoproterenol is a positive chronotropic and inotropic agent. Administration may result in tachyarrhythmias and premature ventricular contractions. These effects are most likely to result from the stimulation of which receptor system? Why could activation of this receptor system cause tachyarrhythmias and PVCs?

    a. The β-2 receptor system mediates most of the increased heart rate and force of contraction. The resultant hypertension with reflex activation of the parasympathetic system causes the arrhythmias.
    b. The α adrenergic receptor system is activated by isoproterenol and causes the observed effects.
    c. The β-1 receptor system is activated by isoproterenol and produces the increase in heart rate and force of contraction. cAMP levels are increased by isoproterenol as is phosphorylation of troponin and phospholamban. These proteins are likely to be important in mediation of positive inotropism. Tachyarrhythmias

    and PVCs could occur because of increased normal automaticity in latent pacemaker fibers.
    d. Isoproterenol is the most selective cholinergic muscarinic agonist. Therefore it would cause the increase in heart rate noted and would, through increasing cGMP, produce increased force of heart contraction.

3. Consider the following mechanism of action: the drug binds to neuronal storage vesicles and destroys them. Choose the drug(s) that both act(s) in this matter and has the associated physiologic result.

    a. Botulinum toxin: ptosis, dysphagia, dyspnea
    b. Nicotine: positive chronotropic response
    c. Reserpine: hypotension
    d. Prazosin: hypotension
    e. Propranolol: negative chronotropic response

4. A 70-year-old male patient was brought to the hospital suffering from chest pain. Just before becoming symptomatic he had taken his morning medication, which consisted of metoprolol and an aspirin tablet. His medical history documented several previous myocardial infarctions and a coronary artery by-pass procedure performed several years earlier. On this occasion, he was diagnosed as having a severe myocardial infarction with significant loss of myocardial mass. Shortly after admission the patient's condition worsened, and he now presents in cardiogenic shock. He is given IV dobutamine to improve cardiac output. What happens?

    a. Cardiac output increases as dobutamine stimulates cardiac β receptors.
    b. Cardiac output does not increase. Increasing dobutamine levels increase peripheral resistance.
    c. Cardiac output increases only at higher than expected dobutamine levels, but no effect on peripheral resistance is observed.
    d. Cardiac output does not increase with dobutamine, but it does with dopamine.

5. An anesthetized experimental animal whose myocardial activity and level of blood pressure are being recorded and has received an injection of hexamethonium would respond to:

    a. cervical vagus nerve stimulation by cardiac slowing and fall in blood pressure.
    b. methoxamine injection by rise in blood pressure and reflex bradycardia.
    c. cervical vagus nerve stimulation by cardiac slowing and no change in blood pressure.

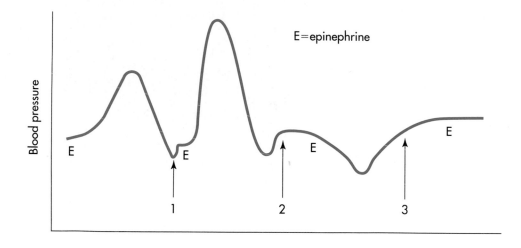

Fig. 2.11 Blood pressure tracing in an anesthetized cat. Continuous infusion of drugs 1, 2, and 3 are started at the times indicated by the arrows. Epinephrine is injected at each time indicated by E.

d. methacholine injection by cardiac acceleration and rise in blood pressure.

e. isoproterenol injection by cardiac excitation and fall in blood pressure.

6. A normotensive 65-year-old female began experiencing dyspnea upon exertion associated with chest pain. The chest discomfort was determined to be angina pectoris. In order to improve her exercise tolerance, medication was prescribed. Consider each drug and rationale and select the most appropriate.

a. Scopolamine: the muscarinic agonistic effects would reduce heart rate and therefore reduce oxygen demand.

b. Phentolamine: hypotension associated with phentolamine would reduce myocardial work and prevent ischemic symptoms.

c. Isoproterenol: increased β_1-receptor stimulation would increase cardiac output and therefore increase coronary perfusion resulting in decreased angina symptoms.

d. Phenoxybenzamine: because of its long action, phenoxybenzamine is the preferred treatment for angina. The decrease in blood pressure from α-receptor blockade is long-term and decreased myocardial work is because of reduced afterload.

e. Metoprolol: reduced effects of adrenergic nerve activity and circulating catecholamines on the heart result in reduced rate and inotropy. Both factors reduce myocardial oxygen demand and therefore may increase exercise tolerance and reduce anginal events.

7. Which of the following causes reflex bradycardia?

a. Isoproterenol
b. Terbutaline
c. Phentolamine
d. Clonidine
e. Methoxamine

8. Which of the following causes a competitive block of uptake I?

a. Tyramine
b. Clonidine
c. Isoproterenol
d. Cocaine
e. Oxymetazoline

9. Refer to Fig. 2.11. Compound 1 could be:

a. Doxazosin
b. Propranolol
c. Phenoxybenzamine
d. Cocaine
e. Acetylcholine

10. Refer to Fig. 2.11. Compound 2 could be:

a. Doxazosin
b. Atropine
c. Propranolol
d. Acetylcholine
e. Phenylephrine

11. Refer to Fig. 2.11. Compound 3 could be:

a. Acetylcholine
b. Atropine
c. Propranolol
d. Tyramine
e. Trimethaphan

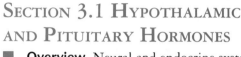

Chapter 3

Endocrine Pharmacology

SECTION 3.1 HYPOTHALAMIC AND PITUITARY HORMONES

■ **Overview** Neural and endocrine systems of the hypothalamus and pituitary gland mediate neuroendocrine control of metabolism, growth, and aspects of reproduction. Secretion of anterior pituitary hormones is regulated by hypothalamic hormones carried to the adenohypophysis by the hypothalamic-hypophyseal portal system. Hypothalamic hormones are small peptides that regulate release of hormones of the anterior pituitary. Target gland hormones inhibit hypothalamic-pituitary release of their respective tropic hormones. Neurotransmitters such as serotonin, norepinephrine (NE), and dopamine influence secretion of hypothalamic hormones by peptidergic neurones of the median eminence. Fig. 3.1 summarizes the regulation of secretion of hypothalamic and anterior pituitary hormones. Tables 3.1 and 3.2 list the hormones and their relative sizes and Table 3.3 indicates the links between the hypothalamic, pituitary, and target organ hormones.

Hormones of the posterior pituitary are synthesized in the hypothalamus and transported to the posterior lobe by neurosecretory fibers.

Therapeutic preparations of pituitary or hypothalamic peptide hormones may be synthetic or are isolated from animal or human sources. They are used in hormone deficiency states as diagnostic tools or in pharmacologic doses for achieving hormonal effects normally absent at physiologic blood levels.

Peptide hormones are administered intravenously (IV), subcutaneously (SQ), intramuscularly (IM), or intranasally. Inactivation in plasma, liver, kidney, or tissues is usually rapid. Some analogs possessing long half-lives are available, including octreotide (somatostatin analog), leuprolide, and nafarelin (GnRH analogs).

■ **Growth Hormone-releasing Hormone** Growth hormone-releasing hormone (GHRH) or sermatorelin is administered IV, IM, SQ, or intranasally. When given IV, GHRH has a half-life of 7 minutes. It is used clinically as a diagnostic agent to evaluate the ability of the pituitary somatoroph to produce growth hormone (GH). An analog of GHRH, sermorelin, is available.

■ **Somatotropin Release-inhibiting Hormone** (SRIH or somatostatin) inhibits GH release but has no therapeutic utility because of lack of specificity and short half-life. The SRIH analog octreotide has a much longer half-life and is used SQ or orally to treat acromegaly.

■ **Growth Hormone** (GH or somatotropin) is synthesized and stored in pituitary somatotrophs. Human growth hormone, somatotropin, for therapeutic use is produced by recombinant DNA technology and a biosynthetic form, somatrem

Posterior Pituitary Hormone

Oxycytocin
Vasopressin

Long-acting Analogs

Octreotide
Leuprolide
Nafarelin

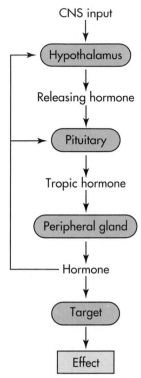

Fig. 3.1 The hypothalamic-pituitary-peripheral gland systems involve the release of a series of hormones beginning with central nervous system (CNS) regulation of secretion of releasing hormones from the hypothalamus that stimulate the pituitary to release tropic hormones, which act on peripheral endocrine glands to release their hormones. The hormones from the peripheral glands exert feedback control on the hypothalamus and pituitary.

is available. They are administered IM or SQ; active blood levels persist for up to 36 hours. GH is cleared by the liver.

- **Pharmacodynamics** GH has both metabolic and anabolic actions. It increases amino acid transport into tissues, enhances protein synthesis, and decreases lipolysis, at least initially. Some time after administration, GH exerts an insulin-antagonistic effect in the periphery with impaired glucose uptake and increased lipolysis. Thus GH is diabetogenic in patients with diabetes mellitus. This hormone also stimulates the synthesis of somatomedins, insulin-like growth factors, in the liver. These promote cartilage

Table 3.1   *Hypothalamic Regulatory Hormones*

HORMONE	ABBREVIATION	STRUCTURE
Growth hormone–releasing hormone, sermatorelin	GHRH	40 or 44 amino acids
Somatotropin release-inhibiting hormone, somatostatin	SRIH	14 amino acids
Thyrotropin-releasing hormone, protirelin	TRH	3 amino acids
Corticotropin-releasing hormone	CRH	41 amino acids
Gonadotropin-releasing hormone, gonadorelin	GnRH, LHRH	10 amino acids

Table 3.2 *Anterior Pituitary Hormones*

HORMONE	ABBREVIATION	STRUCTURE
Growth hormone	GH	191 AAs
Thyrotropin	TSH	glycoprotein
Adrenocorticotropin	ACTH	39 AAs
Follicle-stimulating hormone	FSH	glycoprotein
Luteinizing hormone	LH	glycoprotein
Prolactin	PRL	glycoprotein

synthesis and bone growth. In GH deficiency, somatomedin production is inadequate resulting in hypopituitary dwarfism. Hypersecretion of GH from pituitary tumors leads to acromegaly. Control of GH secretion and action is shown in Fig. 3.2.

- ● **Pharmacotherapeutics** GH is used for replacement therapy in children deficient in this hormone. Only human GH is effective in this condition. It is contraindicated in patients with closed epiphyses.

- ■ **Thyrotropin-releasing Hormone** Thyrotropin-releasing hormone (TRH or protirelin) is administered IV. It has a plasma half-life of 4 to 5 minutes.

  - ● **Pharmacodynamics** TRH stimulates pituitary production of thyrotropin (TSH), which in turn stimulates the thyroid to release thyroxine (T_4). TRH is used diagnostically to distinguish between primary hypothyroidism when thyrotropin levels are high and the response to TRH is large and secondary hypothyroidism when levels are low and fail to rise in response to TRH. In tertiary (hypothalamic) hypothyroidism, baseline TSH levels may be low and the TSH response may be delayed. Fig. 3.3 shows the negative feed-back effects of triiodothyronine (T_3) and thyroxine (T_4) on the TSH response to TRH in healthy subjects.

- ■ **Thyroid-stimulating Hormone** TSH has a half-life of approximately 1 hour when administered IM or SQ.

Table 3.3 *Links Among Hypothalamic, Pituitary, and Target Gland Hormones*

HYPOTHALAMIC	PITUITARY	TARGET ORGAN	TARGET ORGAN HORMONES
GHRH (+)	GH (+)	Liver	Somatomedins
SRIH (−)			
CRH (+)	ACTH (+)	Adrenal cortex	Glucocorticoids
			Mineralocorticoids
			Androgens
TRH (+)	TSH (+)	Thyroid	T_4, T_3
GnRH or LHRH (+)	FSH (+)	Gonads	Estrogen
	LH (+)		Progesterone
			Testosterone
Dopamine (−)	Prolactin (+)	Breast	
PRH (+)			

(+) = Stimulant; (−) = Inhibitor
GHRH, Growth hormone-releasing hormone; *GH,* growth hormone; *SRIH,* somatotropin-releasing inhibiting hormone; *CRH,* corticotropin-releasing hormone; *ACTH,* adrenocorticotropin hormone; *TRH,* thyrotropin-releasing hormone; *TSH,* thyroid stimulating hormone; *GnRH* or *LHRH,* gonadotropin-releasing hormone; *FSH* or *LH,* follicle-stimulating hormone, *PRH,* prolactin-releasing hormone.

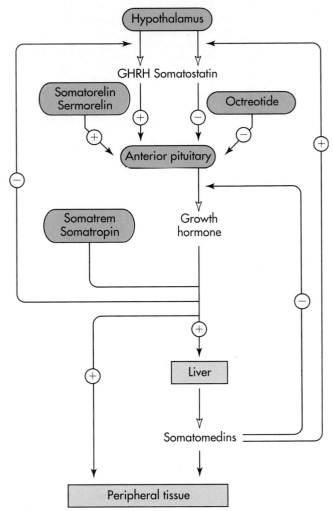

Fig. 3.2 Schematic showing the regulation of growth hormone secretion and effects of growth hormone. Synthetic peptides used as drugs are shown in red. *(Adapted from Rang et al:* Pharmacology, *New York, 1995, Churchill Livingstone.)*

- **Pharmacodynamics** TSH stimulates thyroid cell adenylyl cyclase, increasing iodine uptake and the production of thyroid hormones.

- **Pharmacotherapeutics** TSH is used primarily to promote uptake of ^{131}I in the treatment of thyroid carcinoma. Commercial TSH is derived from bovine pituitaries.

- **Corticotropin-releasing Hormone** Corticotropin-releasing hormone (CRH) stimulates the release of adrenocorticotropin (ACTH) from the pituitary. It is typically administered IV. It is used diagnostically to distinguish Cushing's disease caused by a pituitary tumor from ectopic ACTH-producing tumor cells. Ovine CRH, which differs from human CRH by seven amino acids, is used because it is more potent and longer lasting than the human hormone.

- **ACTH** or adrenocorticotropin administration increases the production of cortisol, mineralocorticoids, and androgens. It is used primarily in assessing adrenocortical responsiveness. Commercial ACTH is derived from porcine pituitaries or is a synthetic derivation of the human hormone (cosyntropin). It is administered IM and displays a half-life of less than 20 minutes.

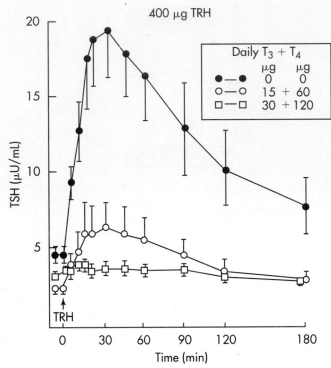

Fig. 3.3 Effect of $T_3 + T_4$ administration on the TSH response to TRH (Protirelin) in healthy subjects.

- **Pharmacodynamics** ACTH acts on the adrenal cortex to stimulate adenylyl cyclase and activate the conversion of cholesterol to pregnenolone, the rate-limiting step in steroid hormone production. It stimulates the release of glucocorticoids, and slightly increases the release of mineralocorticoids and androgens.

- **Pharmacotherapeutics** ACTH is used to diagnose adrenal insufficiency (Addison's disease). In this case, plasma cortisol or urinary 17-hydroxycorticosteroids are measured before and after administration of ACTH, as discussed further in Section 3.3. The levels of endogenous ACTH are increased in primary and decreased in secondary adrenal insufficiency.

■ **Gonadotropin-releasing Hormone** Gonadotropin-releasing hormone (GnRH/LHRH) or gonadorelin regulates release of follicle-stimulating hormone (FSH) and luteinizing hormone (LH). It is administered IV or SQ. The analogs leuprolide and nafarelin are given SQ, IM, or intranasally. The half-lives of GnRH and the analogs are 4 minutes and 3 hours, respectively.

- **Pharmacodynamics** GnRH and its analogs bind to receptors on pituitary gonadotrophs. Pulsatile IV administration of GnRH stimulates FSH and LH secretion. Continuous administration of GnRH or depot formulations of the analogs inhibits gonadotropin release.

- **Pharmacotherapeutics** GnRH is used for the diagnosis of hypogonadism and to stimulate pituitary function in delayed puberty and cryptorchidism.

Half-lives

Gonodorelin = 4 minutes
Leuprolide = 3 hours
Nafarelin = 3 hours

■ **Follicle-stimulating Hormone and Luteinizing Hormone** Follicle-stimulating hormone and luteinizing hormone (FSH and LH) are available as partially catabolized forms extracted from urine of post menopausal women.

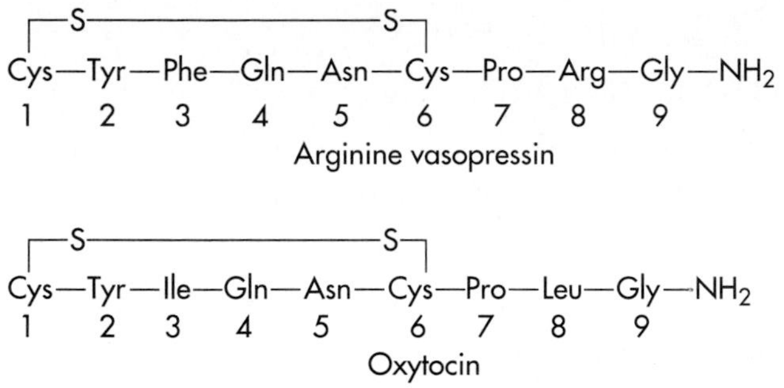

```
    ┌─S──────────────S─┐
Cys─Tyr─Phe─Gln─Asn─Cys─Pro─Arg─Gly─NH₂
 1   2   3   4   5   6   7   8   9
          Arginine vasopressin
```

```
    ┌─S──────────────S─┐
Cys─Tyr─Ile─Gln─Asn─Cys─Pro─Leu─Gly─NH₂
 1   2   3   4   5   6   7   8   9
              Oxytocin
```

Fig. 3.4 Structures of arginine vasopressin and oxytocin.

Urofollitropin (human FSH) and **menotropin** (human menopausal gonado-tropins, hMG), which have both FSH and LH activity, are used to treat infertil-ity in women by stimulating ovarian follicular growth and maturation. They are used in conjunction with a luteinizing hormone, human chorionic gonado-tropin (hCG), to induce ovulation and implantation. A glycoprotein similar in structure to LH, hCG is obtained from the urine of pregnant women. The gonadotropins are administered IM.

▪ **Prolactin and Bromocriptine** Prolactin, the principal hormone responsible for lactation, has no therapeutic use. Hyperprolactinemia, due to impaired transport of dopamine to the pituitary, can produce galactorrhea. Prolactin secretion can be inhibited with bromocriptine, a dopamine receptor agonist. Bromocriptine stimulates pituitary GH release in normal patients and, paradoxically, suppresses GH release in acromegalics.

▪ **Posterior Pituitary Hormones** Oxytocin and vasopressin are structurally simi-lar nonapeptides (Fig. 3.4).

● Oxytocin

— *Pharmacokinetics* Oxytocin is administered IV and is rapidly catabo-lized, with a half-life of 5 minutes.

— *Pharmacodynamics* Oxytocin causes sustained contraction of the uterus by altering transmembrane ionic currents in myometrial smooth muscle. Sensitivity to oxytocin increases during pregnancy. Oxytocin also causes contraction of myoepithelial cells surrounding mammary alveoli leading to milk ejection.

— *Pharmacotherapeutics* Oxytocin is given by IV infusion to induce labor in mild preeclampsia, uterine inertia, and incomplete abortion. It is also used IM to control postpartum uterine hemorrhage after delivery of the placenta. A nasal puff formulation may be used to induce lactation.

— *Adverse effects* Adverse effects include uterine rupture, water intoxi-cation, and fetal death.

● **Vasopressin** A deficiency in vasopressin leads to diabetes insipidus. Both vasopressin and its longer-acting synthetic analog, **desmopressin**, are used to treat this condition. Vasopressin is administered IV, IM, or intranasally. Desmopressin is given only intranasally. Vasopressin acts at V_1 vasopressin receptors to cause vasoconstriction and at V_2 vasopressin receptors to in-hibit diuresis.

Vasopressin Receptor/ Second Messenger

V_1 = Ca^{2+}; polyphosphoinosi-tides
V_2 = cAMP

SECTION 3.2 THYROID AND ANTITHYROID DRUGS

■ Thyroid Hormones (THs)

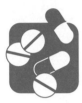

- **Overview** Normally the thyroid secretes thyroxine (T_4) and triiodothyronine (T_3) in sufficient amounts to maintain normal growth, development, body temperature, and energy levels. As shown in Fig. 3.5 ingested iodide is actively transported into the gland (iodide trapping) where it is oxidized to a form that iodinates tyrosine residues in thyroglobulin to yield monoiodotyrosine (MIT) and diiodotyrosine (DIT) (iodide organification). Coupling of MIT and DIT yields T_4 and T_3 which are stored in thyroglobulin. T_4 and T_3 are released from the thyroglobulin by proteolysis. Deiodination of T_4 to T_3 occurs in the periphery. Control of thyroid function is by way of the hypothalamic-pituitary axis, with TRH stimulating release of TSH, and TSH stimulating adenylyl cyclase in the gland to increase synthesis, and release of T_4 and T_3. They in turn provide negative feedback to inhibit TRH release and TSH synthesis and release. The blood iodide concentration also influences the level of iodide uptake and thyroid hormone synthesis.

- **Pharmacokinetics** The major carrier of THs is thyroxine-binding globulin (TBG) (Table 3.4). Total amounts of plasma THs and the concentrations of unbound hormones, vary independently. Pregnancy or estrogens elevate TBG leading to a rise in total and bound TH, but the concentration of free hormone and the steady-state elimination remain normal, and the patient is euthyroid. The major route of metabolism of TH is deiodination, which occurs in the liver and kidney and involves microsomal enzymes. Table 3.4 summarizes TH kinetics.

- **Pharmacodynamics** Binding sites for T_3 are present in the nucleus, mitochondria, and plasma membrane of TH-responsive cells indicating multiple sites of action. After THs enter the cell T_4 is deiodinated to T_3, which binds to a specific receptor associated with DNA in the nucleus, leading to synthesis of new protein (Fig. 3.6). The affinity of T_4 for TH receptors is 10 times lower than the affinity of T_3.

Location of TH Receptors
Nucleus
Mitochondria
Plasma membrane

■ Disorders of Thyroid Function
A TH deficiency in adults leads to hypothyroidism, myxedema (severe hypothyroidism), and myxedema coma, a

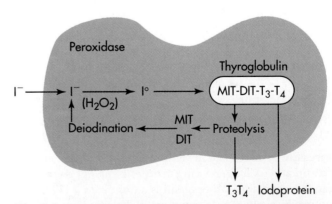

Fig. 3.5 Hormone synthesis in the thyroid gland. *I°*, Oxidized iodine; *MIT*, monoiodotyrosine; *DIT*, diiodotyrosine; *T₃*, triiodothyronine; *T₄*, thyroxine.

Table 3.4 *Thyroid Hormone Kinetics*		
	T_4	T_3
Total serum concentration	4-11 µg/dL	80-180 ng/dL
Concentration of free	1.5 ng/dL	0.2-0.6 ng/dL
Amount free	0.03%	0.3%
Amount produced per 24 hr	80 µg	30 µg
Half-life	8 days	1 day
Biologic activity	1	5
Oral absorption	75%-90%	95%

medical emergency. A congenital deficiency of TH must be treated from birth or cretinism will result. Endemic cretinism occurs when dietary iodine is inadequate. Nontoxic goiter is any enlargement of the thyroid without hyperthyroidism and results from insufficient TH to cause feedback inhibition of TRH and TSH release. This results in increased levels of TSH, leading to hypertrophy of the thyroid. Table 3.5 summarizes the etiology of hypothyroidism.

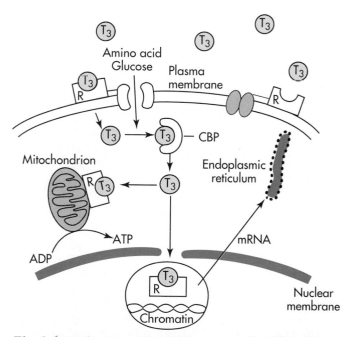

Fig. 3.6 Mechanism of thyroid hormone action. Thyroid hormone (in this case triiodothyronine, T_3) binds to receptor proteins (*R*) on the cell surface and increases the uptake of glucose and amino acids. T_3 also enters the cell, where it reacts with cytoplasmic binding proteins (*CBP*) and receptors on mitochondria and chromatin. In the nucleus, the T_3-receptor complex leads to the synthesis of new proteins. *(Adapted from Katzuns: Basic and clinical pharmacology, East Norwalk, CT, 1995, Appleton & Lange.)*

Table 3.5   *Etiology and Pathogenesis of Hypothyroidism*

CAUSE	PATHOGENESIS	GOITER	DEGREE OF HYPOTHYROIDISM
Hashimoto's thyroiditis	Autoimmune destruction of thyroid	Present early, absent later	Mild to severe
Drug-induced*	Blocked hormone formation	Present	Mild to moderate
Radiation, ^{131}I	Destruction of gland	Absent	Severe
Congenital (cretinism)	Athyreosis or ectopic thyroid, iodine deficiency	Absent or present	Severe
Secondary (TSH deficit)	Pituitary or hypothalamic disease	Absent	Mild

*Iodides, lithium, fluoride, and thiocarbamides.

Hyperthyroidism, or thyrotoxicosis, results from excess TH. It may be caused by an autoimmune disorder in which thyroid-stimulating immunoglobulin (TSI) stimulates the TSH receptor on the thyroid gland, resulting in Grave's disease or diffuse toxic goiter. Toxic nodular goiter is caused by thyroid adenoma. Thyrotoxic crisis, or thyroid storm, is a life-threatening form of hyperthyroidism caused by unrelated medical problems in patients with untreated hyperthyroidism.

- **Pharmacotherapeutics** Hypothyroidism is treated with TH given orally. Synthetic T_4, levothyroxine, is the preferred form because of its longer half-life. Also, T_4 is converted to T_3 in the periphery. Use of T_3, liothyronine, should be avoided in patients with cardiac disease because of its greater potency and consequent risk of cardiotoxicity. IV T_4 or T_3 is used for myxedema coma. Hyperthyroidism is treated with antithyroid drugs or surgery.

■ **Antithyroid Drugs**

- **Overview** A reduction in thyroid activity and the effects of excess TH can be reduced by using agents, such as thiocarbamides (Fig. 3.7) or iodides that interfere with the production of these hormones. It can also be achieved by glandular destruction with radiation (^{131}I) or surgery and by agents that modify tissue response to TH (e.g., propranolol).

- **Thiocarbamides**

  — *Pharmacokinetics* Propylthiouracil, carbimazole, and methimazole

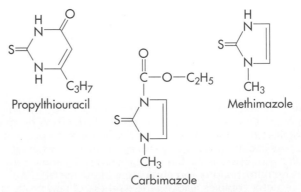

Fig. 3.7 Structure of thiocarbamides.

are orally absorbed, concentrated in the thyroid, and eliminated through the kidneys. Plasma half-life is 1 to 6 hours, but the duration of action may be longer. The onset of action of the thiocarbamides is slow because depletion of stores of T_4 takes 3 to 4 weeks. Methimazole is the active metabolite of carbimazole formed in vivo. Thiocarbamides cross the placenta and may affect the fetus. They are also secreted into the milk of lactating females.

— *Pharmacodynamics* Thiocarbamides reduce TH biosynthesis by inhibiting iodination of tyrosyl residues in thyroglobulin and the coupling of MIT and DIT. Propylthiouracil also inhibits the peripheral conversion of T_4 to T_3.

— *Adverse effects* Adverse effects include pruritic rash, arthritic manifestations, and agranulocytosis. An increase in TSH levels caused by reduction of T_4 and T_3 may lead to goiter.

— *Pharmacotherapeutics* These drugs are used in the treatment of hyperthyroidism associated with Grave's disease or nodular goiter. Onset of action is 3 to 4 weeks because stores of T_4 must be depleted. The goal of therapy is to achieve and maintain euthyroidism in anticipation of spontaneous remission.

● **Iodides** In high concentrations iodide temporarily blocks TH synthesis. In this case a solution of iodine in potassium iodide is administered orally. The iodine is reduced to iodide in the intestine before absorption, and the iodide immediately blocks TH synthesis, perhaps by inhibiting the proteolysis of thyroglobulin. Iodides decrease the vascularity, size, and fragility of the gland. The block lasts 2 to 4 weeks.

— *Adverse effects* Adverse effects that are rare and reversible include acneiform rash and swollen salivary glands.

— *Pharmacotherapeutics* Iodides are used to reduce the vascularity of the thyroid gland before surgery and in conjunction with thiocarbamides and propranolol in the treatment of thyrotoxic crisis.

● **Anion inhibitors** Included are the monovalent anions perchlorate (ClO_4^-) and thiocyanate (SCN^-) which block iodide uptake by the thyroid by competing with it for the iodide transport mechanism. These agents are no longer used for this purpose because of toxicity, but they are still used for short-term diagnostic testing of organification.

● **Radioactive iodine** ^{131}I emits x-rays and β-particles and has a half-life of 5 to 8 days. ^{131}I is concentrated in the thyroid gland and incorporated into the iodoamino acids emitting β-radiation that destroys the gland. Tracer doses of ^{131}I are used in the diagnosis of thyroid function with x-rays quantified by external detection. The response of the thyroid to TSH is evaluated by the accumulation of ^{131}I, which may be given orally.

— *Adverse reactions* Adverse reactions include permanent hypothyroidism. Radioactive iodine is contraindicated in pregnancy.

● **Propranolol** Propranolol, an adrenoceptor antagonist, is used to counteract the symptoms of thyrotoxicosis. These include tachycardia, tremor, and palpitations, all signs of sympathetic nerve stimulation.

Thiocarbamides
Propylthiouracil
Carbimazole
Methimazole

Adverse Effects
Pruritic rash
Arthritic manifestation
Agranulocytosis
Goiter

Anion Inhibitors
Perchlorate
Thiocyanate

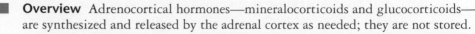

Glucocorticoids
Cortisol
Corticosterone

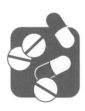

SECTION 3.3
ADRENOCORTICOSTEROIDS

■ **Overview** Adrenocortical hormones—mineralocorticoids and glucocorticoids—are synthesized and released by the adrenal cortex as needed; they are not stored.

The glucocorticoids cortisol (hydrocortisone) and corticosterone are produced in the zona fasciculata, with their synthesis under the positive control of ACTH released from the pituitary. The synthesis is also under negative feedback control of circulating cortisol acting on its receptors in the hypothalamus and pituitary to inhibit the release of ACTH. (Fig. 3.8). Chronic suppression of ACTH leads to atrophy of the hypothalamic-pituitary-adrenal axis.

Cortisol (Fig. 3.9) has both mineralocorticoid and glucocorticoid activity. Chemical modifications of the structure have yielded synthetic corticosteroids that are devoid of mineralocorticoid activity, have enhanced antiinflammatory activity, have increased potency, and have increased duration of action. The 11-keto forms of corticosteroids are not active but are converted in vivo to the active 11-hydroxy forms. Table 3.6 lists some of the most commonly used natural and synthetic glucocorticoids and mineralocorticoids and their relative antiinflammatory and mineralocorticoid activities.

■ **Pharmacokinetics** Cortisol and the synthetic corticosteroids are well absorbed after oral administration and circulate bound to cortisol-binding globulin. Cortisol (11-hydroxy) and cortisone (11-keto) are interconverted in the liver. Biotransformation of corticosteroids is by oxidation, reduction, and conjugation. Urinary metabolites include 17-hydroxycorticosteroids, which are quantified to measure glucocorticoids. Inasmuch as synthetic glucocorticoids are resistant to metabolism, they display a longer duration of action.

■ **Basic Pharmacology** Glucocorticoids influence the function of most cells in the body. They have permissive actions that are not dose-related, as well as dose-related effects. The former include responses of vascular and bronchial smooth muscle to catecholamines, which occur only in the presence of glucocorticoids. In addition, the lipolytic responses of fat cells to catecholamines and growth hormone require the presence of glucocorticoids.

Dose-related effects of glucocorticoids are observed on carbohydrate, protein, and fat metabolism. In the fasting state these effects contribute to maintaining the supply of glucose to the brain. Formation of glucose is stimulated by increasing gluconeogenesis, by diminishing glucose use in the periphery, and by promoting the storage of glucose as glycogen, resulting in a diabetic-like state characterized by hyperglycemia and glycosuria. Excessive doses of glucocorticoids induce protein catabolism in peripheral tissues leading to muscle wasting, atrophy of lymphoid tissue, osteoporosis, and a negative nitrogen balance. The distribution of fat is promoted by increased lipogenesis leading to a rounded face (moon facies), trunkal obesity, and buffalo hump (Cushing's habitus).

Glucocorticoids inhibit fibroblasts, causing loss of connective tissue and a thinning of the skin. They affect CNS activity by impairing cognitive function, inducing behavioral changes, and causing euphoria.

Glucocorticoids have antiimmune effects and cause a reduction and redistribution of circulating leukocytes. This increases susceptibility to infection.

The antiinflammatory response to glucocorticoids is due to reduction in inflammatory mediators such as interleukins 1 and 2 and a stabilization of lysosomal membranes. Synthesis of proinflammatory leukotrienes and prostaglandins is reduced by glucocorticoids because they stimulate the production of lipocortin, an endogenous inhibitor of phospholipase A_2, and they inhibit the expres-

**Major Clinical Features
of Cushing's Syndrome**

Obesity
Facial plethora
Hirsutism
Hypertension
Muscle weakness
Psychologic symptoms
Polyuria-polydipsia
Back pain
Striae
Edema

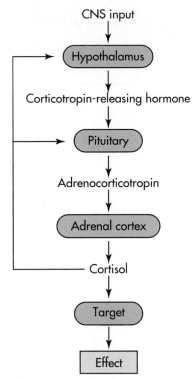

Fig. 3.8 Regulation of cortisol synthesis and release.

sion of an inducible, cyclooxygenase, cox-2, in inflammatory cells. The glucocorticoids are the most potent antiinflammatory drugs available.

The mineralocorticoids aldosterone, deoxycorticosterone, and corticosteroids with mineralocorticoid activity bind to mineralocorticoid receptors in the cytoplasm of cells, inducing the reabsorption of sodium by the distal renal tubules.

Mineralocorticoids
Aldosterone
Deoxycorticosterone

■ **Pharmacodynamics** Glucocorticoids enter cells and act by modifying gene expression (Fig. 3.10). They bind to cytoplasmic glucocorticoid receptors; the hormone-receptor complex binds to glucocorticoid-response elements on various genes to increase or decrease their expression. In addition, cell-surface receptors may mediate the fast feedback inhibition of ACTH release by glucocorticoids.

■ **Adverse Effects** Glucocorticoid therapy is associated with a number of undesirable side effects, especially when they are administered systemically for pro-

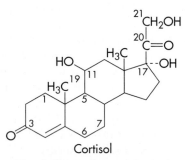

Cortisol

Fig. 3.9 Structure of cortisol.

Table 3.6   *Some Commonly Used Corticosteroids*

AGENT	ACTIVITY*	
	ANTIINFLAMMATORY	SALT-RETAINING
Short-acting Glucocorticoids		
Hydrocortisone (cortisol)	1	1
Cortisone	0.8	0.8
Prednisone	4	0.3
Prednisolone	5	0.3
Methylprednisolone	5	0
Meprednisone	5	0
Intermediate-acting Glucocorticoids		
Triamcinolone	5	0
Paramethasone	10	0
Long-acting Glucocorticoids		
Betamethasone	25–40	0
Dexamethasone	30	0
Mineralocorticoids		
Fludrocortisone	10	250
Desoxycorticosterone acetate	0	20

*Potency relative to hydrocortisone.

Adverse Effects of Corticosteroids

Edema
Hypokalemic alkalosis
Weight gain
Glycosuria
Negative nitrogen balance
Osteoporosis
Cushing's habitus
Peptic ulceration
Myopathy
Increased infection
Inhibition of growth
Cataracts
Psychoses

Mineralocorticoid Effects

Sodium retention
Increased blood pressure
Edema
Loss of potassium

Nonendocrine Diseases Treated with Corticosteroids

Arthritis
Status asthmaticus
Allergic disease
Collagen disease (systemic lupus erythematosus)
Ocular diseases

longed periods of time at high doses, and the clinical picture may resemble that of Cushing's syndrome. The mineralocorticoid effects of corticosteroids cause sodium and fluid retention, a rise in blood pressure, edema, and loss of potassium. This leads to hypokalemic hypochloremic alkalosis.

Contraindications to the use of corticosteroids are sudden cessation of therapy (must be tapered off to avoid adrenal insufficiency) and herpes simplex of the eye (progression of the disease may be masked, and irreversible clouding of the cornea may occur).

■ **Pharmacotherapeutics** The adrenal corticosteroids are used to suppress inflammatory and immune responses in diseases such as arthritis, and asthma, and in collagen and ocular diseases. Although not curative, they are effective in reducing symptoms. Routes of administration are oral, parenteral, and topical.

These drugs are also used to treat adrenal insufficiency and congenital adrenal hyperplasia. Hypocorticism may be primary, from destruction of the adrenal gland, or secondary, resulting from pituitary malfunction. The IV injection of ACTH on three successive days is used to distinguish primary from secondary hypocorticism. Urinary 17-hydroxycorticosteroids are measured each day and compared with levels before ACTH administration. Patients with secondary adrenal insufficiency exhibit an increase in urinary steroids on the second or third day. Patients with primary adrenal insufficiency show no response. **Metyrapone,** an 11-β-hydroxylase inhibitor, is used to confirm pituitary-dependent hypocorticism. It inhibits cortisol biosynthesis and increases release of 11-deoxycortisol, which can be measured in the urine. In normal patients, metyrapone treatment will result in an increase in ACTH release, because cortisol levels will be reduced, and there will be an increase in 11-deoxycortisol. In patients with pituitary-dependent hypocorticism there will be no increase in 11-deoxycortisol. Adrenal insufficiency requires daily therapy with cortisol and a potent mineralocorticoid.

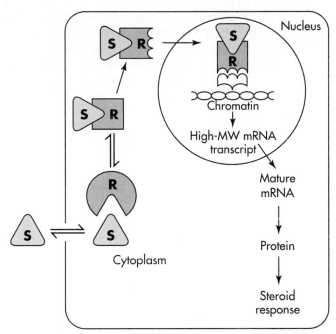

Fig. 3.10 Mechanism of action of glucocorticoids. Gluco-corticoid, estrogen, progesterone, and thyroid cytosolic receptors belong to the same supergene family, and all these hormones act similarly via gene transcription to mediate their effects.

Adrenal hyperfunction caused by partial deficiency of 21-hydroxylase results in overproduction of ACTH and adrenal androgens leading to virilization in female children and macrogenitosomia in male children. It is treated with a glucocorticoid and, where salt-losing tendency is present, a mineralocorticoid.

Glucocorticoids are used for diagnostic purposes in Cushing's syndrome. This is adrenal hyperplasia caused by a pituitary tumor or tumor of the adrenal gland, resulting in excessive corticoid secretion that causes Cushing's habitus. In the glucocorticoid suppression test a potent glucocorticoid such as dexamethasone is administered. Urinary 17-hydroxysteroids will be reduced in patients with pituitary-dependent hypercorticism. Little effect will be observed in patients with tumor of the adrenal cortex.

SECTION 3.4 SEX STEROIDS

■ **Overview** The natural and synthetic estrogens, progestins, and androgens are used to treat endocrine disorders such as hypogonadism. Synthetic estrogens and progestins are used in oral contraceptive combined preparations, and synthetic progestins are used for contraception by progestin only. The use of contraceptive agents differs from that of other drugs because it involves prolonged administration to normal individuals. Oral contraceptives are the most widely used of all drugs requiring a prescription. Estrogen and progesterone receptor antagonists are employed for the treatment of disorders of ovulation and as a postcoital contraceptive and abortifacient, respectively.

■ **Estrogens**

● **Overview** Estrogens are required for the normal maturation of the female, stimulating development of primary and secondary sex characteristics. The most active endogenous estrogen is 17-β-estradiol, followed by estrone and estriol. Estradiol and estrone are used in commercial preparations, as are equine estrogens, which are isolated from stallion urine. Equine estrogens differ from human estrogens in having unsaturation in steroid ring B. Many synthetic estrogens have been synthesized, some of which have enhanced bioavailability. Several nonsteroidal compounds with estrogenic activity are used clinically. **Diethylstilbestrol** is probably the most important of this group. Commonly used natural and synthetic estrogens are listed in Box 3.1.

Box 3.1

ESTROGENS

1. Synthetic Estrogens
Ethinyl estradiol
Mestranol

2. Nonsteroidal Estrogens
Diethylstilbestrol

3. Commonly Used Natural Estrogens
Estradiol
Estrone
Equine estrogens

● **Pharmacokinetics** Estrogens are readily absorbed through skin, mucous membranes, and the gut. Naturally occurring estrogens circulate in association with sex hormone-binding globulin (SHBG) and albumin. Estradiol, as well as synthetic estrogens, is converted in the liver to conjugated metabolites, which are excreted in bile. Because significant amounts of estrogen are reabsorbed from the intestine, orally administered compounds have a high ratio of hepatic to peripheral effects.

● **Pharmacodynamics** Estrogens diffuse into target cells and bind to cytosolic estrogen receptors; initiates or regulates gene transcription, altering the production of several proteins. Steroid receptors occur mainly in reproductive tissues and in the hypothalamus and pituitary with smaller numbers in tissues such as liver. Liver metabolism is affected by estrogens, resulting in higher circulating levels of SHBG, thyroxine-binding globulin, renin substrate, and fibrinogen. This results in an increase in the circulating levels of estrogen, thyroxine, and testosterone. Estrogens enhance the coagulability of blood by increasing the concentration of circulating clotting factors and they antagonize the action of parathyroid hormone on bone, decreasing the rate of bone resorption.

● **Adverse effects** Nausea, breast tenderness, and hyperpigmentation are common adverse effects associated with estrogen therapy. Estrogens also increase the frequency of migraine headaches, cholestasis, and hypertension. Continuous exposure to estrogens leads to hyperplasia of the endometrium which is usually associated with abnormal bleeding patterns. The risk of endometrial cancer is increased in patients taking estrogens but may be reduced with the concomitant administration of a progestin.

● **Pharmacotherapeutics** The major use of estrogens is in contraception. In addition, estrogens are administered as replacement therapy for patients

Table 3.7 *Therapeutic Progestational Agents*

	Route	Duration of Action
Progesterone in oil	IM	1 day
Medroxyprogesterone	PO	1-3 days
	IM	4-12 weeks
Norethynodrel	PO	1-3 days
Norethindrone	PO	1-3 days
Ethynodiol diacetate	PO	1-3 days
L-Norgestrel	PO	1-3 days
	SQ	5 years

IM, Intramuscularly; *PO,* per OS; *SQ,* subcutaneously.

who are estrogen-deficient because of failure of the ovaries to develop, castration, or menopause. Estrogens reduce the hot flushes, atrophic vaginitis and inappropriate sweating of menopause and decrease the risk of osteoporosis. Routes of administration are oral, IM, and transdermal.

■ **Antiestrogens** Clomiphene and tamoxifen are nonsteroidal agents that are competitive, partial agonists at the estrogen receptor. Clomiphene is orally active and is excreted slowly from an enterohepatic pool. It blocks estrogen receptors in the hypothalamus and pituitary, disrupting the normal feedback inhibition of GnRH and gonadotropin secretion. This results in ovarian stimulation and ovulation. Clomiphene may cause ovarian hyperstimulation and multiple births. Tamoxifen is used to treat hormone-dependent breast cancer.

Antiestrogens
Clomiphine
Tamoxifen

■ **Progestins**

● **Overview** Progesterone is the major progestin in humans. Its secretion from the corpus luteum during the second half of the menstrual cycle causes development of a secretory endometrium. Its concentrations are greatly increased during pregnancy, when it acts to suppress uterine contractility. Progesterone is ineffective orally because of extensive first-pass metabolism, but it can be effective when injected IM in oil. A number of synthetic progestational agents that are orally active and that display a longer duration of action from progesterone are available. Table 3.7 lists commonly used progestins. The synthetic progestins may also have some estrogenic or androgenic activity.

● **Pharmacokinetics** Progesterone is rapidly absorbed by any route and is almost completely metabolized in one passage through the liver. The inactive metabolites are excreted in the urine. The plasma half-life of progesterone is about 5 minutes. The synthetic progestins are also metabolized to inactive products that are excreted mainly in the urine.

● **Pharmacodynamics** Progestins bind to progesterone receptors in the cell nucleus and cytoplasm with the ligand-receptor complex activating gene transcription. Progesterone causes proliferation of mammary gland acini and induces the maturation and secretory changes in the endometrium that follow ovulation.

● **Adverse effects** Progestins, alone and in combination oral contraceptives, increase blood pressure and lower plasma high-density lipoprotein (HDL) levels.

Progestins
Increase blood
  pressure
Decrease HDL

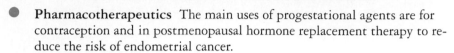

	ESTROGEN	PROGESTIN
Loestrin	Ethinyl estradiol	Norethindrone
Demulen	Ethinyl estradiol	Ethynodiol diacetate
Ovulen	Mestranol	Ethynodiol diacetate
Ortho-novum	Ethinyl estradiol	Norethindrone
Lo/Ovral	Ethinyl estradiol	DL-Norgestrel

Table 3.8 *Commonly Used Combined Oral Contraceptives*

Antiprogestin
Mifepristone

Mechanisms
Estrogens
   Inhibit FSH
Progestins
   Inhibit LH

Estrogenic Side Effects
Nausea
Mastalgia
Headache
Weight gain
Breakthrough bleeding
Skin pigmentation

- **Pharmacotherapeutics** The main uses of progestational agents are for contraception and in postmenopausal hormone replacement therapy to reduce the risk of endometrial cancer.

■ **Antiprogestins** Mifepristone (RU486) is a steroid derivative that is a weak partial agonist at progesterone receptors. Mifepristone facilitates luteolysis, menstruation, and uterine motility and causes embryo detachment. It is used orally in combination with prostaglandins as an abortifacient in early pregnancy.

■ **Hormonal Contraception**

- **Overview** Combined oral contraceptives consist of an estrogen and a progestin (Table 3.8). When properly administered these contraceptives reduce the risk of pregnancy to less than 1%. Other oral preparations contain only progestin and are used to avoid the side effects produced by the estrogen in combined preparations. Depot, and an implantable formulation of a progestin are also available for estrogen-free, long-term contraception.

- **Pharmacodynamics** Estrogen and progestin in combined oral contraceptives inhibit circulating levels of FSH and LH, respectively. The estrogen inhibits ovulation and the progestin induces physiologic withdrawal bleeding. Combination agents also render cervical mucous spermicidal and inhibit coordinated tubal and uterine contractions. These actions play a major role in the contraceptive effectiveness of continuous progestin treatment even when ovulation is not inhibited.

- **Adverse effects** Life-threatening adverse effects associated with contraceptives include cardiovascular disorders such as venous thromboembolism, myocardial infarction, stroke, and hypertension. Patients taking oral contraceptives have increased blood concentrations of certain clotting factors. Risk of cardiovascular disorders is greater in women 35 years of age or older who are heavy smokers. Cholelithiasis can also occur, and psychologic depression is observed in some patients. Mild to moderate adverse effects are similar to the manifestations of early pregnancy and are almost entirely caused by the estrogenic component. These include nausea, mastalgia, headache, weight gain, breakthrough bleeding, and increased skin pigmentation.

  Contraception with progestin alone can be achieved with small doses administered orally. There is a high incidence of abnormal bleeding with this therapy. Subcutaneous implantation of levonorgestrel capsules (Norplant) allows continuous diffusion of small quantities of progestin into the blood for as long as 5 years. Medroxyprogesterone acetate (Depoprovera) injected IM every 1 to 3 months also achieves long-lasting contraception but has a risk of permanent infertility.

■ **Postcoital Contraceptives** "Morning after" contraception occurs with short-term administration of high doses of estrogens alone or in combination with progestins. Treatment is begun within 72 hours of coitus and is effective 99% of the time. A single large dose of mifepristone is also an effective postcoital contraceptive. Diethylstilbestrol is used only in this way and is never prescribed to women who may be pregnant because of the risk of vaginal carcinoma in female offspring.

■ **Androgens**

● **Overview** Androgens are synthesized in the testis, ovary, and adrenal cortex. In human males, the most important androgen secreted by the testis is testosterone. The normal function of androgens is to induce the changes and growth that occur during puberty. Androgens cause accelerated development of primary and secondary sex characteristics and have remarkable growth-promoting activity, causing rapid increases in height, skeletal muscle development, and body weight.

● **Pharmacokinetics** Circulating testosterone is bound to SHBG and serum albumin. It is ineffective by mouth because it is metabolized in the liver by oxidation of the 17-hydroxyl group yielding inactive products. Synthetic derivatives such as methyltestosterone have an alkyl substituent on the 17 position and are effective orally because their substitution retards metabolism. Testosterone esters, injected IM in oil, are absorbed slowly and are more active than testosterone.

● **Pharmacodynamics** Testosterone is converted to dihydrotestosterone in most target tissues. Both forms bind to the cytosolic androgen receptor, and initiate and modify gene transcription by the same mechanisms as other steroids (see Fig. 3.10) leading to growth, differentiation, and protein synthesis.

● **Pharmacotherapeutics** Androgens are used to replace or augment androgen secretion when testicular function is deficient, as in hypogonadism or hypopituitarism (Table 3.9).

● **Adverse effects** Adverse effects include enhancement of epiphyseal closure in children and jaundice. The use of large doses of androgens by athletes to promote muscle development can lead to hepatic carcinoma and impotence in males and masculinization in females.

Section 3.5 Pancreatic Hormones and Antidiabetic Drugs

■ **Overview** The major hormones of the endocrine pancreas are insulin, the storage and anabolic hormone of the body that is present in β-cells, and glucagon, the hyperglycemic factor that mobilizes glycogen stores and is present in α-cells.

Diabetes mellitus is the most important disease of the endocrine pancreas. Type I, insulin-dependent diabetes mellitus (IDDM), is an autoimmune disease characterized by loss of β-cells whereas in type II, non-insulin-dependent diabetes mellitus (NIDDM), the β-cells are desensitized to glucose challenge, and peripheral tissues are resistant to insulin. Type I occurs in genetically predisposed individuals after infection or environmental insult. Acutely, it is characterized by hyperglycemia, ketoacidosis, azoturia, reduced plasma volume, coma, and circulatory collapse. The long-term outcome includes microvascular complications, particularly in the eye and kidney, ulceration, gangrene, and athero-

Postcoital Contraceptives

Conjugated estrogens (equine estrogens plus estrone)
Ethinyl estradiol
Diethylstilbestrol
Norgestrel plus ethinyl estradiol
Mifepristone

Pancreatic Hormones

Insulin
Glucagon

Diabetes Mellitus

Type I—IDDM
Type II—NIDDM

Table 3.9   *Androgen Preparations for Replacement Therapy*

	ROUTE OF ADMINISTRATION
Testosterone propionate	IM, sublingual
Testosterone cypionate	IM
Methyltestosterone	Oral, sublingual
Fluoxymesterone	Oral

IM, Intramuscularly.

Table 3.10   *Characteristics of Types of Diabetes*

	INSULIN-DEPENDENT, TYPE I	NON–INSULIN-DEPENDENT, TYPE II
Synonyms formerly used	Juvenile onset	Adult or maturity onset
	Ketosis prone	Ketosis resistant
Age of onset	Usually below 25	Usually over 40
Type of onset	Usually sudden	Usually gradual
Presentation	Polyuria, polydipsia, poly-phagia, acidosis	Often asymptomatic
Nutrition	Often thin	Usually overweight
Control of diabetes	Difficult	Easy
Ketoacidosis	Frequent	Seldom, unless under stress
Insulin requirement	Always	Often unnecessary
Control by oral agents	Never	Frequent
Control by diet alone	Never	Frequent
Complications	Frequent	Frequent

sclerosis. These complications are due directly to elevated plasma glucose. Table 3.10 summarizes the characteristics of the two types of diabetes mellitus. Fig. 3.11 outlines the metabolic effects of insulin deficiency.

Diabetes is milder in NIDDM patients. Circulating insulin is sufficient to prevent ketoacidosis but is subnormal or inadequate because of tissue insensitivity to insulin. Most NIDDM patients are obese. Obesity generally results in impaired insulin action and is a common risk factor for NIDDM.

Control of type I diabetes is achieved by administration of insulin, whereas NIDDM may be controlled with diet to reduce obesity, by oral antidiabetic drugs, or by insulin.

Release of insulin in normal subjects is triggered by glucose and vagal stimulation. It is inhibited by catecholamine stimulation of α-adrenoceptors. Enteric hormones such as cholecystokinin and gastrin, β-adrenoceptor stimulation, and amino acids amplify glucose-induced release of insulin.

Insulin is a small protein that contains two peptide chains linked by disulfide bridges. It is synthesized by the β-cells as preproinsulin, which is cleaved to yield the insulin precursor, proinsulin. Proinsulin is packaged in granules where it is hydrolyzed into insulin and C-peptide. Insulin is stored in granules in the β-cells as crystals containing two atoms of zinc and six molecules of insulin. Porcine insulin differs from human insulin by one amino acid; bovine insulin differs by three amino acids and is more hydrophobic.

Insulin Release

↑ By glucose
↑ By leucine
↑ By vagal stimulation
↓ By catecholamines on α-adrenoreceptors

Amplify Glucose-Induced Release

Cholecystokinin
Gastrin
β-adrenoreceptor stimulation
Arginine

Insulin Deficiency

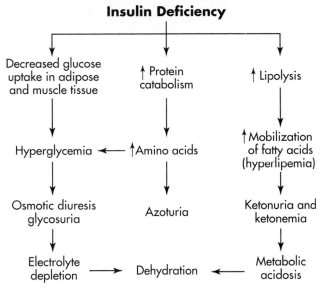

Fig. 3.11 Metabolic effects of insulin deficiency.

Pharmacology of Insulin

- **Pharmacokinetics** Insulin is administered SQ, or in acute hyperglycemia, IV. The circulating half-life of insulin is 3 to 5 minutes. Insulin is removed from the blood by the liver and kidney.

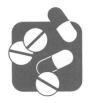

- **Insulin preparations** Commercial insulin is bovine or porcine in origin or human made by modification of porcine insulin or by recombinant DNA technology. Three principal therapeutic forms of insulin are (1) short-acting with rapid onset, (2) intermediate-acting, (3) long-acting with slow onset (Table 3.11). Regular insulin, also called crystalline zinc insulin, a short-acting soluble form, is the only type used IV or in infusion pumps. The longer-acting insulins are suspensions of insulin precipitates with zinc (lente and untralente) or a combination of insulin with protamine (NPH). After SQ injection proteolytic enzymes degrade protamine to permit absorption of insulin. Human recombinant, porcine, or bovine insulins can be used for each insulin form except ultralente. Only bovine insulin is sufficiently hydrophobic to provide the delayed, sustained-releasing form of ultralente insulin.

- **Pharmacodynamics** Insulin receptors are located on liver, muscle, and adipose tissue where they promote glucose uptake. The insulin receptor consists of two heterodimers with an extracellular alpha subunit that is the receptor recognition site, and a beta subunit that spans the membrane and contains a tyrosine kinase. Binding of insulin to its receptor is accompanied by autophosphorylation of the beta subunit and phosphorylation of other proteins within the cell. This constitutes the second message and leads to translocation of the glucose transporter to the cell surface and stimulation of the activity of key enzymes such as kinases and phosphatases. The effect of insulin on the liver is to reverse the catabolic features of insulin deficiency and to promote glucose storage as glycogen. In muscle, insulin increases protein and glycogen synthesis, whereas it increases triglyceride storage in adipose tissue.

Table 3.11 *Insulin Preparations*

| PREPARATIONS | APPEARANCE | ACTION, HOURS | | |
		ONSET	PEAK	DURATION
R Regular insulin	Clear	0.3-0.7	2-4	5-8
I Isophane insulin	Cloudy	1-2	6-12	18-24
I Lente insulin	Cloudy	1-2	6-12	24-28
L Ultralente insulin	Cloudy	4-6	16-18	20-36

R, Rapid acting; *I*, intermediate acting; *L*, long acting.

- **Adverse effects** The major adverse effect of insulin is hypoglycemia. This results from the administration of excessive insulin, not taking a regular meal at the expected time, stress, illness, surgery, or unaccustomed exercise. When the fall in blood glucose is rapid, the symptoms are those of autonomic hyperactivity and include sweating, tachycardia, palpitations, and hunger. Headache, confusion, coma, and other CNS symptoms follow. Immediate treatment is oral or IV glucose or IM glucagon.

- **Immunopathology** Insulin antibodies may be formed during insulin therapy, but true allergy is rare. When allergy to bovine insulin occurs, a change to porcine or human insulin is usually satisfactory. When IgG anti-insulin antibodies develop, the dosage of insulin should be increased, or another species of insulin should be used.

    Lipodystrophy (lipoatrophy or lipohypertrophy) may develop in areas where insulin is repeatedly injected and may be reduced by alteration of injection sites.

- **Diet and exercise** Diet is the cornerstone of treatment of both type I and type II diabetic patients. Calories must be controlled, and ideal body weight must be maintained. Regular exercise improves insulin sensitivity and lowers blood glucose. Alcohol should be avoided because it causes hypoglycemia by inhibiting hepatic gluconeogenesis.

■ **Oral Hypoglycemic Drugs**

- **Overview** In the United States the only oral medications for treating hyperglycemia in patients with NIDDM is the class of compounds known as sulfonylureas, which increase release of endogenous insulin and improve its peripheral effectiveness. There are two generations of sulfonylurea hypoglycemic agents. The older generation of drugs tends to be less potent than those developed since the mid-1980s (e.g., glyburide and glipizide) as indicated in Table 3.12.

- **Pharmacokinetics** Oral hypoglycemic drugs are absorbed from the gastrointestinal tract and are partially bound to plasma proteins. Chlorpropamide is excreted unchanged by the kidney and has a long half-life. Acetohexamide is rapidly metabolized to more active metabolites. Tolbutamide and tolazamide are metabolized in the liver. Glipizide and glyburide have short plasma half-lives but prolonged duration of biologic action.

- **Pharmacodynamics** The sulfonylureas stimulate pancreatic β-cells to release insulin by binding to a receptor associated with a K^+ channel in the

Table 3.12 *Sulfonylureas*

SULFONYLUREA	CHEMICAL STRUCTURE	DAILY DOSE	DURATION OF ACTION (HOURS)
Tolbutamide	H_3C—〈 〉—SO_2—NH—C(=O)—NH—$(CH_2)_3$—CH_3	0.5-2 g	6-12
Tolazamide	H_3C—〈 〉—SO_2—NH—C(=O)—NH—N〈 〉	0.1-1	10-14
Acetohexamide	H_3C—C(=O)—〈 〉—SO_2—NH—C(=O)—NH—〈 〉	0.25-1.5 g	12-24
Chlorpropamide	Cl—〈 〉—SO_2—NH—C(=O)—NH—$(CH_2)_2$—CH_3	0.1-0.5 g	Up to 60
Glyburide	Cl / OCH3 〈 〉—C(=O)—NH—$(CH_2)_2$—〈 〉—SO_2—NH—C(=O)—NH—〈 〉	0.00125- 0.02 g	10-24
Glipizide	H_3C—[pyrazine]—C(=O)—NH—$(CH_2)_2$—〈 〉—SO_2—NH—C(=O)—NH—〈 〉	0.005-0.03g	10-24*

*Elimination half-life considerably shorter.

β-cell membrane (Fig. 3.12). K^+ efflux is inhibited by these drugs, leading to Ca^{2+} influx and release of insulin.

Chronic administration of sulfonylureas reduces serum glucagon levels.

The sulfonylureas have an extrapancreatic effect to promote the action of insulin on its target tissues, especially muscle. This is probably due to an increase in the number of insulin receptors.

● **Adverse effects** The most serious consequence associated with sulfonylureas is hypoglycemia. These drugs are contraindicated in pregnancy.

● **Drug interactions** The actions of the sulfonylureas are antagonized by drugs that impair the release or action of insulin and potentiated by drugs that compete for liver enzymes, for plasma protein binding, or that interfere with urinary excretion of the sulfonylureas (Table 3.13).

A disulfiram-like action (alcohol-induced flush) may occur in patients receiving chlorpropamide and tolbutamide.

● **Pharmacotherapeutics** Sulfonylureas are used only for the treatment of NIDDM.

■ **Glucagon** Glucagon is a 29-amino-acid polypeptide that is identical in all mammals. It is synthesized in the α-cells of the pancreas. Glucagon is rapidly inactivated in plasma and degraded in the liver. Glucagon stimulates adeny-

Disulfiram-like Effect

Chlorpropamide
Tolbutamide

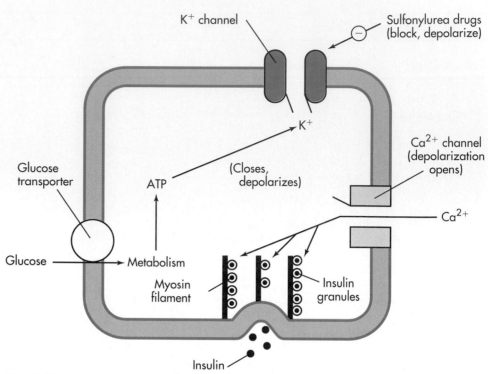

Fig. 3.12 Control of insulin release by the pancreatic β-cell. Glucose uptake and metabolism by the β-cell increases the intracellular concentration of ATP, which blocks ATP-sensitive K⁺-channels, causing depolarization of the cell and opening of voltage-dependent Ca²⁺ channels. Increased intracellular Ca²⁺ results in insulin secretion. Sulfonylurea hypoglycemic drugs block the ATP-dependent K⁺-channel, depolarizing the membrane and causing insulin release. *(Adapted from Katzung: Basic and clinical pharmacology, Norwalk, CT, 1995, Appleton & Lange.)*

lyl cyclase in the liver, facilitating the catabolism of stored glycogen, increasing gluconeogenesis, and thereby raising blood glucose. The major clinical use is for the treatment of severe hypoglycemia. Commercial preparations consist of bovine or porcine glucagon. Glucagon is typically administered IM.

Table 3.13   *Sulfonylureas—Drug Interactions*

	MECHANISM
Drugs Antagonizing Sulfonylureas	
Diazoxide	Inhibit release or action of insulin
Phenytoin	
Propranolol	
Corticosteroids	
Drugs Potentiating Sulfonylureas	
Sulfonamides	Displace from plasma protein
Salicylates	
Phenylbutazone	
Chlorampheniccol	Competition for liver enzymes
Phenylbutazone	
Salicylates	Interfere with urinary secretion
Probenecid	
Phenylbutazone	

SECTION 3.6 HORMONES REGULATING CALCIUM METABOLISM

■ **Overview** Calcium and phosphorus are the major mineral constituents of bone and two of the most important minerals for general cellular function. **Parathyroid hormone** and **vitamin D** are the principal regulators of calcium and phosphorus metabolism. **Calcitonin** also contributes to calcium homeostasis. Parathyroid hormone (PTH) is a single-chain polypeptide hormone produced in the parathyroid gland and stored there in secretory granules. Secretion is regulated by the concentration of ionized serum calcium. Vitamin D, a secosteroid hormone, is a prohormone synthesized in the skin or obtained from the diet as D_3 (cholecalciferol) or as a structurally related plant-derived supplement, D_2 (ergocalciferol). The structural difference among these drugs is of no physiologic consequence. Vitamin D is metabolized in vivo to active forms that, together with PTH, control calcium and phosphorus concentrations in serum through their action on absorption from the gut and from bone and on excretion in the urine. Both hormones increase input of calcium and phosphorus from bone into the serum; vitamin D also increases the absorption of calcium and phosphorus from the gut. Parathyroid hormone reduces urinary calcium excretion and increases urinary phosphorus excretion, whereas vitamin D decreases both. These actions are summarized in Table 3.14.

Calcitonin is a single-chain polypeptide secreted by the parafollicular cells of the thyroid. Biosynthesis and secretion are regulated by plasma calcium. When plasma calcium levels are high, calcitonin levels increase, lowering serum calcium and phosphorus. Calcitonin is less critical for calcium homeostasis than PTH and vitamin D, but in high concentrations reduces serum calcium and phosphorus by stimulating their renal excretion and inhibiting bone resorption.

■ **Parathyroid Hormone**

● **Pharmacokinetics** PTH is administered parenterally and has a short plasma half-life. It is cleared by the kidney and liver.

● **Pharmacodynamics** PTH regulates calcium and phosphorus flux across cell membranes in bone and kidney, increasing serum calcium and decreasing serum phosphate. The actions of PTH on bone and kidney are mediated by cAMP. In the kidney, PTH simulates the production of $1,25(OH)_2D$ (calcitriol).

● **Pharmacotherapeutics** The only clinical use of PTH is in the diagnosis of pseudohypothyroidism, a disorder characterized by organ resistance to the hormone. Administration of bovine PTH is either IV or IM.

■ **Vitamin D**

● **Pharmacokinetics** Vitamin D is administered orally and is absorbed from the small intestine. Bile is essential to the absorption process. Vitamin D is hydroxylated in the liver to $25(OH)D$ (calcifediol), which is converted in the kidney to $1,25(OH)_2D$ (calcitriol) and $24,25(OH)_2D$ (Fig. 3.13). Vitamin D and its metabolites circulate bound to a vitamin D-binding protein. It is rapidly cleared from the blood by the liver into the bile. Excess vitamin D is stored in adipose tissue for long periods.

● **Pharmacodynamics** Vitamin D is a positive regulator of calcium homeostasis, maintaining normal plasma concentrations of calcium and phosphate by facilitating their absorption from the gut and bone and decreasing their urinary excretion. Calcitriol is the most potent vitamin D metabolite.

Regulators of Calcium
Parathyroid Hormone
Vitamin D
Calcitonin

Regulators of Phosphorus
Parathyroid Hormone
Vitamin D

Table 3.14	Actions of Parathyroid Hormone and Vitamin D on Gut, Kidney, and Bone	
	PTH	**VITAMIN D**
Intestine	Increased calcium and phosphate absorption by increased 1,25(OH)$_2$D production	Increased calcium and phosphate absorption by 1,25(OH)$_2$D
Kidney	Decreased calcium excretion, increased phosphate excretion	Calcium and phosphate excretion may be decreased by 25(OH)D and 1,25(OH)$_2$D
Bone	Calcium and phosphate resorption increased by high doses; low doses may increase bone formation	Increased calcium and phosphate resorption by 1,25(OH)$_2$D; bone formation may be increased by 24,25(OH)$_2$D
Net effect on serum levels	Serum calcium increased, serum phosphate decreased	Serum calcium and phosphate both increased

- **Adverse effects** Overdosage of vitamin D causes serious toxicity. The syndrome termed hypervitaminosis D is associated with hypercalcemia and nephrocalcinosis.

- **Pharmacotherapeutics** Vitamin D and its commercially available metabolites are used orally for prophylaxis or cure of nutritional and metabolic rickets, osteomalacia, and hypoparathyroidism (Table 3.15). Treatment of hypoparathyroidism requires high doses of vitamin D or the vitamin D analog dihydrotachysterol. The latter is more effective because it bypasses renal mechanisms of metabolic control.

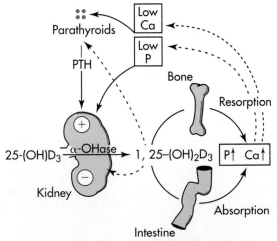

Fig. 3.13 Regulation of 1,25(OH)$_2$D$_3$ biosynthesis. Solid arrows indicate a positive effect; broken arrows refer to a negative feedback. *PTH,* Parathyroid hormone.

Table 3.15 *Vitamin D and Its Clinically Available Metabolites and Analog*

CHEMICAL NAME	ABBREVIATION	GENERIC NAME
Vitamin D_3	D_3	Cholecalciferol
Vitamin D_2	D_2	Ergocalciferol
25-Hydroxyvitamin D	$25(OH)D_3$	Calcifediol
1,25-Dihydroxyvitamin D_3	$1,25(OH)_2D_3$	Calcitriol
Dihydrotachysterol	DHT	Dihydrotachysterol

■ Calcitonin

- **Pharmacokinetics** Calcitonin is administered parenterally and has a short plasma half-life. Clearance occurs through the kidney.

- **Pharmacodynamics** The principal effect of calcitonin is to lower serum calcium and phosphate. This is brought about by direct inhibition of bone resorption by osteoclastic and osteocytic cells.

- **Adverse effects** Calcitonin is nontoxic.

- **Pharmacotherapeutics** Calcitonin reduces hypercalcemia in patients with hyperparathyroidism and vitamin D intoxication and is effective in Paget's disease, which is characterized by increased skeletal remodeling. Human (**Cibacalcin**) and salmon (**Calcimar**) calcitonin are available.

MULTIPLE CHOICE REVIEW QUESTIONS

1. A 71-year-old female has been eating poorly since her husband died two years ago. She was being treated for depression by both her primary care physician and a psychiatrist. Generally, she had been in good health, although she had been taking phenytoin for seizure control for five years. Over the past few months she began experiencing muscle spasms, including facial grimacing and carpopedal spasm. Her blood workup showed a calcium level of 7.2 mg/dl (8.9-10.4) and a phosphate level of 4.4 mg/dl (2.6-4.4). Which of the following is the best explanation?

   a. Inadequate dietary vitamin D.
   b. Inadequate sunlight.
   c. Phenytoin reduces calcium absorption.
   d. Phenytoin reduces vitamin D levels by hepatic enzyme induction.
   e. All of the above.

2. Choose the incorrect statement concerning growth hormone (GH, somatotropin).

   a. Before epiphyseal closure, excessive growth hormone results in gigantism.
   b. Growth stimulation is mediated directly by growth hormone.
   c. Growth hormone may produce an antiinsulin effect.
   d. Growth hormone stimulates incorporation of amino acids into protein.
   e. Growth hormone is secreted by somatotrophs.

3. Which of the following agents increases serum levels of growth hormone in a normal individual?

   a. LevoDOPA
   b. Cyproheptadine
   c. Clonidine
   d. Phentolamine
   e. A & C

4. Long-term treatment with corticosteroids may result in which of the following side effects?

   a. Hypertension
   b. Hyperglycemia
   c. Moon facies
   d. Truncal obesity
   e. All of the above

5. Choose the correct statement(s) concerning modulation of insulin release.

   a. Phentolamine decreases plasma insulin.
   b. Propranolol decreases insulin release.
   c. Vagal nerve stimulation inhibits insulin release.
   d. Most gastrointestinal hormones inhibit insulin release.
   e. All of the above are false.

6. All of the following may be presenting symptoms of diabetes mellitus except:

   a. polydipsia.
   b. oliguria.
   c. polyphagia.
   d. diabetic coma.
   e. neuropathy.

7. The polyuria associated with hyperglycemia in a diabetic patient most closely parallels the mechanisms of action of which of the following diuretic agents?

   a. Furosemide
   b. Bumetanide
   c. Acetazolamide
   d. Mannitol
   e. Chlorothiazide

8. A diabetic may experience hypoglycemia from:

   a. an overdose of insulin.
   b. unaccustomed exercise.
   c. failure to eat breakfast.
   d. over-indulgence in alcohol.
   e. all of the above.

9. How is insulin cleared?

   a. Hepatic
   b. Renal
   c. Both
   d. Neither

10. Which of the following drugs is classified as a second generation sulfonylurea?

    a. Acetohexamide
    b. Chlorpropamide
    c. Glipizide
    d. Tolazamide
    e. Tolbutamide

11. Glyburide achieves the same therapeutic effect as tolbutamide but does so at a dosage that is 100-fold less. One may conclude that:

   a. glyburide is more efficacious than tolbutamide.

   b. glyburide is more potent than tolbutamide.

   c. glyburide is equipotent when compared with tolbutamide.

   d. glyburide is less efficacious than tolbutamide.

   e. none of the above.

12. Which agents may be useful in the treatment of thyrotoxicosis?

   a. Iodide

   b. Methimazole

   c. Propylthiouracil

   d. Glucocorticoids

   e. All of the above

PART 2

Drugs Acting on Organ Systems

Chapter 4

Autacoid, Renal, Respiratory, and Gastrointestinal Drugs

SECTION 4.1 HISTAMINE, SEROTONIN, AND RELATED AGENTS

■ **Overview** Histamine and serotonin are produced in the body and are seldom used as therapeutic or diagnostic agents. However, drugs influence both systems, leading to a beneficial effect, or in some cases, adverse effects and toxicities. Therapeutic uses for drugs that modify the histamine or serotonin systems include the treatment of cardiovascular, gastrointestinal (GI), central nervous system (CNS), and inflammatory disorders.

■ **Histamine**

● **Occurrence** Histamine is most highly concentrated in the lungs, skin, and the mucosa of the gastrointestinal tract. Principal storage sites include mast cells and basophils, where histamine is co-localized with heparin in granules. Histamine is also present in the brain, where it may serve a neurotransmitter-like function.

● **Biotransformation** Histamine is formed by decarboxylation of histidine, an amino acid, by histidine decarboxylase (Box 4.1). This process occurs primarily in the tissues in which histamine is stored. Histamine is initially metabolized by diamine oxidase and histamine-N-methyltransferase. The acid metabolites have no appreciable biologic activity, and they are excreted in the urine (Box 4.1).

Box 4.1

● **Release** The release of histamine from mast cells may occur by either an exocytotic or nonexocytotic process. During mast cell activation products such as peptides, enzymes, and lipid mediators, are released with histamines and contribute to the physiologic response. Thus symptoms in allergic and anaphylactic responses are due to a host of agents, only one of which is histamine, released from activated mast cells.

With immediate hypersensitivity reactions (IgE-associated), histamine is released in response to a sensitizing antigen. In addition to protein antigens, drug-associated macromolecular complexes may initiate this type of release. Histamine release can also occur in response to cell injury, such as after trauma, low temperatures, bee stings, and toxins.

A class of agents known as *histamine liberators* includes basic drugs such as morphine, curare, and codeine, as well as larger molecules such as compound 48/80 (a basic amine-polymer), radiocontrast media, and dextrans.

● **Mechanism of action** The actions of histamine are exerted through H_1 and H_2 receptors on the cell surface. Some actions within the brain have been ascribed to H_3 receptors which may regulate histamine release (autoreceptor).

HISTAMINE METABOLISM
Histidine
↓ Histidine decarboxylase
Histamine
↓ Diamine oxidase
Imidazole Acetic acid
↓ Methyl transferase
Methyl imidazole Acetic acid

Box 4.2

MODIFICATION OF HISTAMINE

Histamine Release
Stimulate: morphine
Block: cromolyn

Histamine Receptors
Block H_1: pyrilamine
Block H_2: ranitidine

Act on Opposing Receptors
Stimulate: epinephrine

Receptor	Location
H_1	Smooth muscle
	Endothelium
	Brain
H_2	Gastric mucosa
	Cardiac muscle
	Mast cells
	Brain

Second Messengers

H_1	Phosphoinositides
H_1	cGMP
H_2	cAMP

Box 4.3

EXAMPLES OF HISTAMINE ANTAGONISTS

Histamine H_1 Antagonists
Alkylamines
  Chlorpheniramine
  Brompheniramine
Ethanolamines
  Dimenhydrinate
  Diphenhydramine
Ethylenediamines
  Triplenamine
  Pyrilamine
Phenothiazines
  Promethazine
Piperazines
  Hydroxyzine
  Meclizine
Piperdines
  Azatidine
  Cyproheptadine
Second generation
  Astemizole
  Terfenadine
  Loratidine

Histamine H_2 Antagonists
Cimetidine
Raniditine
Famotidine
Nizatidine

Histamine receptor subtypes are not uniformly distributed throughout the body. The H_1 receptors are present on vascular, intestinal, and bronchiolar smooth muscle and capillaries, whereas H_2 sites are localized to gastric secretory cells, vascular smooth muscle cells, and heart tissue. H_1 receptor-mediated affects predominate when both types of receptors are present.

Different second messenger pathways are coupled to H_1 and H_2 receptors. The H_1 receptors are coupled to the phosphatidyl inositol cycle and in some cases to cyclic guanosine monophosphate (cGMP) generation. The H_2 receptors are associated with adenylyl cyclase and the formation of cyclic adenosine monophosphate (cAMP). Several chemicals can modify the actions of histamine (Box 4.2).

- **Pharmacodynamics**

  — *Cardiovascular system* Exogenously administered histamine decreases blood pressure and increases heart rate. The blood pressure effect is due to dilation of blood vessels and capillaries, whereas the rise in heart rate is due to a baroreceptor reflex response to the fall in peripheral resistance and to a direct chronotropic effect on the heart. These effects are mediated by H_1 and H_2 receptor activation, with the H_1 site being more important for cardiovascular responses.

    Injection of histamine subdermally causes a triple response consisting of an initial *redness* from capillary dilation, a subsequent broader reddish area, called a *flare*, which results from an axon reflex dilatation of arterioles, and an edematous swelling, called a *wheal*, which is secondary to an increase in capillary permeability. This injection is also associated with pain and itching.

    Some of the cardiovascular components of allergy and anaphylaxis are due to liberation of histamines.

  — *Smooth muscle* Histamine causes smooth muscle contraction in the gastrointestinal tract and bronchioles by way of H_1 receptors. The effects on the respiratory tract are more pronounced in individuals with bronchial asthma.

  — *Exocrine glands* Glandular secretions in the nasal and bronchiolar mucosa are stimulated by histamine, which can lead to respiratory symptoms.

  — *Gastric glands* Histamine is a potent stimulant of gastric acid and pepsin secretion. These effects are mediated by H_2 receptors.

  — *Sensory nerve endings* The pain and itching caused by injection of histamine into the skin are due to sensory nerve stimulation.

Antagonists of Histamine H_1 Receptors

- **Mechanism of action** Histamine H_1 receptor antagonists are competitive blockers of histamine and are the classic antihistamines that have been available for prescription and over-the-counter use for many years. They are classified on the basis of the chemical modification of their ethyl amine side chain. A more recent pharmacologic classification is based on whether the drugs are sedating. Newer antihistamines do not cross the blood-brain barrier, so they tend to be less sedating than older agents. A representative list of some antihistamines is shown in Box 4.3.

  Histamine H_1 receptor antagonists block most of the actions of histamine with the exception of gastric acid stimulation, which is mediated by H_2 receptors.

- **Pharmacotherapeutics** Antihistamines are usually well absorbed orally and are effective in providing symptomatic relief of allergies such as rhinitis urticaria. They are ineffective in the treatment of bronchial asthma because of the number of other mediators involved in the pathogenesis of this condition. Most antihistamines have a half-life of 4 to 6 hours. None is generally more efficacious or safer than the others, although there is considerable individual variation in patient response.

     These compounds are sometimes used in the treatment of motion sickness (**dimenhydrinate, cyclizine,** and **meclizine**) and as sedatives.

- **Adverse effects** The adverse effects of antihistamines are due in part to their ability to antagonize adrenergic, cholinergic, and serotonergic receptors. The antimuscarinic effects of antihistamines are common and primarily responsible for the xerostomia associated with these agents.

     A feature common to many of the classic antihistamines is their tendency to cause sedation. This action is sometimes used therapeutically to aid patients in sleeping. Generally, however, sedation is an undesirable effect with these drugs.

     For some, particularly infants, antihistamines may stimulate the CNS. The CNS effects in general are less common with newer antihistamines, such as **terfenadine, loratidine,** and **astemizole,** which do not readily penetrate the CNS.

     Toxic effects from overdosage of H_1 receptor antihistamines are rare in adults. In children, CNS stimulation may lead to excitement, hallucinations, ataxia, and possible convulsions. Coma and cardiorespiratory collapse may follow seizures.

- **Drug interactions** Because they are CNS depressants, H_1 receptor antihistamines enhance the depressant effects of alcohol and other CNS depressants.

     The concurrent use of terfenadine and erythromycin has led to serious cardiac arrhythmias because of inhibition of conversion of terfenadine to its therapeutically active metabolite. Other drugs that inhibit drug metabolism should be used with care in patients taking terfenadine and astemizole.

Antagonists of Histamine H_2 Receptors

- **Mechanism of action** H_2 receptor antagonists compete with histamine at receptors located primarily in the stomach. These agents reduce the gastric acid secretion induced by histamine and gastrin, and partially reverse that produced by acetylcholine. They have little affinity for H_1 receptors.

- **Pharmacotherapeutics** The approved histamine H_2 blockers are **cimetidine, ranitidine, nizatidine,** and **famotidine.** Although they differ with respect to their metabolism, the pharmacologic effects are similar. They are used in the treatment of peptic ulcers.

- **Adverse effects** Although cimetidine has few serious adverse effects, it displays some antiandrogen effects, including gynecomastia. The other histamine H_2 antagonists, although more potent than cimetidine, are equally free of adverse effects.

- **Drug interactions** Cimetidine inhibits cytochrome P-450-mediated drug metabolism in the liver. The other histamine H_2 blockers do not share this property.

Triple Response
Red spot
Flare
Wheal

Treatment of Motion Sickness
Dimenhydrinate
Cyclizine
Meclizine

Multiple Actions
Antihistamine
Antiadrenergic
Anticholinergic
Antiserotonergic

Less Sedating
Terfenadine
Loratidine
Astemizole

H_2 Antagonists
Cimetidine
Ranitidine
Famotidine
Nizatidine

- **Inhibitors of histamine release** Drugs that inhibit histamine release from mast cells, but do not block histamine receptors, include **cromolyn** sodium, which is used prophylactically to control bronchial asthma.

■ Serotonin

- **Occurrence** Serotonin, also known as 5-hydroxytryptamine (5-HT), is widely distributed in nature, being present in animals, plants, and insects. In humans, most serotonin is located in enterochromaffin cells of the gastrointestinal tract.

  Serotonin is also present in platelets and in CNS neurons, where it serves as a neurotransmitter.

- **Biotransformation** Serotonin is synthesized from dietary tryptophan by the enzymes tryptophan hydroxylase and 5-hydroxytryptophan decarboxylase. In the brain, because tryptophan levels do not saturate enzyme activity, increased levels of the amino acid elevate 5-HT in the CNS (Box 4.4).

Box 4.4

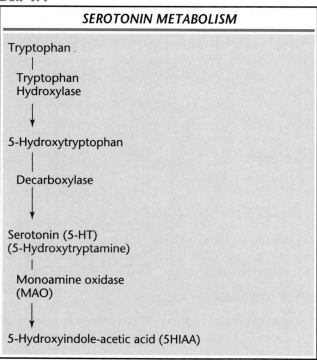

SEROTONIN METABOLISM

Tryptophan
|
Tryptophan
Hydroxylase
↓
5-Hydroxytryptophan
|
Decarboxylase
↓
Serotonin (5-HT)
(5-Hydroxytryptamine)
|
Monoamine oxidase
(MAO)
↓
5-Hydroxyindole-acetic acid (5HIAA)

Extracellular 5-HT is accumulated and stored in platelets. Serotonin is metabolized by monoamine oxidase (MAO) excreted in the urine as 5-hydroxyindole acetic acid (5HIAA). Elevation of serotonin levels is partly responsible for the pharmacologic response to MAO inhibitors.

- **Release and uptake** Stored 5-HT is released from platelets after their destruction or stimulation by thrombin. The active neuronal uptake of 5-HT is inhibited by transport blockers, including some antidepressants. Inhibition of neuronal accumulation increases the extracellular concentration of 5-HT.

  Serotonin accumulation into storage granules in platelets and neurons is inhibited by reserpine, which blocks the storage of a host of monoamines.

- **Mechanism of action** There are numerous serotonin receptor subtypes, many of which are located within the CNS. These receptors influence a variety of second messengers, including phosphatidyl inositides, calcium, and cAMP. The actions of serotonin can be modified in a number of ways (Box 4.5).

Box 4.5

MODIFICATION OF SEROTONIN
Serotonin Metabolism Activate: tryptophan Inhibit: monoamine oxidase inhibitors **Serotonin Uptake** Inhibit vesicle uptake: reserpine Inhibit surface membrane uptake: fluoxetine **Serotonin Release** Platelet activation: thrombin **Serotonin Receptors** Activate: LSD (also antagonist) Inhibit: methysergide

LSD, Lysergic acid diethylamide.

- **Pharmacodynamics**
  - *Cardiovascular* Serotonin has complex effects on the cardiovascular system. Included are direct vasoconstrictor effects, vasodilator effects in skeletal muscle, and baroreceptor reflex effects. 5-HT may either increase or decrease blood pressure. It also causes aggregation of platelets as it is released from these cells.
  - *Gastrointestinal* Serotonin has both direct and indirect effects on the gastrointestinal tract. The increase in motility caused by 5-HT is associated with the diarrhea characteristic of metastatic carcinoid tumors, which derive from enterochromaffin cells and the excessive secretion of 5-HT. There is an increased urinary excretion of 5HIAA in this condition.
  - *Nervous system* Serotonin has numerous actions in the peripheral and central nervous systems. It also modulates the release of a number of pituitary hormones.

Serotonin Receptor Antagonists

- **Mechanism of action** Serotonin receptor antagonists are competitive inhibitors of this substance. Some are full antagonists at some 5-HT receptors and partial agonists at others.

- **Pharmacotherapeutics** Serotonin receptor antagonists have been used in the treatment of migraine headaches, carcinoid syndrome, and in dumping syndromes after gastrointestinal surgery.

  Methysergide is a 5-HT receptor antagonist used in the prophylactic treatment of migraine headaches. It is thought to act primarily by blocking the action of 5-HT on cerebral blood vessels. A unique side effect of methysergide therapy is retroperitoneal fibrosis.

Serotonin Antagonists
Methysergide
Cyproheptadine
LSD (also agonist)

Ergot Alkaloids
Methylergonovine
Ergonovine
Ergotamine
Methysergide
LSD

Cyproheptadine is a 5-HT receptor antagonist that also blocks histamine H_1 receptors. It is used in the treatment of allergic disorders, especially urticaria.

Lysergic acid diethylamide (LSD) has agonist and antagonist properties at different classes of 5-HT receptors. It and a number of other related compounds are potent hallucinogens.

■ **Ergot Alkaloids** Ergot alkaloids act at a number of neurotransmitter receptors, including 5-HT, α-adrenoceptors, and dopamine receptors. These naturally occurring alkaloids are produced by a fungus that grows on grains. Ingestion causes ergotism, which is characterized by prolonged vasospasm, which, if untreated, may lead to ischemia and gangrene. Other actions of ergot alkaloids include hallucinations, uterine smooth muscle stimulation, and alterations in the circulating levels of prolactin.

● **Mechanism of action** Ergot derivatives may act as agonists at 5-HT and dopamine receptors and as either agonists or antagonists at α-adrenoceptors.

● **Pharmacotherapeutics** **Methylergonovine** and **ergonovine** are used clinically to reduce postpartum hemorrhage. This effect is due to uterine contraction.

Ergotamine is used for the acute management of migraine headaches. Its effectiveness is probably related to its vasoconstrictor action, although this may be unrelated to its effects on 5-HT receptors. Ergotamine is not used in obstetric patients.

● **Adverse effects** Nausea, vomiting, and diarrhea are common adverse effects. Ergotamine is much more toxic than ergonovine and methylergonovine and can cause excessive vascular contraction and hallucinations at higher doses.

● **Drug interactions** Because ergot alkaloids are metabolized in the liver, blood levels are increased in patients with hepatic disease or a drug-induced decrease in hepatic function or enzyme activity.

SECTION 4.2 POLYPEPTIDES

■ **Overview** Polypeptides are amino acid-containing substances. Naturally occurring polypeptides are typically not used as therapeutic agents because they have short half-lives and affect an array of biologic systems. However, endogenous peptide systems are targets for drugs that may modify their function by influencing the synthesis, release, receptors, or metabolism of these peptides. Progress has been made in producing nonpeptide chemicals that interact with receptors for polypeptides, enhancing the clinical use of polypeptide receptor agonists and antagonists.

■ **Angiotensin** Angiotensin peptides are proteolytic products derived from a plasma substrate, angiotensinogen, an α_2-globulin secreted by the liver. Angiotensin II, the most active vasoconstrictor of the angiotensin family, is sometimes just called angiotensin.

● **Biochemistry** **Renin,** the enzyme that initiates angiotensin generation, is produced from its precursor, **prorenin,** and released by the kidney. The initial enzymatic product, angiotensin I, is a decapeptide with little intrinsic biologic activity. Angiotensin I is rapidly converted to the biologically active octapeptide, angiotensin II, by the action of angiotensin converting enzyme (ACE), a dipeptidyl peptidase. In some tissues, even smaller angiotensin peptides displaying biologic activity are produced, such as angiotensin III, a heptapeptide.

Angiotensin peptides are rapidly metabolized by peptidases, termed angiotensinases. This accounts for the short half-life (minutes) of these peptides. The formation and destruction of angiotensins is given in Fig. 4.1.

● **Regulation of renin** Multiple factors regulate renin secretion and in turn modify plasma angiotensin levels. These include blood pressure within the kidney, intrarenal salt concentration, and the sympathetic nervous system.

Drugs that diminish renin secretion include those acting centrally to decrease sympathetic outflow, such as clonidine, and those that act in the periphery to interfere with β-adrenergic activity, such as propranolol. Vasodilators, such as minoxidil, increase renin secretion by causing a baroreceptor-induced increase in sympathetic activity. Diuretic agents may also increase plasma renin levels. Direct vasoconstrictors generally cause a decrease in plasma renin because of a reflex-mediated decrease in sympathetic activity.

Plasma levels of angiotensin are also modified by enhancing the release of angiotensinogen from the liver. This may occur in some patients treated with estrogens and can lead to hypertension.

● **Mechanism of action** Angiotensin reacts with cell surface receptors coupled to second messenger systems. There are two major types of angiotensin receptors: type 1 (AT1) and type 2 (AT2). So far, AT1 receptors appear to be more prominent in mediating the actions of angiotensin in humans.

The AT1 receptors are coupled by G proteins to at least two second

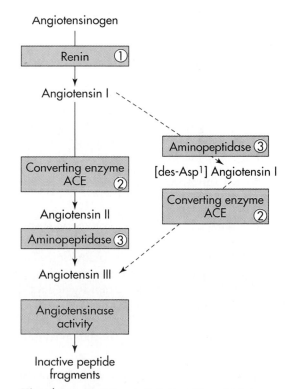

Fig. 4.1 Formation and destruction of angiotensins. ACE, angiotensin converting enzyme.

messenger systems. In some tissues phosphatidyl inositide breakdown yields IP_3, which increases intracellular calcium. In other tissues AT1 receptors are coupled through G_i proteins to adenylyl cyclase, thereby inhibiting the production of cAMP.

- **Pharmacodynamics**

  — *Cardiovascular system* Angiotensin II is an extremely potent vaso-constrictor. It raises blood pressure directly by contracting vascular smooth muscle. This effect is transient because of its rapid metabolism and therefore observed only after intravenous (IV) administration.

    Although angiotensin stimulates the isolated heart, in intact animals and humans the reflex decrease in sympathetic activity induced by its vasopressor effect usually results in bradycardia.

    Aldosterone secretion is stimulated by angiotensin II and angiotensin III. This is produced by low doses of angiotensin and is thought to be one of its physiologic effects. Aldosterone promotes an increase in intravascular volume through salt and water retention. Nevertheless, angiotensin produces hypertension in adrenalectomized animals.

- **Other actions** Through direct actions on the CNS, angiotensin stimulates thirst, the sympathetic nervous system, and the adrenal medulla.

■ **Antagonists of the Renin-Angiotensin System** Inhibition of the conversion of angiotensin I to angiotensin II by ACE inhibitors is a major approach for the treatment of hypertension. Detailed pharmacology is discussed in Chapter 5.

Treatment with ACE inhibitors has been shown to prevent myocardial infarction and restenosis of occluded blood vessels. This is thought to be related to possible actions of angiotensin on the growth of vascular smooth muscle and related cells.

Angiotensin Antagonist
Saralasin

An antagonist of angiotensin receptors is **saralasin,** a peptide analog of angiotensin II. Saralasin has practical limitations as a therapeutic agent because it must be given parenterally, has an extremely short half-life, and has some partial agonist activity. More recent approaches to interfering with the renin-angiotensin system include the development of nonpeptide antagonists of angiotensin receptors and inhibitors of renin. Clinical studies are ongoing with both types of agents. The most studied is **losartan,** an angiotensin II, AT1 receptor antagonist that is converted in the body to an active metabolite.

■ **Kinins** The kinins are naturally occurring vasodilator polypeptides. **Kallidin** and **bradykinin** are the major members of this class.

- **Biochemistry** Kallikreins, which are proteolytic enzymes, occur in tissues and body fluids and act on a plasma α-2 globulin (kininogen) to release the decapeptide kallidin or the nonapeptide bradykinin. Kallidin is converted in some tissues to bradykinin. Other enzymes, such as trypsin, may also generate these peptides. The kinins are rapidly degraded by tissue kininases, such as dipeptidyl peptidase (kininase II), which is identical to ACE. Thus bradykinin degradation is inhibited by ACE inhibitors such as **captopril,** which may partially explain some of the nonangiotensin-related effects of the ACE inhibitors.

ACE Inhibitors
Captopril
Enalapril

- **Mechanism of action** The kinins react with G protein-coupled plasma membrane receptors associated with second messenger systems such as cAMP or calcium. These receptors mediate a variety of effects, depending on the type of receptor and the coupling system. Some responses to kinins are mediated by the release of prostaglandins and nitric oxide from endothelial cells.

- **Pharmacodynamics**

    — *Cardiovascular system* The most prominent effects of systemically administered kinins are vasodilation and reflex tachycardia. Although potent dilators of arterioles, the kinins may cause contraction of veins. Locally produced or injected kinins are associated with increases in capillary permeability and may induce some of the signs of inflammation.

    — *Other actions* Bradykinin and kallidin contract extravascular smooth muscle, including gastrointestinal, bronchiolar, and uterine tissue. These actions are independent of innervation. The kinins are involved in inflammatory reactions and induce pain by actions on nerve endings and by releasing cytokines.

- **Pharmacotherapeutics** The kinins have been implicated in a wide variety of pathologic conditions, including hypertension, inflammation, carcinoid syndrome, angioneurotic edema, and pancreatitis. Although there are some experimental inhibitors of kinin synthesis and receptors, none has been found to be clinically useful. The cough associated with ACE inhibitors is thought to be related to a decrease in the metabolism of kinins.

■ **Vasopressin** Vasopressin is also known as arginine vasopressin or antidiuretic hormone (ADH).

Vasopressin is a nonapeptide synthesized in the hypothalamus and stored in the posterior pituitary gland. The major therapeutic use of ADH and its derivatives is in the treatment of diabetes insipidus.

- **Pharmacodynamics** Vasopressin acts on two receptors, subtypes V1 and V2. The former is associated with vasoconstrictor effects and the latter is associated with the antidiuretic effect by increasing water reabsorption in the kidneys. This effect on the kidneys is associated with an increase in intracellular cAMP.

- **Pharmacotherapeutics** Because of stability and receptor selectivity, the most frequently used vasopressin analog is **desmopressin (DDAVP)**, which is administered by intranasal or subcutaneous (SQ) routes.

    Alcohol and a number of CNS active drugs inhibit the secretion of ADH.

SECTION 4.3 EICOSANOIDS

■ **Overview** The term *eicosanoids* refers to the number of carbon atoms (20) in various arachidonic acid metabolites. Many of these metabolites have profound effects on the organs in which they are formed. The two major routes of arachidonic acid metabolism are through the cyclooxygenase and lipoxygenase pathways (Fig. 4.2). Drugs that affect the synthesis of these metabolites or that act on the corresponding receptors are widely used as therapeutics or are under investigation.

■ **Occurrence, Biotransformation, and Release** Arachidonic acid is released from membrane phospholipids by the action of phospholipase A2 and some other hydrolases (Fig. 4.2). Subsequent metabolism of arachidonic acid depends on the tissue, resulting in a differential appearance of the various metabolites.

    Substances derived from cyclooxygenase metabolism include prostaglandins, thromboxanes, and prostacyclin. Products of lipoxygenase metabolism are straight chain fatty acid derivatives, including leukotrienes.

■ **Cyclooxygenase Products** Prostaglandins were named for the prostate gland, which was once thought to be the main source of these substances. They are now known to be produced throughout the body, particularly in allergic and inflammatory conditions. There are numerous structurally related prostaglandins.

The prostaglandin nomenclature is based on the degree of unsaturation of the carbon bonds in the long side chain and the substituents on the ring structure. The major prostaglandins are PGE_1, PGE_2, PGD_2, and $PGF_{2\alpha}$. These substances have diverse actions on vascular and other smooth muscle and serve as signals in inflammatory conditions.

Prostacyclin (PGI_2), which is produced by vascular endothelial cells, is an important vasodilator and reduces platelet aggregation.

The major active thromboxane product, TXA_2, is a potent vasoconstrictor and accelerates platelet aggregation. TXA_2 is rapidly converted to a more stable and much less active metabolite TXB_2.

The products resulting from the action of cyclooxygenase have short half-lives and act primarily on the tissues in which they are synthesized.

■ **Lipoxygenase Products** The major products of lipoxygenase metabolism include the leukotrienes LTB_4, LTC_4, LTD_4, and LTE_4. These appear to be impor-

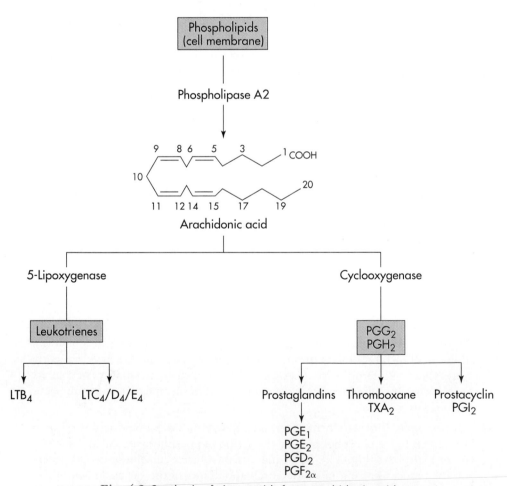

Fig. 4.2 Synthesis of eicosanoids from arachidonic acid.

tant in chemotaxis, bronchoconstriction, and allergic reactions. Other lipoxygenase products include the hydroxyeicosatetaraenoic acids (HETEs), which have also been implicated in inflammation.

Products of lipoxygenase metabolism also have short half-lives. No lipoxygenase agonists or antagonists have been approved for clinical use.

■ Eicosanoids

- **Mechanism of action** The eicosanoids act on numerous cell surface receptors coupled to a variety of second messengers. In general, vasodilators and inhibitors of platelet activation increase cAMP production, and smooth muscle contraction and platelet aggregation arc associated with phosphoinositide metabolism and increases in intracellular calcium.

- **Pharmacodynamics**

  — *Cardiovascular system* PGE_2 and PGI_2 are potent vasodilators. PGE_1 is active in maintaining the patent ductus arteriosus before birth. $PGF_{2\alpha}$ and TXA_2 are vasoconstrictors. Platelet aggregation is inhibited by PGI_2 and activated by TXA_2.

  — *Bronchiolar smooth muscle* Bronchoconstriction has been found with $PGF_{2\alpha}$ and leukotrienes of the C, D, and E series. These agents have been implicated in asthma.

  — *Other smooth muscle* Stimulation of uterine and gastrointestinal smooth muscle is observed with a variety of prostaglandins, particularly $PGF_{2\alpha}$.

  — *Inflammatory reactions* Prostaglandins such as PGE_2 have been shown to cause pain and sensitize nerve endings to other hyperalgesics. In addition, LTB_4 and various HETEs promote the accumulation of proinflammatory cells through chemotactic effects.

  — *Gastric cytoprotection* Protection against gastric ulcer production, cytoprotective effect, has been found with PGE_2 and PGI_2.

Vasodilators
PGE_2
PGI_2

Vasoconstrictors
$PGF\alpha\alpha$
TXA_2

- **Pharmacotherapeutics** Prostaglandins appear to have limited therapeutic use because of their short half-lives and generalized actions.

  Both PGE_2 and $PGF_{2\alpha}$, **dinoprostone** and **dinoprost**, respectively, have been used for inducing abortions. Longer-acting analogs, such as **carboprost**, are used for the same purpose.

  Alprostadil, PGE_1, is used in patients with certain cardiac anomalies to maintain the patent ductus arteriosus.

  Misoprostol, an analog of PGE_1, is used as a cytoprotective, antisecretory agent in the prevention of gastric ulcers, particularly those aggravated by treatment of nonsteroidal antiinflammatory drugs (NSAIDs).

- **Adverse effects** Nausea, vomiting, and especially diarrhea are common adverse effects associated with prostaglandins. Fever is sometimes found as well. Treatment with $PGF_{2\alpha}$ (dinoprost trimethamine) may induce bronchoconstriction.

■ Inhibitors of Eicosanoid Synthesis

- **Cyclooxygenase inhibitors** Aspirin and **NSAIDs** inhibit cyclooxygenase. This decreases production of a variety of eicosanoids and is thought to account for their therapeutic use.

- **Mechanism of action** Aspirin is unique in producing an irreversible inhibition of cyclooxygenase through acetylation of the enzyme. Thus, depending on the dose, there is a decreased production of prostaglandins, prostacyclin, and thromboxanes. Some doses of aspirin may have a more profound effect on thromboxane synthesis than on the synthesis of prostaglandin or prostacyclin. This underlies the use of small doses in the prophylactic treatment of cardiovascular disease. All other NSAIDs are reversible inhibitors of this enzyme.

● **Inhibition of arachidonic acid release** One of the proposed mechanisms of the antiinflammatory actions of glucocorticoids is that these steroids induce the synthesis of lipocortins, proteins that inhibit phospholipase A_2, decreasing arachidonic acid release. A second postulated mechanism of action of glucocorticoids is inhibition of the synthesis of cyclooxygenase. Whether these mechanisms are relevant to the broad array of actions associated with the glucocorticoids remains to be seen.

● **Pharmacotherapeutics** Inhibitors of cyclooxygenase are widely used as analgesics and antiinflammatory agents.

● **Adverse effects** A number of adverse effects are associated with the use of cyclooxygenase inhibitors. Particularly prominent is the induction or exacerbation of peptic ulcers. This is the rationale for the use of misoprostol in patients treated with NSAIDs.

SECTION 4.4 DIURETICS

■ **Overview** One of the major functions of the kidney is to maintain a constant extracellular environment by regulating the excretion of water and electrolytes. *Diuretics* are drugs that act on the renal tubules to correct abnormal electrolyte or water metabolism. Their efficacy is related primarily to their ability to diminish the reabsorption of tubular Na^+ and water. Diuretics are classified according to their chemical structure, potency of effect on Na^+ transport, as well as their mechanism and sites of action in the nephron (Box 4.6, Fig. 4.3, and Table 4.1).

Box 4.6

DIURETICS
Carbonic anhydrase
inhibitors
Acetazolamide
Osmotic diuretics
Mannitol
Loop diuretics
Furosemide
Ethacrynic acid
Bumetanide
Thiazides
Hydrochlorothiazide
Benzoflumethiazide
K$^+$-sparing diuretics
Amiloride
Triameterene
Aldosterone antagonists
Spironolactone
ADH Antagonists
Demelcocycline

Table 4.1 *Diuretics Divided by Tubular Action Site and Potency*

Nephron Portion	Diuretic	% Maximum Filtered Na$^+$ Excreted	Potency
Proximal tubule	Acetazolamide	3-5	Mildly potent
	Mannitol	3-10	Moderately potent
Ascending Limb of Loop of Henle	Furosemide	20-25	Very potent
	Ethacrynic acid	15-25	Very potent
	Bumetanide	20-25	Very potent
	Torsemide	20-25	Very potent
Distal tubule Early portion	Thiazides	5-8	Moderately potent
	Metolazone	5-8	Moderately potent
	Indapamide	5-8	Moderately potent
Distal tubule Late portion	Spironolactone	2-3	Mildly potent
	Triamterene	2-3	Mildly potent
	Amiloride	2-3	Mildly potent

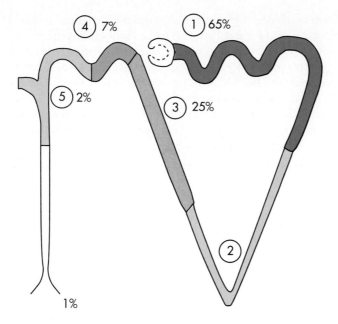

1. Carbonic anhydrase inhibitors
2. Osmotic diuretics
3. Loop diuretics, mercurials
4. Thiazides
5. Potassium-sparing diuretics, aldosterone antagonists

Fig. 4.3 Diagram representing the nephron. *(Modified from Wilcox CS: Diuretics. In Breener BM and Rector FC, editors:* The kidney, *W.B. Saunders Co., 1991.)*

Renal Physiology

● **Tubular function** Fluid filtered across the glomerulus flows through a series of tubules, each of which performs somewhat different functions. In all portions of the nephron, the most abundant active transport system is associated with Na^+-K^+ATPase (Na^+ pump) and is located exclusively on the basolateral membrane (Fig. 4.4). During each cycle, three Na^+ ions are transported out of the cell and two K^+ ions are taken up by the cell. Approximately 70% of Na^+ transport by the kidney involves active transport. The remaining 30% is transported passively.

● **Proximal tubules** Carbonic anhydrase in the brush border of the proximal tubules promotes the reabsorption of much of the filtered HCO_3^- by Na^+-H^+ exchange.

The preferential reabsorption of HCO_3^- and H_2O increases the concentration of Cl^-, resulting in electrical and osmotic gradients that cause the passive reabsorption of Na^+ and H_2O as they follow Cl^- across the tubular cells. Thus Na^+-H^+ exchange plays a central role in the reabsorption of $NaHCO_3$, $NaCl$, and H_2O. Angiotensin II, norepinephrine, dopamine, glomerular filtration rate, and peritubular capillary hemodynamics are factors controlling this transport system.

- **Loop of Henle (LH)** In the thin descending limb of the LH the dominant process is H_2O reabsorption. The thick ascending limb is relatively impermeable to H_2O and, as a result, Na^+ reabsorption leads to a progressive reduction in the tubular Na^+ concentration. The Na^+ entry is primarily mediated by a Na^+-K^+-Cl^- carrier. Because the concentration of luminal K^+ is much lower than that of Na^+ and Cl^-, K^+ is recycled into the lumen through K^+ channels. This movement of K^+ promotes the passive reabsorption of Na^+, Ca^{++}, and Mg^{++}. Transport in this region depends on tubular flow and pressure natriuresis (Fig. 4.5).

- **Distal tubule (DT)** also called the diluting segment, DT reabsorbs Na^+ by way of a Na^+-Cl^- carrier that is flow dependent. This is the site at which Ca^{++} reabsorption (Ca^{++}-ATPase and Na^+/Ca^{++} enchanger) is regulated by parathyroid hormone.

- **Collecting tubules (CT)** The Na^+ reabsorption in the CT occurs by Na^+ channels. This process makes the lumen electronegative, promoting the secretion of K^+ and H^+ from the cell into the lumen. Aldosterone and atrial natriuretic peptide regulate this transport. The CTs respond to antidiuretic hormone (ADH), which increases H_2O reabsorption, leading to the excretion of a concentrated urine. The secretion of H^+ leads to the acidification of the urine.

Individual Classes of Diuretics

- **Carbonic anhydrase inhibitors**

    — *Mechanism of action* Carbonic anhydrase is found in red blood cells, kidney, intestine, ciliary body, choroid plexus, and glial cells. Carbonic

Prototype of Carbonic Anhydrase Inhibitors

Acetazolamide
Methazolamide
Both have an unsubstituted sulfonamide group that is required for CA inhibition.

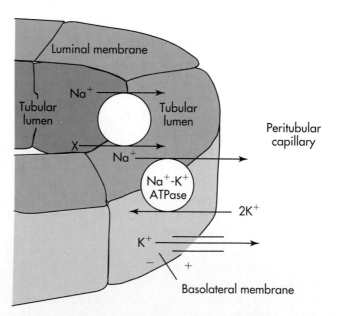

Fig. 4.4 Schematic representation of the general mechanism of tubular Na^+ reabsorption performed by Na^+-K^+ ATPase (the Na^+ pump). *(Adapted from Rose BD: I. Renal function and disorders of water and sodium balance. In Scientific American Medicine, Nephrology 3:10, 1992.)*

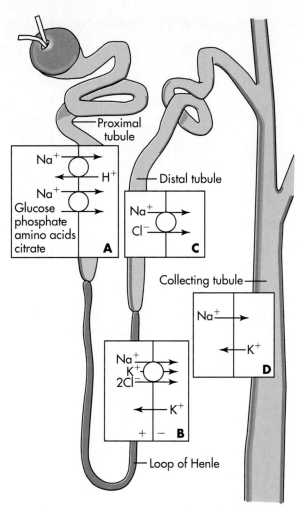

Fig. 4.5 Diagram representing the various mechanisms by which luminal Na^+ enters different nephron segments. **A,** The proximal tubule reabsorbs HCO_3^- and other solutes via specific cotransport with Na^+. **B,** Thick ascending loop of Henle reabsorbs Na^+ by a Na^+-K^+-$2Cl^-$ transporter, which competes for Cl^- binding sites. Passive reabsorption of Na^+, Ca^{++}, and Mg^{++} occurs in this segment. **C,** The distal tubule has Na^+ and Cl^- binding sites. **D,** Na^+ enters the collecting tubule through Na^+ channels located in the luminal membrane. *(Adapted from Rose BD: I. Renal function and disorders of water and sodium balance. In Scientific American Medicine,* Nephrology 3:10, 1992.)

anhydrase inhibitors block proximal tubular HCO_3^- reabsorption at various stages. Thus at the brush border they block the catalytic dehydration of the luminal carbonic acid. They also decrease the intracellular formation of H^+ required for countertransport with Na^+ and decrease peritubular HCO_3^- exit. Therefore the administration of carbonic anhydrase inhibitors induces brisk alkaline diuresis, increases the excretion of Na^+, K^+, and HCO_3^-, and phosphate, and decreases

Carbonic Anhydrase Inhibitor Toxicity

Abnormal taste
Paresthesia
Gastrointestinal distress
Malaise
Decreased libido
In patients with liver disease, carbonic anhydrase inhibitors may increase the levels of ammonia and precipitate encephalopathy.

titratable acid and ammonia. These effects lead to metabolic acidosis (Box 4.7).

Box 4.7

CARBONIC ANHYDRASE INHIBITOR MECHANISM OF ACTION
Slow the following reaction catalyzed by carbonic anhydrase: $H^+ + HCO_3^- \rightarrow H_2O + CO_2$

— *Pharmacokinetics* Carbonic anhydrase inhibitors are readily absorbed from the gastrointestinal system and eliminated by tubular secretion. They bind tightly in tissues to carbonic anhydrase. Compared with acetazolamide, methazolamide has less plasma protein binding, a longer half-life (14 hours versus 5 hours), and a greater lipid solubility, favoring its penetration into aqueous humor and cerebrospinal fluid. Therefore methazolamide is normally preferred, particularly for treating glaucoma.

— *Clinical use* Carbonic anhydrase inhibitors have limited usefulness as diuretics because of the development of metabolic acidosis and other adverse effects. They are used primarily to induce short-term alkaline diuresis in conjunction with $NaCO_3^-$ infusion to increase the excretion of weak acids such as phenobarbital, salicylates, urate, and cysteine. They are sometimes used to treat glaucoma to diminish the transport of HCO_3^- and Na^+ by the ciliary processes and for acute mountain sickness.

Prototype of Osmotic Diuretics

Mannitol
Structurally resembles glucose

● **Osmotic diuretics**

— *Mechanism of action* **Mannitol** is freely filtered at the glomerulus but poorly reabsorbed by the tubules. Mannitol retains water in the lumen, increasing the osmotic concentration and diminishing tubular fluid reabsorption, primarily at the proximal convoluted tubules. Reabsorption of water is also diminished in the descending limb of the LH and in the CT.

— *Pharmacokinetics* Mannitol is not absorbed from the gastrointestinal tract. After IV infusion it is distributed throughout the extracellular space, filtered freely, and poorly reabsorbed. Its half-life is normally 30 to 60 minutes.

— *Clinical use* Mannitol is useful in the prophylactic treatment of acute renal failure because it has the following effects:
  1. It expands the extracellular volume.
  2. It maintains renal blood flow and glomerular filtration.
  3. It increases tubule fluid flow.
  4. It reduces renal edema.
  5. It redistributes blood to the relatively hypoxic inner cortical and outer medullary regions.
  6. It scavenges free radicals.

Although overly aggressive therapy for cerebral edema is dangerous, mannitol is used to treat this condition.

Mannitol and furosemide are useful additions to saline diuresis in preventing cisplatin toxicity.

● **Loop diuretics**

— *Mechanism of action* Loop diuretics inhibit the Na^+-K^+-$2Cl^-$ carrier at the thick ascending limb of the loop of Henle. This inhibition induces pronounced diuresis, 25% excretion of filtrated Na^+, and an increase in K^+ and H^+ excretion. Loop diuretics also increase the excretion of Ca^{++} (up to 30%) and Mg^{++} (more than 60%) by impairing the active reabsorption of Ca^{++} and the passive reabsorption of Mg^{++} in the cortical ascending loop of Henle.

There are two classes of loop diuretics. The first, represented by **furosemide,** inhibits salt transport rapidly, completely, and reversibly when applied from the tubule lumen. The second class, represented by **ethacrynic acid,** inhibits transport when applied from the tubule lumen but has a delayed onset of action or incomplete reversibility. This class of diuretics retains some action when applied from the basolateral side. In addition, furosemide, bumetanide, and torsemide have secondary effects in the proximal tubule. Furosemide has a modest carbonic anhydrase inhibitory effect, whereas bumetanide inhibits the sodium phosphate cotransporter (Box 4.8).

Box 4.8

CLINICAL INDICATIONS OF LOOP DIURETICS
1. Moderate to severe edema caused by congestive heart failure, cirrhosis, nephrotic syndrome 2. Acute left ventricular failure (IV) 3. In combination with saline infusion to manage hyponatremia or hypercalcemia 4. To increase K^+ and H^+ excretion in patients with distal renal tubular acidosis

— *Pharmacokinetics* Loop diuretics are well absorbed when administered by mouth. Furosemide's bioavailability is 50% to 70%, and it binds extensively to plasma albumin. Approximately half of an oral dose is eliminated unchanged by the kidneys, where it is secreted by a probenecid-sensitive transport mechanism in the proximal tubule. The simultaneous administration of indomethacin or other NSAIDs reduces the responsiveness of the tubule to furosemide. Reduced dietary salt intake and repeated furosemide administration during salt restriction diminishes the natriuretic effect of furosemide.

— *Adverse effects* The loop diuretics cause hyponatremia, hypokalemia, hypomagnesemia, and metabolic alkalosis. They increase the plasma concentration of urate and cholesterol and may impair carbohydrate tolerance. At high doses the danger of ototoxicity is present, especially in patients with impaired renal function.

Adverse Effects of Mannitol

Expansion of extracellular volume
Hemodilution
Expansion acidosis from the dilution in HCO_3^- extracellularly
Pulmonary edema
Central nervous system depression
Severe hyponatremia can develop and require urgent hemodialysis to remove excess mannitol

Prototypes of Loop Diuretics

Sulfonamide derivatives
  Furosemide
  Torsemide
  Bumetanide
Phenoxyacetic acid derivative
  Ethacrynic acid
Torsemide is a new long-acting loop diuretic effective as an antihypertensive agent. Administered once daily in low doses, it does not cause hypokalaemia or increased blood sugar, or result in dyslipidemia. It is therapeutically attractive due to its antihypertensive efficacy with once-daily administration, low incidence of adverse side effects, and sustained improvement of the cardiovascular risk profile.

Clinical Use of Loop Diuretics

Clinical use of loop diuretics is reserved for those patients refractory to more conservative measures.

Prototypes of Thiazides

Water-soluble
  Hydrochlorothiazide
Lipid-soluble, more potent,
  and longer acting
  Benzoflumethiazide

- Thiazides

  — *Mechanism of action* Thiazides inhibit the coupled reabsorption of Na^+/Cl^- at the distal tubules. This inhibition results in approximately 3% to 5% excretion of filtered Na^+ and an increase in Cl^-, K^+, and H^+ excretion. Thiazides also impair maximal urinary dilution. The combination of increased NaCl excretion with impaired dilution predisposes patients to hyponatremia. Thiazide therapy produces a sustained reduction in renal Ca^{++} excretion, which is accompanied by a small rise in serum Ca^{++}. Thiazides also increase Mg^{++} excretion and reduce urate clearance.

  — *Pharmacokinetics* Thiazides are readily absorbed from the gastrointestinal tract. They are extensively bound to plasma proteins. The water-soluble thiazides, such as hydochlorothiazide, are eliminated by the kidney. The lipid-soluble thiazides, such as benzoflumethiazide, are extensively metabolized and display a more prolonged action than water-soluble thiazides.

  — *Adverse effects are given in Box 4.9.*

Box 4.9

ADVERSE EFFECTS OF THIAZIDES
Hypokalemia and Hypomagnesemia Can be serious in patients with a) Cardiac failure who are receiving digitalis b) Cirrhosis or poorly compensated edema c) Myocardial ischemia or arrhythmias **Mild Chronic Hyponatremia** Usually asymptomatic, but is serious and requires urgent therapy **Impaired Carbohydrate Tolerance** Therefore this therapy should be avoided in patients with diabetes mellitus, obesity, or hyperlipidemia

Prototypes of K⁺-Sparing Diuretics

Do not interact with aldosterone receptor:
  Amiloride
  Triamterene
Competitive antagonists of aldosterone:
  Spironolactone

  — *Clinical use* Thiazides are among the drugs of choice for the treatment of hypertension in patients with well-preserved renal function. They are ineffective when used alone in patients whose creatinine clearances are less than 20 to 30 ml/min and in patients with severe edema. Such individuals require loop diuretics. Thiazides are also used in the management of hypercalciuria, nephrolithiasis, and diabetes insipidus.

- K⁺-sparing diuretics and aldosterone antagonists

  — *Mechanism of action* These diuretics act in the distal tubule and the cortical collecting duct, where they inhibit Na^+-K^+ ATPase, inducing a modest natriuresis and a reduction in the excretion of K^+ and H^+.

  — *Pharmacokinetics* Triamterene is well absorbed from the gastrointestinal tract and rapidly hydroxylated to derivatives that retain some diuretic activity. Both the drug and its metabolites are excreted by the kidney, with half-lives of 3 to 5 hours. Triameterene accumulates in cirrhosis because of decreased hydroxylation and biliary secretion, and in renal disease because of decreased renal excretion.

Spironolactone is converted to active metabolites, is readily absorbed orally, and is bound to plasma proteins. It has a half-life for elimination of 20 hours and requires 24 to 48 hours to achieve maximal natriuresis.

— *Clinical uses* These drugs are used when modest or limited diuresis is required such as with poorly compensated edema or cirrhosis. They are most effective in primary and secondary hyperaldosteronism.

— *Adverse effects* Hyperkalemia is a potentially lethal complication associated with K^+-sparing diuretics. The risk is directly related to dose and increases considerably in patients with renal failure or in those receiving K^+ supplements. Hyperchloremic metabolic acidosis is another potential adverse effect, as is formation of renal stones, especially with triameterene. This agent can cause acute renal failure when given with indomethacin, even in normal subjects. Spironolactone can cause gynecomastia or androgenic effects, such as hirsutism or postmenopausal bleeding.

● **Antidiuretic hormone antagonists**

— *Mechanism of action* Antidiuretic hormone (ADH) facilitates reabsorption from the collecting ducts by activating adenylyl cyclase. Antagonists of ADH, such as **demeclocycline** and **lithium** ions, inhibit the action of the hormone at some point distal to the generation of cAMP.

— *Clinical use* The ADH antagonists are used primarily in the treatment of conditions characterized by an excessive secretion of the hormone or of ADH-like peptides.

— *Adverse effects* Demeclocycline, like other tetracyclines, causes abnormalities of bone and teeth in young children.

● **Diuretic resistance** When there is an inadequate clearing of edema or antihypertensive response is blunted despite the fact that a normally effective dose of diuretic is being administered, an effort should be made to determine whether the edema is due to inappropriate renal Na^+ and fluid retention rather than to lymphatic or venous obstruction. Other possibilities for drug resistance include the level of NaCl and fluid intake, inadequate drug reaching tubule lumen in the active form, and a decreased renal response (Table 4.2).

Section 4.5 Bronchodilators and Other Agents Used for Asthma

■ **Immunopathologic Considerations** Asthma is mediated by macrophage-induced antigenic sensitization of T-cell lymphocytes, which results in B-cell lymphocyte stimulation with formation of antigen-specific IgE, which subsequently attaches to specific receptors on airway mast cells and circulatory basophils. After reexposure the antigen bridges between adjacent antigen-specific IgE molecules on the surface of respiratory tract mast cells. This activates the mast cells, initiating the following sequence of events:

1. Energy-dependent Ca^{++} entry into the cell

Definition

Asthma is a disease characterized by an increased responsiveness of the trachea and bronchi to various stimuli and manifested by a widespread narrowing of the airways that changes in severity either spontaneously or as a result of therapy.

Table 4.2   *Common Causes of Diuretic Resistance*

CAUSE	EXAMPLE
Incorrect diagnosis	Venous or lymphatic edema
Inappropriate NaCl or fluid intake	
Inadequate drug reaching tubule lumen in active form:	
Noncompliance	
Dose inadequate or too frequent	
Poor absorption	Uncompensated CHF
Decreased renal blood flow	CHF, cirrhosis, elderly
Decreased functional renal mass	ARF, CRF, elderly
Proteinuria	Nephrotic syndrome
Decreased renal response	
Low GFR	CHF, cirrhosis, ARF, CRF, elderly
Decreased effective ECFV	Edematous conditions
Activation of RAA axis	Edematous conditions
Nephron adaptation	Prolonged diuretic therapy
NSAID	Indomethacin, aspirin

CHF, Congestive heart failure; *ARF,* acute renal faulure; *CRF,* chronic renal failure; *GFR,* glomerular filtration rate; *ECFV,* extracellular fluid volume; *RAA,* renin-angiotensin-aldosterone; *NSAID,* nonsteroidal antiinflammatory drug.

Incidence

Asthma affects nearly 2% of the population.

Nearly 10 million Americans suffer from asthma. It is especially troublesome in childhood, and the most frequent cause of absence from school and work.

Education

Patient education as to the nature of the disease and treatment is perhaps the single most important non-drug treatment.

2. Elevation of intracellular cAMP
3. Changes in cell-surface charge
4. Release of preformed mediators and generation of unstored mediators including histamine, tryptase, neutral proteases, leukotrienes C_4 and D_4, prostaglandin D_2, eosinophil chemotactic factor, and neutrophil chemotactic factor

As a result, there is activation of airway afferent nerve endings, an increase in endothelial and epithelial cell permeability, and an increase in airway smooth muscle contraction and mucus cell secretion. These physiologic changes lead to the characteristic symptoms associated with asthma, including bronchospasm, mucus hypersecretion, airway epithelial cell damage, and airway immune-inflammatory reaction (Fig. 4.6).

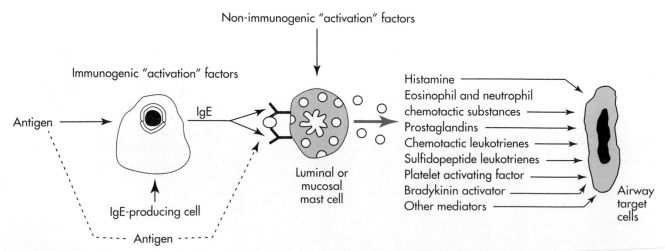

Fig. 4.6 Schematic representation of the factors involved in the early events leading to airway allergen sensitization. *(Modified from Sell S:* Immunology and immunopathology and immunity, *New York, 1992, Elsevier.)*

Drugs used to treat asthma are classified into two groups according to their mechanisms of action. One class includes drugs aimed at correcting the bronchospasm by acting on the adrenoceptors on the tracheobronchial smooth muscle to dilate the bronchi by a direct action. Drugs used as bronchodilators include β_2-adrenoreceptor agonists, xanthines, and muscarine-receptor antagonists. The other class is characterized by drugs that act mainly as inhibitors of the immune-inflammation, such as corticosteroids and cromolyn sodium. These agents inhibit or prevent the inflammatory phase of asthma.

■ Bronchodilators

● **β-Adrenergic agonists** The adrenergic drugs used for the management of acute and chronic asthma are **epinephrine, isoproterenol,** and a group of adrenoceptor agonists including **albuterol** and **terbutaline** that are relatively selective for β_2-adrenoceptors. The latter group of agents has become the backbone of modern bronchodilator therapy.

— *Chemistry* Epinephrine and isoproterenol are catechols and substrates for catechol-O-methyltransferase (COMT). They have relatively short-acting activity. Albuterol and terbutaline are tertiary butyl derivatives that are not substrates for COMT and therefore have a longer duration of action.

— *Pharmacodynamics* Their action in the lung is the result of relaxation of bronchial smooth muscle, an effect induced by the activation of β_2-adrenoceptors. They also induce tachycardia, anxiety, and tremor.

   In severe acute episodes of bronchospasm and status asthmaticus, **epinephrine** is administered SQ. Within 5 to 15 minutes, epinephrine induces bronchodilation and pulmonary vasoconstriction, resulting in a reduction in pulmonary edema. Improvement of pulmonary function is maintained for up to 4 hours. The cardiovascular effects of epinephrine represent the sum of both α- and β-adrenoceptor stimulation, including increased heart rate, cardiac output, and stroke volume; an elevation of systolic pressure; and a decline in diastolic pressure and systemic vascular resistance.

   Isoproterenol is administered almost exclusively by inhalation. Its response is almost instantaneous, and the improvement of pulmonary function lasts up to 3 hours. Since isoproterenol has equal affinity for both β_1- and β_2-adrenoceptors, it has equal capacity to induce bronchodilation and cardiac stimulation.

   Terbutaline and **albuterol** are relatively selective for β_2-adrenoceptors and theoretically are capable of producing bronchodilation with minimal cardiac stimulation. Their maximum effect is within 30 minutes and lasts 4-6 hours.

   Salmeterol and **formoterol,** two newer compounds, appear to extend the duration of action to 10-12 hours and maintain β_2-selectivity. The place of these compounds in routine asthma therapy has not yet been well-defined. The use of these compounds is clearly advantageous for patients with nocturnal asthma and for those whose symptoms are not well controlled by the use of antiinflammatory agents. In patients who require higher dosing schedules, they may reduce the amount of inhaled steroids.

— *Pharmacokinetics* Epinephrine and isoproterenol are essentially ineffective orally because they are rapidly metabolized in the intestine and

Bronchodilators

β-Adrenergic Agonists
   Epinephrine
   Isoproterenol
   Albuterol
   Terbutaline
   Salmeterol
   Formoterol
Xanthine Drugs
   Theophylline
   Aminophylline
Anticholinergic Agents
   Ipratropium bromide

Mechanism of Action

The therapeutic effects of β-adrenergic agonists are mediated by
a. cAMP that induces bronchial smooth muscle relaxation and bronchodilation.
b. Stimulation of β_2-adrenoceptors, resulting in relaxation of smooth muscles.
c. Stimulation of ciliary movements, resulting in increased mucociliary clearance.
d. Inhibition of the release of mediators from mast cells.

Receptor Selectivity

Drug	Adrenoceptors
Epinephrine	α & β
Isoproterenol	β
Albuterol	β_2
Terbutaline	β_2

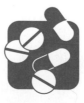

liver. However, when isoproterenol is given by inhalation, the metabolic patterns observed after inhalation administration are similar to those after oral administration suggesting that most of the dose delivered by inhalation is swallowed and inactivated in the GI tract, with only about 10% of the dose getting directly into the lungs.

Terbutaline and albuterol are effective after oral administration or by inhalation. Terbutaline is not completely absorbed from the GI tract, while albuterol is well-absorbed.

All β-adrenergic agonists appear in the urine as sulfate conjugates and as the unchanged drug.

Tolerance to β-Agonists

Continual treatment with β-agonists can induce tolerance, manifested by a decrease in the peak and duration of bronchodilation and becoming maximal within two weeks. It may extend to all β-adrenergic drugs. IV administration of corticosteroids can restore responsiveness within one hour.

Theophylline's Actions

Induces smooth muscle relaxation.
Cardiac stimulation.
It has a moderate bronchoprotective effect in pretreatment before exercise and histamine challenge.
It attenuates the early- and late-phase responses to allergen exposure by its modest antiinflammatory properties.
It increases cardiac output and lowers venous pressure.
Although it is a weak bronchodilator compared with β-adrenergic agents, its main advantage is its long duration of action. This effect is particularly useful in the management of nocturnal asthma.

— *Clinical uses* Epinephrine is used extensively for the management of acute asthma attacks. Isoproterenol is used mainly by inhalation for the management of bronchospasm, and IV for asthma or as a stimulant in cardiac arrest. Albuterol, terbutaline, and other β$_2$-agonists are the drugs of first choice for treatment of acute attacks of bronchostenosis.

— *Adverse effects* Patients treated with epinephrine may complain of feeling anxious or nervous. Some may experience hand or upper extremity tremors, and many may complain of palpitations. Epinephrine is dangerous at high doses, especially in patients with coronary artery disease, arrhythmias, or hypertension. An overdose may result in extreme hypertension and cerebrovascular accidents, pulmonary edema, angina, and ventricular arrhythmias, including ventricular fibrillation. Isoproterenol at recommended doses is not associated with severe adverse effects; however, it may cause tachycardia, dizziness, nervousness, and arrhythmias.

Oral administration of β$_2$-adrenoceptor agonists may result in muscle tremor because of their direct stimulation of β$_2$-adrenoceptors in skeletal muscle. This effect is more prominent at the initiation of therapy, but gradually disappears. These compounds can also cause tachycardia and palpitations in some patients. When administered by inhalation, β$_2$-agonists produce only minor side effects. Recent epidemiological studies suggest that the use of β$_2$-adrenoceptor agonists is associated with overall deterioration in disease control and a slight increase in asthma mortality. This finding may be due to the fact that some patients rely too heavily on bronchodilator therapy to control acute symptoms at the expense of antiinflammatory therapy necessary to control the underlying disease process.

● **Xanthine drugs** Methylxanthines include theophylline, theobromine, and caffeine. The xanthine employed in clinical medicine is **theophylline,** which is often used in the conjugate form, **aminophylline.** A new compound, **enprofylline,** is under study. The bronchodilator action of this group of drugs is less than that observed with β$_2$-agonists.

— *Mechanism of action* The relaxant effect on smooth muscle induced by methylxanthines has been attributed to inhibition of **phosphodiesterase,** which results in an increase in cAMP, causing bronchial smooth muscle relaxation and bronchodilation. The inhibition of phosphodiesterase induced by methylxanthines occurs at very high doses; therefore, it is unlikely that this action alone is responsible for the relaxation of the smooth muscle. Other mechanisms that may contribute to their antiasthmatic action include antagonism of

Table 4.3 *Factors That Can Decrease Theophylline Clearance and Magnitude of Effect*

FACTOR	PERCENTAGE DECREASE IN CLEARANCE
Heart failure	60
Liver disease (cirrhosis, acute hepatitis)	30-75
	Increase in serum half-life of 70%
Viral respiratory disease	10-15
Renal failure	20
High-carbohydrate, low-protein diet	Modest
Dietary xanthines	50
Troleandmycin	25
Erythromycin	40 (23-100)
Cimetidine	34
Oral contraceptives	25
Allopurinol	40 in smokers, 20 in nonsmokers
Propranolol	Increase of 145% in serum half-life

adenosine receptors, inhibition of mediator release, increased sympathetic activity, alteration in immune cell function, and reduction in respiratory muscle fatigue.

— *Pharmacokinetics* Xanthine drugs are given either orally or by slow IV injection of a loading dose followed by IV infusion. Absorption of theophylline from the GI tract is virtually complete. The rate of absorption varies greatly depending on the formulation. Slow releasing preparations peak after 6 to 8 hours, making once or twice daily dosing schedules possible. Aminophylline is the preparation used for IV administration. Oxidation and demethylation of theophylline take place in the liver. Its average serum half-life in nonsmoking adults is approximately 7 to 9 hours. Its clearance is accelerated in children, cigarette smokers, and persons taking phenytoin or on a high protein, low carbohydrate diet. Such conditions as heart failure, liver disease, and severe respiratory obstruction slow the metabolism of theophylline. Factors that influence theophylline's clearance are given in Tables 4.3 and 4.4.

Theophylline in Asthma Care

Despite its limitations, theophylline
  Is easy to use when compliance with inhaled medications is difficult.
  Is effective in treating nocturnal symptoms because of its long duration of action.
  Is a useful adjunct to inhaled antiinflammatory agents.
  Reduces the need for frequent courses of oral glucocorticoids.
Serum concentrations should be used as a guide for safety.

Table 4.4 *Factors That Can Increase Theophylline Clearance and Magnitude of Effect*

FACTOR	PERCENTAGE INCREASE IN CLEARANCE
Smoking	
Tobacco	50
Marijuana	50
Tobacco and marijuana	90-100
High-protein, low-carbohydrate diet	55
Charcoal-broiled beef	30
Phenobarbital	33
Phenytoin	80
Isoproterenol (intravenous infusion)	20

— *Clinical uses* The main use of theophylline is in the management of asthma. It is also used to relieve dyspnea associated with pulmonary edema that develops from congestive heart failure.

— *Adverse effects* Patients receiving theophylline for the first time complain of nausea and vomiting. These effects are dose related; plasma levels under 15 µg/ml rarely cause these symptoms. The fact that IV administration of theophylline induces similar effects suggests that the nausea and vomiting are the result of CNS action.

When the plasma concentration increases over 40 µg/ml, there is a high probability of seizures; however, nausea will always be a premonitory sign of impending toxicity. A rapid IV infusion of theophylline can cause arrhythmias, hypotension, and cardiac arrest. Since it is not possible to predict blood levels from the dose given, blood levels are often determined by laboratory analysis.

● **Anticholinergic agents** In human airways, the parasympathetic cholinergic pathway originating from the vagus nerve is the main neuronal control. This cholinergic pathway plays a key role in the maintenance of the caliber of the airways and contributes to the airway obstruction of both asthma and chronic obstructive pulmonary disease. Stimulation of these nerve fibers results in release of acetylcholine and activation of muscarinic cholinoceptors, eliciting bronchoconstriction, mucous secretion, and bronchial vasodilation.

Anticholinergic compounds have been used in the treatment of respiratory disorders for centuries. Plants containing atropine, as well as atropine alone, were used in the treatment of asthma; however, their use faded because of atropine's multiple side effects, as well as the introduction of the β_2-adrenoceptor agonists, which possess superior efficacy. Anticholinergics are most useful in exercise-induced asthma.

To improve the clinical use of anticholinergics, quaternary amine derivatives of atropine have been developed. These positive charged compounds induce fewer side effects because of their poor absorption across mucosal surfaces.

Ipratropium bromide is an example of this class of quaternary derivatives. This compound is available only for inhalation and is exclusively locally effective. It is not well-absorbed and does not act at muscarinic receptors other than those present at the bronchi. Its maximum effect is not seen until after 30 minutes or so, but lasts for 3 to 5 hours.

■ **Inhibitors of the Immune-Inflammation**

● **Corticosteroids** Despite many potential side effects, steroids are the most effective antiinflammatory agents available for the treatment of asthma. The introduction of aerosol corticosteroids, by virtue of their local administration and markedly reduced systemic absorption, has been a major innovation in the treatment of asthma. The inhaled corticosteroids are analogues of hydrocortisone.

— *Mechanism of action* The mechanism of improvement of asthma with steroids is unclear. They inhibit the generation of leukotrines B_4, C_4, and D_4, reducing the recruitment and activation of inflammatory cells; and the vasodilators, prostaglandin E_2 and I_2. They also inhibit the allergen-induced influx of eosinophils into the lung. They can up-regulate β_2-receptors, decrease microvascular permeability, and reduce mediator release from eosinophils. The reduction in synthesis of the lymphokine IL-3, which regulates mast cell production, may

Ipratropium Bromide Clinical Uses

Effective in exercise-induced asthma.
Not particularly effective against allergen challenge, but it inhibits the increase of mucus secretion that occurs in asthma and appears to increase the mucociliary clearance of bronchial secretions.
Has no effect on the late inflammatory phase of asthma.
In combination with β_2-agonists, the dose of the sympathomimetic drug can often be reduced, resulting in increased duration of bronchodilator action.

Antiinflammatory Agents

Corticosteroids
  Betamethasone
  Dexamethasone
  Triamcinolone acetonide
  Beclomethasone
   dipropionate
  Hydrocortisone
Others
  Cromolyn sodium
  Nedocromil sodium

explain why long-term steroid treatment eventually reduces the early-phase response to allergens and prevents exercise-induced asthma.

The effects of the steroids take several hours to days to develop; thus, they are not used for quick relief of acute epidoses of bronchospasm.

— *Pharmacokinetics* They can be given parenterally, orally, and by local administration. **Prednisone** and **prednisolone** are absorbed rapidly when given orally, with peak concentrations reached within 1 to 2 hours.

— *Clinical uses* Corticosteroids are particularly useful for the treatment of both acute and chronic asthma in both children and adults. However, inhaled corticosteroids are not effective in the relief of acute episodes of severe bronchospasm. Systemic corticosteroids are used for the treatment of asthma that does not respond to theophylline, β_2-adrenoreceptor agonists, or aerosol corticosteroids; they are also used along with other treatments in the control of status asthmaticus. The decision to initiate systemic steroid use can be difficult. Steroids may be lifesaving if the disease is progressing and may shorten the course of the illness regardless of its status. The general rule is to use high doses initially in an attempt to control the disease and then to taper the drug rapidly within 5 to 7 days to avoid side effects.

— *Adverse effects* The adverse effects range from minor to severe and life-threatening. Their severity depends on the route, dose, and frequency of administration, as well as the specific agent.

Inhaled steroids are generally well-tolerated. Their side effects include sore throat, oral candidiasis (treated by stopping the drug, reducing the dose, or giving nystatin drops), and allergic symptoms such as atopic dermatitis or allergic rhinitis. Washing the mouth out after each use may reduce the incidence of oral candidiasis. Potential adverse effects of systemic administration include adrenal suppression, Cushing's disease, growth retardation, cataracts, osteoporosis, CNS effects and behavioral disturbances, and increased susceptibility to infection.

● **Cromolyn sodium** This compound and the related drug **nedocromil sodium** are not bronchodilators. Their use is prophylactic only and plays no role in acute asthma attacks.

— *Mechanism of action* The mechanism of action is not fully understood. It prevents the release of mediators of bronchoconstriction from mast cells, probably by blocking Ca^{++} entry into the cell. Cromolyn inhibits reflex bronchoconstriction, and reduces bronchial reactivity or level of twitchiness in response to histamine, antigen, and cold air. Therefore a patient treated during a pollen season with cromolyn may have less frequent and milder asthma attacks with the use of this drug.

— *Pharmacokinetics* Cromolyn is poorly absorbed from the GI tract. It is given by inhalation, only about 10% is absorbed, and it is excreted unchanged, in bile and urine. Its plasma half-life is about 90 minutes.

— *Adverse effects* Cromolyn is a remarkably benign drug with few side effects, except for distress of the upper respiratory tract resulting in throat and airway irritation, dry mouth, cough, and perhaps reactive bronchospasm. Rare cases of skin rashes, eosinophilic pneumonia, and allergic granulomatosis have been reported.

Absorption of Corticosteroids

Well-absorbed and with many systemic effects:
Betamethasone
Dexamethasone
Poorly absorbed and with fewer systemic effects:
Triamcinolone acetonide
Beclomethasone dipropionate
Flunisolide

Contraindications and Cautions

Care should be taken in transferring patients from systemic to aerosol corticosteroids, as death due to adrenal insufficiency has been reported.
Also, allergic conditions, such as rhinitis, conjunctivitis, and eczema, previously controlled by systemic corticosteroids, may be unmasked when the patients are switched to inhaled corticosteroids.
Special care should be exercised during pregnancy and in patients with systemic fungal infections.

SECTION 4.6 DRUGS USED IN GASTROINTESTINAL DISORDERS

■ **Overview** The GI system, consisting of the digestive tract, the biliary system, and the pancreas, is responsible for processing the fluids, nutrients, and electrolytes entering the body. The digestive tract has five primary functions:

1. Moves ingested products through the system
2. Digests food substances
3. Secretes electrolytes and enzymes to assist digestion
4. Allows for the absorption of nutrients into the bloodstream
5. Excretes indigestible residues

Box 4.10 lists the drugs used in GI diseases.

> **Box 4.10**
>
> ### DRUGS USED IN GASTROINTESTINAL DISEASES
>
> 1. Acid-peptic disease
>   Gastric secretion
>   Mucosal protective agents
>   Promotion of gastrointestinal activity
> 2. Antiemetics
> 3. Laxatives
> 4. Diarrhea
> 5. Gallstones
> 6. Chronic inflammation of the bowel
> 7. Portal-systemic encephalopathy

■ **Drugs Used in Acid-Peptic Disease** The treatment of this condition is aimed at counteracting the effects of acid and pepsin (Fig. 4.7). This can be achieved by suppressing acid secretion, neutralizing acid and protecting tissue from gastric acid, and by inhibiting *H. pylori* with antibacterial agents. Factors that influence ulcer occurrence are given in Box 4.11.

■ **Acid Suppression**

● **Anticholinergic drugs** Although anticholinergic drugs decrease gastric acidity by blocking the effect of acetylcholine on the parietal cells, these drugs have never been proven effective when administered alone. They are rarely prescribed because of their adverse effects, including xerostomia, blurred vision, and urinary retention.

Pirenzepine has fewer adverse effects than traditional anticholinergic agents and is effective in healing duodenal ulcers. Some antidepressant agents, including **doxzepin** and **trimipramine,** have also been effective in the treatment of this condition.

Prototypes of Histamine H$_2$ Antagonists

Cimetidine
Famotidine
Ranitidine
Nizatidine

● **Histamine H$_2$ receptor antagonists** Histamine H$_2$ receptor antagonists interfere with acid secretion by competing with histamine at the H$_2$ receptor site on the parietal cell. This greatly reduces acid secretion (Fig. 4.8).

Cimetidine was the first histamine H$_2$ receptor antagonist. It heals 75% to 90% of duodenal ulcers in 6 weeks, and between 55% and 80% of gastric ulcers. Cimetidine reversibly inhibits microsomal drug metabolism, enhancing the potential for interactions with numerous drugs such as theophylline, anticoagulants, and propranolol.

Box 4.11

FACTORS THAT DO AND DO NOT INFLUENCE ULCER OCCURRENCE

Yes
Male sex
Genetic factors
Cigarettes
Aspirin
Nonsteroidal antiinflammatory drugs
Steroids: high doses, prolonged treatment
Cirrhosis
Chronic obstructive pulmonary diseases
Chronic nephropathy and renal transplantation
Emotional stress

No
Personality
Occupation
Economic status
Diet
Coffee
Alcohol (except in cirrhosis)
Hyperparathyroidism
Inflammatory bowel disease
Rheumatoid arthritis

— *Adverse effects* The adverse effects most commonly associated with cimetidine include allergic reactions. More serious adverse effects include mental confusion, renal disturbances, and abnormalities in liver function. When cimetidine is used for prolonged periods or in large doses, it also has antiandrogenic effects including gynecomastia, impotence, and decreased sperm count.

Ranitidine is a more potent histamine H_2 receptor antagonist than cimetidine and lacks some of its adverse effects. Ranitidine interferes less with hepatic metabolism than cimetidine and inhibits both daytime and nocturnal basal gastric acid secretion, as well as gastric acid secretion stimulated by food and histamine, for up to 13 hours after a single dose.

Famotidine is the most potent of the histamine H_2 receptor antagonists. It heals most duodenal ulcers within 4 to 8 weeks and a smaller proportion of gastric ulcers. It does not interfere with hepatic oxidation and therefore has less potential for drug interactions. Muscle cramps, headaches, and constipation are associated with its use.

Nizatidine is as effective as cimetidine in the treatment of duodenal ulcer. The adverse effects with nizatidine are minor, and it does not interfere with drug metabolism.

Overall, histamine H_2 receptor antagonists have a remarkably good safety record. All drugs are equally efficacious in treating both gastric and duodenal ulcers. They have revolutionized the treatment of these conditions.

● **Gastric pump inhibitors** Gastric pump inhibitors interfere with the generation of H^+ from the parietal cell by blocking the H^+K^+ATPase.

Omeprazole inhibits 50% to 90% of acid secretion while having no effect on gastric emptying. Suppression of gastric acid begins within 1 hour of administration and reaches its maximal effect within 2 hours. Half of

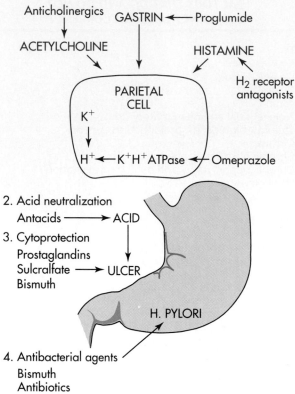

Fig. 4.7 Treatment options for peptic ulcer. *(Adapted from Achkar E: Peptic ulcer disease. In Achkar E, Farmer RG, Fleshler B, editors:* Clinical gastroenterology, *Philadelphia, 1992, Lea & Febiger.)*

the peak effect is still present up to 24 hours after a single dose of omeprazole.

Omeprazole is formulated in a delayed-release hard gelatin capsule containing enteric-coated granules. Only about 50% of the drug reaches the systemic circulation, where 95% is bound to plasma proteins. It is metabolized in the liver and excreted in the urine and feces. Omeprazole tends to achieve quicker healing and more prompt relief than histamine receptor antagonists.

— *Adverse effects* Because omeprazole produces profound hypochlorhydria, significant hypergastrimia is common and intragastric bacterial overgrowth may occur with this agent. The increased levels of gastrin have a trophic effect on the enterochromaffin cells of the stomach, raising concerns about the possibility of inducing carcinoid tumors with long-term treatment. Such tumors have developed in rats given massive doses of omeprazole for prolonged periods of time.

Acid Neutralization In the past, antacids were the most effective treatment for peptic ulcer. Because of the availability of more potent and selective drugs, antacids are prescribed less often, although many patients continue to use them for prompt and temporary relief. Liquid antacids are more effective than tablets.

● **Action** Antacids interact with gastric secretions, releasing anions that par-

The pH of the gastric contents is 1.0 to 3.5.
The pain and discomfort associated with hyperactivity are frequent complaints of patients with peptic ulcers.

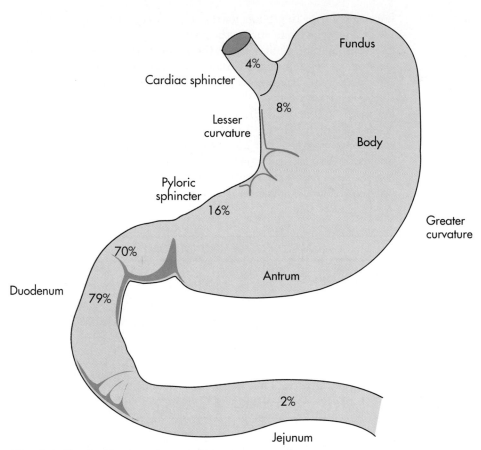

Fig. 4.8 The distribution of peptic ulcers. *(Modified from Kuhn MA: Antacids, histamine H$_2$ antagonists, anti-ulcer drugs, and gastrointestinal stimulants. In Kuhn MA, editor:* Pharmacokinetics: a nursing process approach, ed 3, *Philadelphia, 1994, F.A. Davis.)*

tially neutralize gastric HCl and thereby increase the gastric pH. Antacids do not absorb the acid but generally raise the pH of the stomach above 4.0. Pepsin, a proteolytic enzyme, is suppressed at pH 3 and inactivated above pH 7 to 8. In the bleeding patient, the pH must be above 6.5 for clotting.

● **Antacid classification** Systemic antacids are soluble in gastric contents and are absorbed systemically. The prototype, sodium bicarbonate, is present in Alka-Seltzer, Soda Mint, and Instant Metamucil.

Nonsystemic antacids are insoluble in gastric contents and are not absorbed. These contain Ca^{++}, Al^{+++}, Mg^{++}, or some combination of these ions.

— *Individual agents* Magnesium products are the best overall antacid, whereas aluminum products are the weakest. Calcium and aluminum products tend to cause constipation, and magnesium-based antacids cause diarrhea. The highest neutralizing capabilities are possessed by CaCO$_3$, followed by Mg(OH)$_2$ and Al(OH)$_3$. All three have a duration of action of approximately 30 minutes in a fasting patient and 2 to 4 hours on a full stomach.

— *Clinical uses* The antacids are effective in treating acid indigestion, heartburn, reflux esophagitis, and peptic ulcers. They are also useful in preventing stress ulcers, relieving pain from ulcers, and binding bile salts from reflux into the stomach. They are administered every 1 to 2

Acid-neutralizing capacity is a primary consideration in selecting an antacid. It is expressed in milliequivalents per milliliter (mEq/ml). Milliequivalents of antacid are defined by the mEq of HCl required to keep an antacid suspension at pH 3.0 for 2 hours in vitro. The higher the acid-neutralizing capacity, the more effective the antacid.

hours during waking hours for the first 2 weeks and 1 to 3 hours after meals and at bedtime during the healing stage.

Amphojel and Gelusil are $Al(OH)_3$ antacids used to treat individuals prone to developing PO_4 kidney stones and hyperphosphatemia associated with chronic renal failure. Aluminum binds with PO_4^{3-} in the bowel, forming an insoluble precipitate that is excreted in the feces. Because PO_4^{3-} and Ca^{++} have an inverse relationship, plasma PO_4^{3-} levels fall and Ca^{++} levels rise. Prolonged use of these antacids can lead to hypophosphatemia, with symptoms of anorexia, malaise, and muscle weakness. Also, chronic ingestion of aluminum-containing antacids in chronic renal failure can result in accumulation of aluminum in serum, bone, and brain. Contraindications are listed in Box 4.12.

Box 4.12

ANTACID CONTRAINDICATIONS
In General
In individuals with
Sensitivities to the component's properties
Renal dysfunction because of the possibility of forming urinary calculi
Renal impairment because of accumulation of metal ions
In Particular
Increased Mg may create neurologic cardiovascular and neuromuscular dysfunction. Excessive Ca may result in hypercalcemia, weakness, mental confusion, nausea, vomiting, anorexia, weakness, headache, dizziness, and a change in mental status.

—   *Adverse effects*   Adverse effects of antacids are listed in Box 4.13.

Box 4.13

ADVERSE EFFECTS OF ANTACIDS
In general, antacids are nontoxic.
For All, Most Common
Gastrointestinal: Change in bowel habits
Renal: Hypermagnesemia, hyperphosphatemia
In Particular
$NaHCO_3$ and $CaCO_3$
Renal: Milk-alkali syndrome, characterized by hypercalcemia, alkalosis, and renal failure
Aluminum Compounds
Neurologic: Dialysis dementia in dialysis patients, accumulation of aluminum in serum, bone, and central nervous system, headache, weakness
Gastrointestinal: Constipation, nausea, vomiting
Renal: Alkalosis

■ Protection of the Injured Tissue

● **Cytoprotective agents** Cytoprotection refers to actions that promote healing of the gastrointestinal mucosa without interfering with gastric acid secretion.

—   *Sucralfate* Sucralfate, an aluminum salt of sucrose, binds to the protein substrate of the mucosa and forms a gel that coats the ulcer. Because the gel forms at a low pH, sucralfate should not be administered

Uses of Sucralfate

1. Healing of both gastric and duodenal ulcers
2. Prophylaxis of stress ulcers
3. Relief for oral ulcers and mucosal pain associated with chemotherapy and radiation

with antacids. Sucralfate has a negligible acid-neutralizing capacity, but it does moderately inhibit pepsin activity in gastric juice. It blocks the diffusion of gastric acid across the protective barrier and limits the proteolytic activity of pepsin. Sucralfate also stimulates the synthesis of prostaglandins.

— *Prostaglandins* Prostaglandins are produced naturally and have cytoprotective effects on the GI tract. Prostaglandins increase mucosal blood flow, the thickness of the gastric mucus, and they enhance bicarbonate secretion. Many synthetic prostaglandin analogs (**Misoprostol**) heal 75% to 80% of duodenal ulcers and are protective against agents known to damage the mucosa. Diarrhea has been reported in patients taking prostaglandins. The most serious limitation in their use is their stimulant effect on the uterus.

— *Bismuth compounds* Bismuth compounds have been used effectively in the treatment of both gastric and duodenal ulcers. The exact mechanism of their cytoprotection is not know. These compounds, in combination with **amoxicillin** or **metronidizole**, eradicate *H. pylori*, a bacteria associated with antral gastritis. This organism is also found in a large proportion of patients with duodenal ulcer or gastric cancer. A direct link between *H. pylori* and peptic ulcer has not yet been established because the organism is found in 20% of asymptomatic individuals, an incidence that increases with age.

● **Promotion of gastrointestinal activity** Normal motor function of the stomach depends on a complex interaction between gastric smooth muscle and neurogenic and hormonal modulatory pathways. Disruption of any of these systems can lead to disordered gastric motility. Nonetheless, the precise relationships among disturbed gastric motor function, nausea, vomiting, early satiety, distentions, and bloating remain unknown. Gastroparesis (slow gastric emptying) has a number of potentially correctable causes.

One example is the patient taking medications that slow gastric emptying, such as opioids, anticholinergics, and L-dopa. In diabetic gastroparesis, tighter glucose control may improve gastric motility.

Metoclopramide, a substituted benzamide derivative of procainamide, blocks dopamine receptors and displays both antiemetic and prokinetic effects. The antiemetic effect is due to antagonism of dopamine receptors in the brain, whereas the prokinetic effect is due to inhibition of dopamine on GI smooth muscle. Metoclopramide stimulates the motility of the upper GI tract, increasing the rate of gastric emptying without stimulating gastric, biliary, or pancreatic secretions (Box 4.14).

Adverse Effects of Sucralfate

Minor side effects have been reported, the most frequent being constipation. Others include: dry mouth, diarrhea, nausea, gastric discomfort, indigestion, rash, dizziness, and vertigo.

Prototype of Prostaglandins

Misoprostol

Box 4.14

USES OF METOCLOPRAMIDE
1. Relieves symptoms of acute and recurrent diabetic gastroparesis and gastroesophageal reflux
2. Prevents nausea and vomiting associated with cancer chemotherapy
3. Relieves nausea and vomiting of pregnancy and labor
4. Treats gastric ulcer disease
5. Treats anorexia nervosa
6. May improve lactation because it increases serum prolactin levels
7. Enhances absorption of ergotamine products used in migraine headaches

■ **Antiemetics** Antiemetics prevent or relieve the symptoms of nausea and vomiting by action at the chemoreceoptor trigger zone within the vomiting center of the medulla, the cerebral cortex, or the aural vestibular apparatus in the ear. In general, antiemetics are more useful in preventing vomiting than in halting it.

● **Locally acting antiemetics** Vomiting caused by irritation of the GI mucosa can be treated with locally acting agents (Box 4.15). Such agents soothe the receptors or reduce the reactivity of the irritants. These are temporary measures to allow for healing of the GI tract. Topical anesthetics, such as viscous lidocaine, increase the threshold of the receptor activity to irritants, thereby reducing nausea and vomiting. Antacids, adsorbents, demulcents, and medications that reduce distention act on the stomach mucosa, the receptor centers, or both to make them less sensitive. These preparations are more effective administered between meals. Other protective agents are phosphorylated carbohydrate solution (Emetrol) and cola syrup. These release the GI muscle spasm, permitting fewer afferent impulses to reach the vomiting center.

Box 4.15

CLASSIFICATION OF ANTIEMETICS	
Locally Acting	**Centrally Acting**
Topical mucosal	Antidopaminergic
anesthetics	Phenothiazines
Viscous lidocaine	Anticholinergics
Adsorbents and	Scopolamine
demulcents	Miscellaneous
Kaolin and pectin	Benzequinamide HCl
Activated charcoal	Diphenidol HCl
Bismuth subsalicylate	Timethobenzamide HCl
Attapulgite	Ondanesetron HCl
Cholestyramine	Cannabinoids

● **Centrally acting antiemetics** These compounds inhibit or depress the afferent nerve impulses in the brain, preventing nausea and vomiting.

● **Dopamine receptor antagonists** Phenothiazines, antipsychotic agents, are antiemetics. Phenothiazines decrease the sensitivity of the chemoreceptor trigger zone in the vomiting center in the brain stem to dopamine stimulation. Antiemetic effects are apparent at very low doses of phenothiazines. However, because of their relative toxicity, these drugs are administered only when vomiting cannot be controlled by other means, or when only a few doses will be needed. They are used primarily to control postoperative nausea and vomiting, radiation sickness, nausea and vomiting from cancer chemotherapy, and the nausea and vomiting secondary to ingestion of toxins.

    Metoclopramide (Reglan) is a dopamine receptor antagonist that increases GI motility. It is used to combat the nausea and vomiting associated with antienoplastic agents, to reverse the gastric stasis induced by opioids, and in the treatment of diabetic gastroparesis.

● **Anticholinergics** Scopolamine hydrobromide (Hysocine) is one of the most effective medications for motion sickness. Its use is limited, however, because at pharmacologically active doses, it also causes blurred vision and xerostomia. Scopolamine has a short duration of action and is available in a skin patch formulation that is applied to a hairless area behind the ear. It is used with caution in persons with glaucoma, pyloric obstruction, or urinary obstruction because of its anticholinergic effects.

■ **Laxatives** Laxatives, or cathartics, accelerate the passage of feces through the bowel (Box 4.16).

Box 4.16

CLASSIFICATION OF LAXATIVES BY MECHANISMS OF ACTION

Contact-Stimulant Laxatives
Cascara sagrada
Senna products

Bulk-Forming Agents
Plantago seed (psyllium seed)
Calcium polycarbophil
Methylcellulose

Fecal Softeners
Docusate sodium (Colace)
Docusate calcium (Surfak)
Docusate potassium (Dialose)

Osmotic/Saline Agents
Magnesium salts
Sodium salts
Potassium salts

Lubricants
Mineral oil

Miscellaneous
Glycerine suppository
Lactulose

● **Action** Laxatives promote bowel evacuation by an osmotic action increasing net fluid accumulation within the bowel lumen or by a direct action on mucosal cells to decrease absorption or enhance secretion of water and electrolytes (Fig. 4.9).

● **Contraindications and precautions** Laxatives are contraindicated in persons hypersensitive to any of their ingredients, in patients who have acute symptoms of appendicitis, GI obstruction, or undiagnosed abdominal pain, and in patients suspected of having fecal impaction. Laxatives should be administered cautiously to the elderly, small children, and persons who are acutely ill. Care should also be taken in administering laxatives to patients with cardiac or renal diseases, especially if the preparation contains Na^+ because of the possibility of Na^+ retention, and to patients with renal dis-

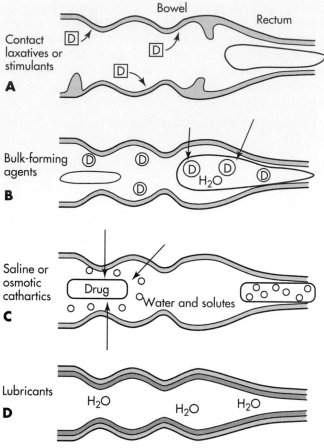

Fig. 4.9 Mechanism of action of laxatives. **A,** Contact laxatives stimulate the intestinal wall inducing an increase in peristalsis. **B,** Bulk-forming agents absorb water into the fecal contents, giving more bulk to the stool. **C,** Saline or osmotic cathartics are osmotically active and pull solutes and water into the bowel, increasing intestinal contents and bulk. **D,** Lubricants lubricate and soften the intestinal contents as well as retard water absorption. *(Adapted from Kuhn MA: Medications for common digestive problems. In Kuhn MA, editor:* Pharmacotherapeutics: a nursing process approach, ed 3, *Philadelphia, 1994, F.A. Davis.)*

ease if the preparation contains Mg^{++} or Ca^{++} because these electrolytes may be retained (Boxes 4.17 and 4.18).

Box 4.17

LAXATIVE USES

1. To treat constipation
2. To prepare patients for diagnostic tests
3. To prevent or decrease colonic absorption of ammonia in patients with hepatic encephalopathy
4. To hasten the excretion of various parasites or poisons
5. In children with congenital or acquired megacolon
6. In geriatric patients with poor muscle tone
7. To provide fresh stool for parasitologic exam
8. To empty the bowel before surgery, colonoscopy, or enema
9. To modify the effluent in patients with an ileostomy or colostomy

Box 4.18

ADVERSE EFFECTS OF LAXATIVES
All laxatives are capable of causing 1. Excessive GI activity such as diarrhea, nausea, and vomiting 2. Perianal irritation because of the frequent stools 3. Abdominal cramps, bloating, and flatulence

● **Contact/stimulant laxatives** These laxatives are obtained from the bark, seed pods, leaves, and roots of a number of plants, including cascara and senna. They increase peristalsis when the laxative comes in contact with the wall of the small or large intestine. They also release prostaglandins and increase the mucosal concentration of cAMP, which, in turn, increases the secretion of electrolytes, enhancing the cathartic effect.

The continuous use of contact/stimulant laxatives can produce *irritable bowel-like diarrhea* that is often severe enough to cause fluid and electrolyte imbalances.

   Castor oil directly stimulates the small intestine smooth muscle and inhibits water and electrolyte reabsorption from the intestinal lumen. It also acts as a hypertonic fluid within the bowel by drawing water into the feces. Glycerin suppositories stimulate the rectal mucosa.

   Castor oil is contraindicated in pregnancy and the cascara sagrada laxatives should not be given to lactating mothers because they are excreted in breast milk.

   Bisacodyl is a synthetic contact/stimulant laxative. Because less than 5% is absorbed from the GI system, it is relatively nontoxic. It is widely used to treat various types of constipation and to evacuate the colon before endoscopy, surgery, and radiologic examinations.

● **Bulk-forming agents,** including natural and semisynthetic cellulose derivatives, are made from agar, natural bran, plantago seed, methylcellulose, and polycarbophil, which absorb water into the fecal contents and expand, giving more bulk to the stool. The increased bulk occurs naturally and promotes peristalsis and natural elimination about 12 to 24 hours after administration. However, several days of administration may be required before achieving the maximal effect. These agents are less likely to be habit forming than other laxatives because of their slower onset and because they evacuate only the descending colon, sigmoid colon, and rectum, rather than emptying the whole bowel (Box 4.19). Bran and dried fruits have the same effect.

Bulk-forming laxatives are the least harmful and do not interfere with the absorption of food.

Box 4.19

USE OF BULK-FORMING LAXATIVES
1. To treat chronic, atonic, or spastic constipation and constipation in the elderly 2. In patients with diverticulosis, irritable bowel syndrome 3. To relieve painful defecation in patients with hemorrhoids Bulk-forming laxatives should always be administered with a full glass of liquid and should be followed by 8 ounces of water to prevent the likelihood of either esophageal or intestinal obstruction or impaction.

● **Fecal softeners** are Na^+, Ca^{++}, or K^+ docusate products. They are not absorbed from the GI tract, and it takes 1 or 2 days before the softened fecal bolus reaches the rectum. The docusate Ca^{++} is thought to be superior to

Uses of Osmotic/Saline Laxatives

Their short duration of action makes them particularly useful for

1. Cleansing the entire gastrointestinal tract for diagnostic tests
2. Flushing poisons or removing parasites

Contraindications and Precautions of Osmotic Laxatives

Should not be used in abdominal pain, fecal impaction, nausea, vomiting of unknown origin, and intestinal obstructions
Mg and K salts contraindicated in patients with renal disease
Should be given cautiously to patients receiving central nervous system depressants

Adverse Effects of Lubricant Laxatives

Anorexia, nausea, vomiting, and nutritional deficiencies
May cause lipid pneumonia in small children and the elderly if accidentally aspirated
Chronic use may decrease the absorption of vitamins A, D, E, and K; food; and bile salts.

the Na^+ and K^+ products. Fecal softeners are administered at bedtime until bowel movements are normal. They are used only when the prevention of constipation is indicated and no cathartic effect is desired.

● **Osmotic/saline agents** are the most rapid acting and powerful of all laxatives. Usually a salt of nonabsorbable anions or cations, they act by increasing the bulk of the intestinal contents and stimulate peristalsis more quickly than do bulk laxatives. They are active within 2 to 6 hours after administration. Included are magnesium citrate and sulfate, Na_3PO_4, and $Mg(OH)_2$. The greater the concentration of the salt, the greater the osmotic effect in the bowel. The magnesium salts increase secretion of cholecystokinin from the duodenum, stimulating the secretion and motility of the small intestine and colon, which may contribute to the cathartic effect. All preparations are taken with water. Lubricant laxatives are used for temporary relief of constipation, to treat tearing of hemorrhoids or fissures, and in patients with cardiac problems, or after surgery. Mineral oil is the only lubricant laxative used today. It lubricates and softens the intestinal contents and retards water absorption. Its onset of action is within 6 to 8 hours after administration.

● **Miscellaneous laxatives** include glycerin suppositories, which promote peristalsis through local irritation of the mucous membranes of the rectum. They are effective within 15 minutes to 1 hour and are often helpful in bowel-retaining regimens and in individuals with intermittent constipation. Lactulose syrup is a synthetic disaccharide analog of lactose that increases the number of bowel movements daily. It acidifies the colon from a normal pH of 7 to pH 5. Because this pH change pulls ammonia into the bowel, it is used in patients with hepatic dysfunction to decrease blood ammonia levels and to reduce the symptoms of hepatic encephalopathy (Box 4.20). Box 4.21 lists contraindications and precautions to the use of lactose syrup.

Box 4.20

HEPATIC ENCEPHALOPHY

Definition: A neuropsychiatric syndrome due to liver disease, usually associated with portal-systemic shunting of venous blood.
Etiology: Fulminating hepatitis due to viruses, drugs, or toxins. Following portacaval shunt or similar anastomoses.
Chronic liver disease.
Symptoms:
 I. Personality change, vacant stare, agitation, difficulty in performing calculations and writing legibly.
 II. Confusion, abnormal sleep patterns, lethargy.
 III. Stupor, disturbances in thought processes, sleepiness.
 IV. Coma.
Management: Eliminate precipitating causes, when possible; bed rest; reduce or eliminate dietary protein; oral neomycin; oral lactulose; prevention of infection.

■ **Drugs Used in Diarrhea** Diarrhea is an acute or chronic condition of excess water elimination from the bowel. It is associated with cramping from intermittent spasm of the intestine, as well as distention from excessive gas production in the bowel. It is usually a self-limiting condition. Diagnostic testing is rarely necessary if diarrhea lasts less than 3 days. If symptoms persist beyond

Box 4.21

┌───┐
│   **LACTOSE SYRUP CONTRAINDICATIONS AND PRECAUTIONS**   │
│   │
│ **It is Contraindicated in**   │
│ Patients on a low-galactose diet because it contains galactose   │
│   │
│ **It is Given With Caution to**   │
│ Pregnant women   │
│ Patients concurrently receiving neomycin because neomycin may reduce or destroy │
│   enough colonic bacteria to interfere with the effective action of lactulose syrup │
│ Diabetic patients because of its high sugar content   │
│   │
│ **Its Adverse Effects Include**   │
│ Flatulence, intestinal cramps, gas, and belching   │
│ Excessive doses may produce diarrhea with hypokalemia and nausea   │
└───┘

this time an examination should be made to identify the cause of the diarrhea and it should be treated (Table 4.5).

Diarrhea is treated with drugs that act locally in the bowel or systematically to decrease the number, consistency, and fluidity of the stools.

Locally acting antidiarrheals directly affect the bowel wall to soothe and reduce irritation of the mucous lining. Examples include adsorbents, which may also have a soothing effect on the irritated mucous membrane, and intestinal flora replacements.

Adsorbents nonspecifically bind gas, toxins, and irritants, inactivating them and facilitating their excretion. They also absorb normal enzymes and nutrients from the bowel. They contribute to the adhesion of the stool but do not necessarily control diarrhea. The most commonly used adsorbents are kaolin and pectin, activated charcoal, salts of bismuth, and attapulgite. All are nontoxic and inexpensive.

Table 4.5   Common Infectious Causes of Diarrhea and Specific Medications

Type of Organism	Medication
E. coli	Neomycin
	Ciprofloxacin
	Colistin sulfate (Coly-mycin S)
	Trimethoprim/sulfamethoxazole (Bactrim)
Shigella	Ampicillin
	Erythromycin
Pseudomonal enterocolitis	Gentamicin
	Polymyxin B
Coagulase-positive staphylococcal enterocolitis	Vancomycin (Vancocin)
	Ciprofloxacin
Acute amebic dysentery	Metronidazole (Flagyl)
	Tetracyclines
Traveler's diarrhea	Ciprofloxacin
	Doxycycline (Vibramycin)
	Ampicillin
	Trimetoprim/sulfamethoxazole (Bactrim)
Salmonellae	Ampicillin
C. difficile	Vancomycin (Vancocin)
	Metronidazole (Flagyl)

Definition

The term *inflammatory bowel disease* denotes two clinically distinct diseases, ulcerative colitis and Crohn's disease, which are chronic, often intermittent, and affect primarily young persons.

Intestinal flora replacements are typically administered to patients receiving antibiotic therapy, which can result in the destruction of bacteria in the bowel and cause diarrhea. The growth of normal intestinal flora is encouraged by ingesting *Lactobacillus acidophilus* found in Bacid or Lactinex, or acidophilus tablets, sweet acidophilus milk, or unpasteurized yogurt. This bacillus also allows the growth of *E. coli*. To assist in the treatment of diarrhea secondary to antibiotic therapy, the diet should be modified to increase carbohydrates containing lactose and dextrose, such as milk, buttermilk, and yogurt, all of which are equally effective in recolonizing the intestine.

◼ Drugs Used to Dissolve Gallstones

Agents used to treat gallstones include chenodiol, monocatanoin, and ursodeoxycholic acid.

- **Chenodiol** is a natural bile salt that decreases cholesterol saturation of bile by reducing the secretion of cholesterol and by increasing the secretion of bile salts. It is typically administered for 9 to 12 months. Adverse effects include diarrhea and possible hepatotoxicity from its breakdown products.

- **Monocatanoin** is a semisynthetic esterified glycerol used when stones of calcium bilirubinate and calcium soaps are resistant to dissolution by oral chenodiol. It is administered through a T-tube, nasobiliary catheter, or percutaneous transhepatic catheter and is considered a contact solvent because it is effective only when in contact with the stone. It is well tolerated if the administration is slow, 3 to 5 ml/hr, and treatment is continued for 7 to 21 days. Diagnostic studies, such as T-tube cholangiograms, are usually performed every 3 to 4 days to assess the extent of dissolution. If the number or size of the stones is unchanged in 7 days, treatment is discontinued. Major adverse effects include diarrhea, nausea, and abdominal pain.

- **Ursodiol** is a naturally occurring bile salt. It suppresses hepatic synthesis and secretion and inhibits intestinal absorption of cholesterol. After repeated dosing a steady-state is achieved within 3 weeks. Gallstone dissolution with ursodiol requires months of therapy. If stone dissolution has not occurred within 12 months, the likelihood of success is greatly reduced.

◼ Drugs Used in Inflammatory Bowel Disease

Ulcerative colitis may involve the distal colon, the rectum, and the sigmoid colon, or the distal to middle descending colon. The primary symptom is rectal bleeding. Although some individuals develop diarrhea, significant abdominal pain and cramping are not usually major clinical features.

- **Treatment** **Sulfasalazine** is of particular value for mild to moderate inflammatory bowel disease. Adverse effects include anorexia, headaches, rash, hemolytic anemia, impaired folate absorption, and abnormalities of sperm. In recent years there have been attempts to separate sulfasalazine into its component parts and to use the therapeutically active 5-aminosalicylic acid (5-ASA) portion, while eliminating the sulfapyridine portion.

  Mesalamine and **olsalazine sodium** are also used in ulcerative colitis. Their exact mechanism of action is unknown, but they are thought to act locally to diminish inflammation by blocking cyclooxygenase and inhibiting prostaglandin production in the bowel mucosa. Oral mesalamine is as effective as sulfasalazine for treatment of mild to moderate ulcerative colitis and may be better tolerated.

  Hypersensitivity to mesalamine or salicylates is the only contraindication for these drugs. Most adverse effects are mild and transient, the most common being abdominal pain, cramps, discomfort, headache, gas, flatulence, eructation, and nausea.

Gallstone Composition

Most gallstones are composed of
Cholesterol, calcium salt of bilirubin, and calcium carbonate
The most common precipitating factors include
Overconsumption of cholesterol and calories
Metabolic and genetic factors
Inadequate exercise
Medications such as birth control
They may affect approximately 10% of the general population of the United States.

Other Drugs Used in Inflammatory Bowel Disease

Corticosteroid agents have been used to treat ulcerative colitis, particularly acute and severe cases. They are effective in achieving short-term remission rapidly.
Antidiarrheal agents are the most frequently used adjunctive drugs, particularly loperamide and diphenoxylate.

Olsalazine sodium is administered to maintain remission of ulcerative colitis. It is contraindicated in persons with salicylate hypersensitivity. The most common adverse effects include pain and cramps, headache and nausea, and dyspepsia.

Crohn's disease is often difficult to differentiate from ulcerative colitis. There are no specific signs or symptoms associated with Crohn's disease. It is typically associated with abdominal pain, diarrhea, and weight loss. Pharmacologic management of Crohn's disease is generally unsuccessful. Surgery is often indicated.

Chapter 5

Cardiovascular Drugs

SECTION 5.1 ANTIHYPERTENSIVE DRUGS

■ **Overview** The objective of the treatment of hypertension is to lower and maintain blood pressure within normal limits with minimal adverse effects. Treatment failures typically occur not because antihypertensive drugs are ineffective but because of patient noncompliance caused by inconvenient dosing or adverse effects. In some cases drug combinations are used to reduce adverse effects and to lower blood pressure in two different ways, which is often more effective than when either drug is used alone.

Nonpharmacologic treatments include dietary salt restriction, weight reduction, and exercise. They should be used to lower blood pressure before or together with antihypertensive therapy.

Antihypertensive drugs include diuretics, sympatholytics, vasodilators, calcium channel blockers, and angiotensin converting enzyme (ACE) inhibitors (Box 5.1).

Box 5.1

ANTIHYPERTENSIVE DRUGS	
Diuretics	α_1-Adrenoceptor antagonist
Thiazides	Prazosin
	Tetrazosin
Sympatholytics	Labetalol
Centrally active	
Clonidine	**Vasodilators**
Guanabenz	Hydralazine
Guanfacine	Minoxidil
Methyldopa	Sodium nitroprusside
Ganglion blocker	Diazoxide
Trimethaphan	
Adrenergic neuron blocker	**Calcium Channel Blockers**
Guanadrel	Verapamil
Guanethidine	Nifedipine
Reserpine	Nicardipine
β-Adrenoceptor antagonist	Diltiazem
Acebutolol	
Atenolol	**Angiotensin Converting Enzyme Inhibitors**
Betaxolol	
Carteolol	Captopril
Metroprolol	Enalapril
Nadalol	Lisinopril
Penbutolol	Ramipril
Pindolol	Fosinopril
Propranolol	
Timolol	

■ **Diuretics**

● **Mechanism of action** Diuretics lower blood pressure primarily by depleting sodium to reduce blood volume and cardiac output. Some diuretics, such as indapamide, are also direct vasodilators.

● **Clinical use** Diuretics used as antihypertensives include chlorothiazide, indapamide, ethacrynic acid, furosemide, amiloride, and spironolactone.

● **Adverse effects** Common adverse effects of diuretics include hypokalemia, impaired glucose tolerance, increased serum lipids, and increased renin secretion.

■ **Sympatholytics**

● **Mechanism of action** Sympatholytics lower blood pressure by reducing sympathetic vasomotor tone through their effect on adrenoceptors in the central and peripheral nervous systems.

Centrally-Acting Sympatholytics

Clonidine
Guanabenz
Guanfacine
Methyldopa

● **Centrally acting sympatholytics** include clonidine, guanabenz, guanfacine, and methyldopa.

— *Mechanism of action* Centrally acting sympatholytics decrease sympathetic tone by stimulating α_2-adrenoceptors in the medulla oblongata. Clonidine, guanabenz, and guanfacine are direct-acting receptor agonists. Methyldopa is converted to α-methylnorepinephrine, a receptor agonist.

All of these agents are active when administered orally. Clonidine can also be given with a transdermal patch.

— *Adverse effects* Methyldopa can cause sedation and a positive Coombs' test. Clonidine can cause sedation and xerostomia.

● **Ganglion blockers** block postganglionic neurons in sympathetic and parasympathetic ganglia. **Trimethaphan,** which is administered intravenously (IV) for the treatment of hypertensive crisis, is the only ganglionic blocker currently in clinical use. Others have been discarded because there are now much safer agents for the long-term management of hypertension.

● **Adrenergic neuron** blocking agents include guanadrel, guanethidine, and reserpine.

Adrenergic Neuron Blockers

Guanadrel
Guanethidine
Reserpine

— *Mechanism of action* These drugs lower blood pressure by preventing the release of endogenous norepinephrine from postganglionic sympathetic nerves. They are administered orally.

— *Adverse effects* Adrenergic neuron blocking agents are associated with postural hypotension, fluid retention, diarrhea, sedation, and psychic depression.

● **β-Adrenoceptor antagonists** are one of the most popular groups of antihypertensive agents. This class includes acebutolol, atenolol, betaxolol, carteolol, metyoprolol, nadalol, penbutolol, pindolol, propranolol, and timolol.

β-Blockers

Acebutolol
Atenolol
Betaxolol
Carteolol
Metoprolol
Nadolol
Penbutolol
Pindolol
Propranolol
Timolol

— *Mechanism of action* These drugs lower blood pressure by blocking β-adrenoceptors. This reduces cardiac output, renin secretion, and sympathetic vasomotor tone, decreasing blood pressure. All of these drugs are usually administered orally.

— *Adverse effects* β-adrenoceptor antagonists can cause depression, aggravate congestive heart failure, and increase bronchospasm in asthmatics.

Vasodilators

Hydralazine
Minoxidil
Sodium
 nitroprusside
Diazoxide

**Calcium
Channel
Blockers**

Verapamil
Nifedipine
Nicardipine
Diltiazem

ACE Inhibitors

Captopril
Enalapril
Lisinopril
Ramipril
Fosinopril

Prodrug

Enalapril
↓
Enalaprilat

- α_1-**Adrenoceptor antagonists** include prazosin and terazosin.
  - *Mechanism of action* These drugs lower blood pressure by blocking vascular α_1-adrenoceptors, dilating both resistance and capacitance vessels. These drugs are administered orally.
  - *Adverse effects* Adverse effects include postural hypotension, drowsiness, dizziness, palpitations, headache, and fatigue.
- **Labetalol** is a unique sympatholytic that lowers blood pressure by blocking both α-adrenoceptors and β-adrenoceptors.

■ **Vasodilators** Vasodilators include hydralazine, minoxidil, sodium nitroprusside, and diazoxide.

- **Mechanism of action** Vasodilators lower blood pressure by relaxing arteriolar smooth muscles, thereby reducing systemic vascular resistance. Because the decrease in blood pressure stimulates reflex tachycardia and increases renin secretion, when used alone the antihypertensive effect of vasodilators diminishes with time. Consequently, vasodilators are most effective when combined with other antihypertensive drugs, such as β-adrenoceptor antagonists, that prevent the reflex effects. Hydralazine and minoxidil are usually given orally, whereas sodium nitroprusside and diazoxide are administered IV for treating hypertensive emergencies.

- **Adverse effects** Common adverse effects include reflex tachycardia, increased renin secretion, and fluid retention. Hydralazine may also induce anginal attacks and myocardial ischemia in patients with coronary artery disease. Sodium nitroprusside may cause headache, palpitations, nausea, vomiting, and sweating.

■ **Calcium Channel Blockers** Calcium channel blockers include verapamil, nifedipine, nicardipine, and diltiazem.

- **Mechanism of action** These drugs lower blood pressure by inhibiting calcium influx in arteriolar smooth muscles, producing vasodilation. The most effective vasodilator is nifedipine, and verapamil has the most profound cardiac effects. Calcium channel blockers are usually given orally.

- **Adverse effects** These drugs are generally very safe, although diltiazem and verapamil may slow atrioventricular (AV) conduction.

■ **Angiotensin Converting Enzyme (ACE) Inhibitors** ACE inhibitors include captopril, enalapril, lisinopril, ramipril, and fosinopril.

- **Mechanism of action** These drugs lower blood pressure mainly by inhibiting peptidyl dipeptidase, the enzyme responsible for the conversion of angiotensin I to angiotensin II, a potent vasoconstrictor.
  All ACE inhibitors are effective orally. Enalapril is a prodrug that becomes active only after conversion in the body to enalaprilat, a metabolite.

- **Adverse effects** These drugs may cause severe hypotension, acute renal failure, dry cough, hyperkalemia, and angioedema.

SECTION 5.2 ANTIANGINAL DRUGS

■ **Overview** Angina pectoris is a strangling chest pain caused by an inadequate coronary blood flow that fails to meet oxygen demands of the heart tissue. In classic angina, or angina of effort, the imbalance occurs when more oxygen is required, such as during exercise. In variant angina, the myocardial supply of oxygen is reduced by spasm or constriction in atherosclerotic coronary vessels. Treatment of either type is aimed at improving coronary blood flow and reducing myocardial oxygen requirements.

Oxygen supply to the heart depends on the delivery and extraction of oxygen by the myocardium. Inasmuch as oxygen extraction is nearly maximal at rest, an increased demand is met by increasing coronary blood flow. The amount of blood flowing through the coronary circulation is determined mainly by the perfusion pressure (aortic diastolic pressure) and the duration of diastole.

Antianginal drugs include nitrates and nitrites, calcium channel blockers, and β-adrenoceptor antagonists (Box 5.2).

Box 5.2

ANTIANGINAL DRUGS
Nitrates and Nitrites
Amyl nitrite
Erythrityl tetranitrate
Isosorbide dinitrate
Nitroglycerin
Pentaerythritol tetranitrate
Calcium Channel Blockers
Diltiazem
Nicardipine
Nifedipine
Nimodipine
Verapamil
β-Adrenoceptor Antagonists
Atenolol
Metoprolol
Propranolol
Nadolol

■ **Nitrates and Nitrites** A major class of agents used to treat angina are the nitrates and nitrites. Included are amyl nitrite, erythrityl tetranitrate, isosorbide dinitrate, nitroglycerin, and pentaerythritol tetranitrate.

● **Basic pharmacology** The nitrates and nitrites cause vasodilation by releasing a nitrite ion, which is metabolized to nitric oxide. The nitric oxide activates guanylyl cyclase, increasing cGMP levels, which relax vascular smooth muscles. Although nitric oxide relaxes all vascular smooth muscle cells, blood vessels are not uniformly affected. Thus, there is a marked relaxation of large veins, which increases venous capacitance, decreasing ventricular preload. Arterioles and precapillary sphincters, on the other hand, are less affected. The drug-induced fall in systemic pressure elicits reflex increases in sympathetic nerve activity, increasing heart rate and myocardial contractility. Although total coronary blood flow may not be increased, it may be redistributed from normal to ischemic areas. Relief of angina is primarily caused by the reduction in the myocardial oxygen requirement that results from the decrease in preload and hypotension.

The nitrates and nitrites also cause relaxation of bronchial, gastrointestinal, and genitourinary smooth muscles.

Because the nitrite ion reacts with hemoglobin to produce methemoglobinemia, large doses of these drugs may cause tissue hypoxia and death. In the treatment of cyanide poisoning, sodium nitrite oxidizes hemoglobin to methemoglobin, which competes with cytochrome oxidase for the cyanide ion.

The chemical composition of these drugs varies from volatile liquids such as amyl nitrite and nitroglycerin to solids such as isosorbide dinitrate. Routes of administration are inhalation, sublingual, oral, and transdermal.

Organic nitrates are rapidly degraded by hepatic organic nitrate reductase, resulting in denitrated derivatives that are excreted by the kidneys.

Tolerance to the therapeutic effects of nitrates and nitrites may develop with prolonged use.

- **Adverse effects** Adverse effects associated with pronounced vasodilation include orthostatic hypotension, tachycardia, and throbbing headaches.

■ **Calcium Channel Blockers** Calcium channel blockers include diltiazem, nicardipine, nifedipine, nimodipine, and verapamil.

- **Basic pharmacology** All of these agents are orally active. After absorption they bind to L-type calcium channels, decreasing transmembrane calcium currents and inducing a long-lasting relaxation of cardiac and smooth muscle cells.

  Vascular smooth muscles, arterioles more so than veins, are most sensitive to calcium channel blockers. However, bronchiolar, gastrointestinal, and uterine smooth muscles are also affected by these agents. Nifedipine is the most effective vasodilator, whereas nimodipine has the highest affinity for cerebral blood vessels.

Strongest Vasodilator
Nifedipine
Strongest Cardiac Effects
Verapamil

  The major effects of calcium channel blockers on the heart are to decrease contractility, reduce impulse generation in the sinoatrial (SA) node, and slow AV node conduction. Verapamil has the strongest cardiac effects.

  Other actions of calcium channel blockers include inhibition of insulin secretion and interference with platelet aggregation.

  All calcium channel antagonists are orally active. Up to 90% of an absorbed dose binds to plasma proteins. Half-lives range from 3 to 6 hours, and the drugs are extensively metabolized in the liver with metabolites excreted in the urine.

- **Adverse effects** Calcium channel blockers may cause serious cardiac depression, including bradycardia, AV block, congestive failure, and cardiac arrest.

■ **β-Adrenoceptor Antagonists** β-Adrenoceptor antagonists include atenolol, metoprolol, propranolol, and nadolol.

- **Basic pharmacology** Although β-adrenoceptor antagonists are generally ineffective in producing coronary vasodilation, they are used to treat angina because they decrease myocardial oxygen needs by lowering blood pressure and reducing cardiac work. These agents are administered orally.

- **Adverse effects** β-Adrenoceptor antagonists should not be used in variant angina because they can slow heart rate and prolong ejection time, increasing left ventricular end-diastolic volume, thereby increasing the myocardial oxygen requirement. These potentially harmful effects can be prevented by concurrent treatment with nitrates.

- **Pharmacotherapeutics** The beneficial effects of antianginal drugs include reduction in myocardial oxygen demand and an increase in coronary blood flow to ischemic areas in the heart. Effective antianginal therapy increases exercise tolerance and decreases the frequency and duration of myocardial ischemia.

■ **Drug Combinations** In some cases angina is most effectively controlled with drug combinations (e.g., β-adrenoceptor antagonists and calcium channel blockers; nitrates and calcium channel blockers). Reflex tachycardia is minimized by combining nitrates with calcium channel blockers, or β-adrenoceptor antagonists. Variant angina is most susceptible to control with nitrates and calcium channel blockers.

Best for Variant Angina
Nitrates
Calcium channel blockers

SECTION 5.3 CARDIAC GLYCOSIDES AND INOTROPIC DRUGS

■ **Overview** The two main types of congestive heart failure (CHF) are low-output failure, which is caused by coronary artery disease, hypertension, or myocardial infarction, and high-output failure, which is caused by hyperthyroidism, beriberi, anemia, or AV shunts. Low-output failure responds to inotropic drugs (Box 5.3), but high-output failure does not.

Box 5.3

INOTROPIC DRUGS
Digitalis
Digitoxin
Digoxin
Ouabain
Bipyrines
Amrinone
Milrinone
β-Adrenoceptor Agonists
Dobutamine
Prenalterol
Albuterol
Pirbuterol
Vasodilators
Angiotensin Converting Enzyme Inhibitors

The major hemodynamic characteristics of CHF are due to subnormal cardiac output which decreases exercise tolerance and causes tachycardia, pulmonary edema, and cardiomegaly. There is also a neurohumoral reflex compensation involving increased sympathetic nerve activity, including an increase in activity of the renin-angiotensin-aldosterone system. Myocardial hypertrophy occurs in CHF to maintain cardiac performance.

The chief factors affecting cardiac performance in CHF are an increase in cardiac preload from increased blood volume and an increase in cardiac afterload from the reflex increase in systemic vascular resistance. There is also an increase in myocardial contractility leading to a reduction in the velocity of muscle shortening, rate of intraventricular pressure development and pump performance, and an increase in heart rate because of reflex tachycardia.

■ **Cardiac Glycosides** The two cardiac glycosides used most commonly for treatment of CHF are **digitoxin** and **digoxin**. A third, ouabain, is most often used experimentally. The cardiac glycosides are composed of an aglycone (genin), which accounts for the biologic activity, attached to three molecules of sugar (digitoxose), which determines the rate of absorption, half-life, and metabolism.

● **Basic pharmacology** The most important effects of digitalis are on the heart, which is affected both mechanically and electrophysiologically.

  Of the mechanical effects, myocardial contractility, also known as stroke volume or positive inotropy, is consistently increased whether the heart is normal or in failure. This effect is mediated by inhibition of the Na^+, K^+-ATPase on myocardial tissue, which increases intracellular sodium and calcium, yielding an increased myocardial contractility (Table 5.1).

  Although bradycardia is also produced by digitalis, the underlying mechanism differs depending on the state of myocardium. Thus, digitalis-induced bradycardia in normal hearts is due to vagal stimulation, whereas in failing hearts it is the result of a reduction in sympathetic tone. In contrast, cardiac output is increased in failing hearts but is unaffected in normal hearts. The different effects on cardiac output are related to differences in effects on sympathetic activity. Thus in CHF the improved cardiac function eliminates the stimulus for increased sympathetic activity, resulting in generalized vasodilation. In normal individuals, there is no increase in sympathetic activity, and therefore digitalis acts directly on blood vessels to cause vasoconstriction, increasing impedance to ventricular contraction. Consequently, cardiac output remains unchanged.

  The effects of digitalis on the electrophysiologic and electrocardiographic properties of the heart are summarized in Table 5.2.

  In normal hearts digitalis acts directly to contract vascular smooth muscle, causing vasoconstriction. However, because of the digitalis-induced reduction in sympathetic activity, the net effect of digitalis on failing hearts is vasodilation.

  Digitalis does not directly affect kidneys, but it does induce diuresis in edematous patients because of improved hemodynamics resulting from the increase in myocardial contractility and cardiac output.

● **Absorption, biotransformation, and excretion** After oral administration, digitoxin is absorbed more readily than digoxin. Although the effects of digoxin appear earlier than digitoxin, they do not persist as long (Table. 5.3).

● **Adverse effects** Digitalis has a narrow margin of safety with therapeutic doses often producing many adverse effects. Adverse effects related to the

Table 5.1	*Cardiovascular Effects of Cardiac Glycosides*	
	MYOCARDIUM	
VARIABLE MEASURED	NORMAL	FAILING
Contractility	↑	↑
Heart rate	↓	↓
Vascular resistance	↑	↓
Cardiac output	—	↑

Table 5.2 *Electrophysiologic Effects of Digitalis Causing its Characteristic ECG Changes*

SITE OF ACTION	ELECTROPHYSIOLOGIC EFFECT	ELECTROCARDIOGRAM CHANGE
AV node	Prolonged refractory period resulting in slowed conduction	Prolonged P-R interval
Ventricle	Changes in phase 2 or 3 or in direction of repolarization	Changes in S-T segment or T wave
Ventricle	Accelerated repolarization	Shortened Q-T interval

heart are the most common and dangerous because digitalis can induce arrhythmias. Adverse gastrointestinal effects, such as anorexia, nausea, vomiting, and diarrhea, are usually the earliest signs of intoxication.

Actions on the brain include stimulation of the medullary chemoreceptor trigger zone, which causes vomiting. These drugs can also cause disorientation and hallucinations, especially in the elderly. There may also be color and visual disturbances.

Treatment of digitalis intoxication includes discontinuing the drugs, oral or IV potassium therapy, and administration of phenytoin, propranolol, or lidocaine to treat arrhythmias.

● **Drug interactions** Quinidine displaces digoxin from tissue binding sites and depresses its renal clearance. These effects may increase plasma glycoside levels sufficiently to cause toxicity. Quinidine may also prolong the half-life of digitoxin.

Catecholamines may sensitize the myocardium to digitalis, and cholestyramine reduces digitalis absorption

● **Clinical use** In addition to CHF, digitalis is used to treat atrial fibrillation to prevent paradoxic ventricular tachycardia because it slows the ventricular rate by inhibiting AV node conduction.

■ **Other Positive Inotropic Drugs** Bipyrines such as **amrinone** and **milrinone** are administered parenterally. These drugs increase myocardial contractility by inhibiting phosphodiesterase, increasing cAMP in the myocardium and enhancing the inward flux of calcium. The bipyrines also relax vascular smooth muscles and therefore are vasodilators. They are less likely than digitalis to produce arrhythmias.

Table 5.3 *Pharmacokinetics of Cardiac Glycosides*

GLYCOSIDE	DIGOXIN	DIGITOXIN
Lipid solubility	Medium	High
Percent oral absorption	75	>90
Percent metabolized	<20	>80 (hepatic)
Excretion	Kidneys	Bile
Half-life (hr)	40	168
Time to peak (hr)	3-6	6-12

β-Adrenoceptor agonists such as **dobutamine** and **prenalterol** increase myocardial contractility. Selective β-adrenoceptor agonists, such as **albuterol** and **pirbuterol,** cause vasodilation by relaxing smooth muscles.

■ **Vasodilators and Angiotensin Converting Enzyme Inhibitors** ACE inhibitors are used to counteract the increased renin-Angiotensin activity brought about reflexly during CHF.

SECTION 5.4 ANTIARRHYTHMIC DRUGS

■ **Overview** Many cardiac rhythm disorders result from abnormalities in impulse generation or propagation through the specialized conduction tissue in the heart. Some arrhythmias occur because of subtle timing abnormalities within this conduction system, and others are due to abnormal impulse initiation or automaticity. Antiarrhythmic drugs influence cardiac automaticity or conduction. Some interact directly with sodium, calcium, or potassium ion channels, altering automaticity and conduction. Others alter the autonomic tone in the heart by diminishing or enhancing adrenergic or cholinergic influences. Box 5.4 lists some antiarrhythmic drugs.

Causes of Arrhythmias
Abnormal automaticity
Abnormal impulse
  conduction

Box 5.4

ANTIARRHYTHMIC DRUGS
Class I (Na⁺ channel blockers)

Class I (Na^+ channel blockers)
Quinidine
Procainamide
Disopyramide
Amiodarone (classes I, II III, IV)
Lidocaine
Tocainide
Mexiletine
Flecainide
Encainide

Class II (β-adrenergic receptor blockers)
Propranolol
Esmolol
Acebutolol

Class III (K^+ channel blockers)
Bretylium
Sotalol

Class IV (Ca^{++} channel blockers)
Verapamil
Diltiazem

Miscellaneous
Adenosine

At therapeutic doses antiarrhythmics terminate an arrhythmia and prevent reinitiation of the disorder. However, because these drugs affect automaticity and conduction, they may also cause arrhythmias.

Myocardial excitation normally originates from pacemaker cells in the SA node and spreads through the specialized conduction system. Arrhythmias are disorders of heart rate or rhythm resulting from changes in automaticity, conduction, or both.

Automaticity resulting from phase-4 depolarization in normal pacemaker cells is responsible for SA-nodal rhythm. The AV node and Purkinje fibers also contain pacemaker cells. In these cells, phase-4 depolarization proceeds more slowly. Because the SA nodal cells are normally the first to reach threshold, AV nodal or other cells exhibiting phase-4 depolarization are themselves depolarized before reaching threshold.

An ectopic focus occurs when any part of the myocardium outside the SA node becomes the pacemaker. Ectopic foci may be due to enhanced automaticity caused by hypoxia, catecholamines, myocardial stretch, or drugs.

Antiarrhythmic drugs reduce automaticity by reducing the slope of phase-4 depolarization at ectopic foci and by reducing the threshold potential.

Some arrhythmias are the result of reentrant excitation within the conduction system. For reentry to occur retrograde conduction and unidirectional block are required. By definition, the initiation point of reentry must no longer be refractory when the retrograde impulse reaches the site. Antiarrhythmics terminate reentry circuits by altering the critical time relationships within the pathway, converting unidirectional blocks to bidirectional blocks or lengthening the refractory period at the initiation site.

Antiarrhythmic Drugs Work By

Reducing automaticity
Altering (usually decreasing) conduction velocity

■ Quinidine

● **Basic pharmacology** Quinidine is an isomer of quinine. Both alkaloids are derived from the bark of the cinchona tree.

Quinidine is well absorbed after oral administration with most of the drug metabolized by the liver. Approximately 20% of an administered dose is excreted by the kidney.

Quinidine is a myocardial depressant. It reduces the excitability and contractility of the heart and prolongs the refractory period, especially in the atria and AV node. Quinidine slows conduction and reduces automaticity. It also suppresses ectopic pacemakers and possesses anticholinergic properties. The anticholinergic effect enhances AV impulse transmission. In the presence of atrial flutter or fibrillation, quinidine may significantly increase ventricular filling rates. Since digitalis enhances vagal tone at the AV node, it antagonizes the effect of quinidine on AV transmission rates.

Quinidine

Myocardial depressant
Decrease conduction velocity
Block sodium channels
Strong antimuscarinic

● **Pharmacotherapeutics**

— *Clinical use* Quinidine is used to treat both atrial and ventricular arrhythmias. It is effective in treating atrial fibrillation and flutter and in suppressing ventricular premature contractions.

— *Adverse effects* The most common adverse effects associated with quinidine are nausea, vomiting, and diarrhea. Cinchonism, a syndrome including tinnitus, deafness, blurred vision, color disturbances, and gastrointestinal upset, may occur. Quinidine may also induce thrombocytopenic purpura. Because it is a myocardial depressant, quinidine may cause sudden death.

Adverse Effects of Quinidine

Cinchonism
Gastrointestinal upsets

— *Drug interactions* Quinidine may increase digoxin blood levels into the toxic range.

■ Procainamide

● **Basic pharmacology** Procainamide is chemically and pharmacologically similar to the local anesthetic procaine. It is well absorbed after oral administration, and it is eliminated by hepatic metabolism and renal excretion. The cardiac effects of procainamide resemble those of quinidine. However, its anticholinergic effect is less than that of quinidine, and procainamide produces less depression of contractility.

Adverse Effects of Procainamide

Lupus-like syndrome
Agranulocytosis (0.5%
  of patients)

Potentiate Procainamide

Amiodarone
Cimefidine
Ranitidine
Trimethoprim

Lidocaine

Administered IV
Emergency treatment of
  ventricular arrhythmias
Central nervous system
  effects include seizures

Phenytoin

Induces drug metabolism

- Pharmacotherapeutics

  — *Clinical use* Procainamide is used to treat atrial and ventricular arrhythmias. It may be effective in atrial fibrillation and flutter and in suppression of ventricular premature contractions.

  — *Adverse effects* Procainamide can produce sufficient myocardial depression to cause sudden death. Extracardiac effects include fever and rash, and in approximately 20% of patients a lupus-like syndrome may develop during long-term use. Procainamide is associated with agranulocytosis in about 0.5% of patients. Toxic levels may accumulate in patients with compromised renal function.

  — *Drug interactions* Plasma concentrations of procainamide and its active metabolite may be increased by coadministration of the following: amiodarone, cimetidine, ranitidine, or trimethoprim.

Lidocaine

- **Basic pharmacology** Lidocaine is used clinically as an antiarrhythmic and local anesthetic. Because it has a substantial first-pass effect lidocaine is administered IV. The short duration of action of lidocaine may necessitate repeat dosing.

  Unlike quinidine and procainamide, lidocaine does not display anticholinergic activity. It acts directly on Purkinje fibers and ventricular muscle to reduce action potential duration and to shorten the refractory period. Conduction velocity is usually unaffected by lidocaine.

  Lidocaine abolishes reentry by converting a unidirectional block to a bidirectional block or by improving slow conduction.

  Lidocaine depresses automaticity in ectopic pacemakers involving Purkinje fibers.

- Pharmacotherapeutics

  — *Clinical use* Lidocaine is administered IV for the emergency treatment of ventricular tachyarrhythmias.

  — *Adverse effects* Lidocaine has few adverse effects at therapeutic levels. Adverse central nervous system (CNS) effects include drowsiness, stimulation, and seizures.

  — *Drug interactions* Propranolol and cimetadine decrease lidocaine clearance. Concurrent use of tocainide or mexiletine may enhance the CNS effects of lidocaine, including seizures.

Phenytoin

- **Basic pharmacology** Phenytoin is given either IV or orally. It is poorly and erratically absorbed from the gastrointestinal tract and is destroyed by hepatic metabolism. Phenytoin is used primarily as an antiepileptic agent, but it also has significant antiarrhythmic properties.

- Pharmacotherapeutics

  — *Clinical use* The cardiac effects of phenytoin resemble those of lidocaine. It shortens the action potential duration and may prevent reentrant arrhythmias. It is also useful in treating digitalis intoxication.

  — *Adverse effects* Prominent adverse effects of pheytoin include drowsiness, vertigo, and ataxia. Death from cardiac arrest may occur after a rapid IV injection.

— *Drug interactions* Phenytoin interacts adversely with many other drugs.

■ **Disopyramide**

- **Basic pharmacology** Disopyramide is well absorbed after oral administration and is metabolized by the liver and excreted in the urine.

- **Pharmacotherapeutics**

    — *Clinical use* Disopyramide is used for treatment of ventricular arrhythmias.

    — *Adverse effects* Disopyramide is an anticholinergic and therefore induces dry mouth, constipation, urinary hesitancy, urinary retention, and gastrointestinal disturbances. It may also aggravate heart failure.

■ **Tocainide**

- **Basic pharmacology** Tocainide is similar to lidocaine except that it is given orally. It shortens the duration of action potentials and refractory periods of the atria, AV node, and ventricles.

- **Pharmacotherapeutics**

    — *Clinical use* Tocainide is effective for the treatment of ventricular arrhythmias and ventricular premature contractions.

    — *Adverse effects* Common adverse effects include nausea, dizziness, tremors, and vomiting. Tocainide causes agranulocytosis in up to 0.2% of patients.

■ **Mexiletine**

- **Basic pharmacology** Mexiletine is similar to lidocaine in terms of its antiarrhythmic properties but is administered orally.

- **Pharmacotherapeutics**

    — *Clinical use* Mexiletine is used to treat ventricular arrhythmias.

    — *Adverse effects* The chief adverse effects associated with mexiletine are nausea and tremors.

■ **Amiodarone**

- **Basic pharmacology** Amiodarone is administered orally. Its antiarrhythmic activity is due to prolongation of action potential duration and refractory period, and by α-adrenoceptor and β-adrenoceptor blockade. Amiodarone suppresses ventricular premature contractions and nonsustained ventricular tachycardia. It prevents recurrences of sustained ventricular tachycardia or fibrillation.

- **Pharmacotherapeutics**

    — *Clinical use* Amiodarone is used to treat life-threatening arrhythmias when less dangerous agents have proven ineffective.

    — *Adverse effects* Amiodarone may cause worsening of a serious arrhythmia and liver injury. Pulmonary toxicity and hepatic dysfunction may occur.

    — *Drug interactions* Amiodarone increases the serum concentrations of digoxin, diltiazem, quinidine, and other drugs commonly used to treat cardiovascular disease.

■ **Flecainide, Encainide, Propafenone**

● **Basic pharmacology** These local anesthetics are antiarrhythmic agents that reduce cardiac conduction velocity and increase the ventricular refractory period.

● **Pharmacotherapeutics**

— *Clinical use* Encainide and flecainide are associated with twice as many deaths as placebo controls when used to treat postmyocardial infarction patients with ventricular arrhythmias. These drugs should be used only to treat life-threatening arrhythmias, such as sustained ventricular tachycardia.

■ **Verapamil and Diltiazem** (calcium channel blockers)

● **Basic pharmacology** These agents are administered orally and are extensively metabolized by the liver.

Calcium blockers reduce the rate of SA nodal discharge, slow conduction through the AV node, and prolong the AV node refractory period.

● **Pharmacotherapeutics**

— *Clinical use* Verapamil and diltiazem are effective in treating paroxysmal supraventricular tachycardia and atrial fibrillation.

— *Adverse effects* Adverse effects include hypotension, dizziness, AV block, and heart failure.

— *Drug interactions* Verapamil increases serum digoxin concentrations and toxicities and can interact with many other drugs.

■ **β-Adrenoceptor Antagonists**

● **Propranolol**

— *Basic pharmacology* Propranolol, acebutolol, and esmolol block the effects of epinephrine and norepinephrine in the heart, slowing conduction. Propranolol and acebutolol are given orally, and esmolol is administered IV.

Esmolol
Short half-life

— *Pharmacotherapeutics*

Clinical use. β-adrenoceptor antagonists are effective in treating supraventricular arrhythmias and in suppressing ventricular premature contractions. They are effective in suppressing digitalis-induced ventricular arrhythmias.

Adverse effects. Propranolol may cause hypotension or cardiovascular collapse. All of these agents may worsen the symptoms of congestive heart failure and should be used with extreme caution, if at all, in patients with bronchospasm and bradyarrhythmias.

SECTION 5.5 HYPOLIPIDEMIC DRUGS

■ **Overview** Lipoproteins are important for transporting plasma cholesterol and triglycerides. Those that are atherogenic include low-density lipoproteins (LDL), intermediate-density lipoproteins (IDL), very-low-density lipoproteins (VLDL), and Lp(a) lipoproteins.

Chylomicrons are the largest lipoproteins. They are formed in the intestine and are normally not present in the serum of fasting patients. They carry dietary triglycerides. VLDL are secreted by the liver and transport endogenous triglycerides from the liver. LDL are formed from IDL, transport endogenous cholesterol, and are sometimes referred to as bad cholesterol. High-density lipoproteins are secreted by the liver, facilitate cholesterol removal from extrahepatic tissues, and are referred to as good cholesterol.

Hyperlipemia is a condition characterized by elevated plasma triglycerides, whereas hyperlipoproteinemia refers more generally to elevated plasma lipoproteins. In both conditions serum lipid is elevated after an overnight fast. Normally, total cholesterol should be below 200 mg/dl. A total cholesterol up to 239 mg/dl is considered borderline high, whereas above 240 mg/dl is considered high. Cholesterol levels are usually unstable and may fluctuate by as much as 50 mg/dl.

■ **Primary Hypertriglyceridemias** Primary chylomicronemia is characterized by increased chylomicrons and elevated VLDL. Patients may have eruptive xanthomas, hepatosplenomegaly, and lipid-laden foam cells in marrow, liver, and spleen. The condition is treated by restricting dietary fat.

Familial hypertriglyceridemia may be severe or moderate and is characterized by increased chylomicrons and VLDL. Patients usually have a centripetal pattern of obesity, eruptive xanthomas, lipemia retinalis, epigastric pain, and overt pancreatitis. It is treated mainly by restricting dietary fat, avoiding alcohol, and reducing body weight. Pharmacotherapy includes niacin, clofibrate, or gemfibrozil.

Drug Treatment
Niacin
Clofibrate
Gemfibrozil

Familial combined hyperlipoproteinemia is characterized by elevated VLDL, LDL, or both. It is associated with a moderate elevation of serum cholesterol and triglycerides, usually without xanthomas. The recommended treatments to prevent coronary atherosclerosis are niacin, clofibrate, or gemfibrozil when VLDL is elevated. If LDL is elevated, niacin, resin, or lovastatin are used. If both VLDL and LDL are increased, niacin alone or combined with resin or lovastatin is preferred.

Familial dysbetalipoproteinemia is characterized by accumulated remnants of chylomicrons and VLDL and reduced LDL levels with increased serum cholesterol and triglycerides. The patients are obese and have impaired glucose tolerance, tuberous or planar xanthomas, hypothyroidism, and increased frequency of coronary atherosclerosis. They are treated with niacin, clofibrate, of gemfibrozil.

Drug Treatment
Niacin
Clofibrate
Gemfibrozil

Box 5.5

HYPOLIPIDEMIC DRUGS
Niacin
Fibric Acid Derivatives Clofibrate Gemfibrozil
Bile Acid–binding Resins Colestipol Cholestyramine
HMG-CoA Reductase Inhibitors Lovastatin Pravastatin Simvastatin
Probucol

■ **Primary Hypercholesterolemia** Familial hypercholesterolemia may be heterozygous or homozygous, resulting in defective LDL receptors. It is characterized by elevated serum LDL and cholesterol. Triglycerides are usually normal in this condition. Patients may have tendinous xanthomatosis, arcus corneae, xanthelasma, and premature coronary atherosclerosis. Heterozygots are treated with niacin, resin, or lovastatin, whereas homozygots receive niacin or probucol.

Lp(a) hyperlipoproteinemia is a familial disorder associated with increased Lp(a) lipoprotein. It is treated with niacin alone or with lovastatin.

Dietary management of hyperlipoproteinemia includes restriction of cholesterol and saturated fat intake, and calories should be provided to achieve and maintain ideal body weight. Total fat calories should be 20% to 25%, saturated fats less than 8%, and cholesterol less than 200 mg/day. The commonly used hypolipidemic drugs are listed in Box 5.5.

■ **Niacin (Nicotinic Acid, Vitamin B)**

● **Basic pharmacology** Niacin is a water-soluble vitamin excreted in the urine. It lowers plasma VLDL and LDL mainly by inhibiting VLDL secretion. It also inhibits hepatic cholesterogenesis.

● **Clinical use** Niacin is most effective in heterozygous familial hypercholesterolemia, especially when combined with bile acid-binding resin. It is also

Drug Treatment
Niacin
Resin
Lovastatin
Probucol

effective in familial combined hyperlipoproteinemia, familial dysbetalipo-proteinemia, and hypercholesterolemia.

- **Adverse effects** Adverse effects are generally mild, consisting of cutaneous vasodilation and a warm sensation with pruritus, dry skin, nausea, and abdominal discomfort. Niacin may elevate serum transminase or alkaline phosphatase, impair glucose tolerance, and cause hyperuricemia. Its use has been associated in rare cases with severe hepatotoxicity.

■ Fibric Acid Derivatives: Clofibrate and Gemfibrozil

- **Basic pharmacology** Clofibrate is the ethyl ester of clofibric acid, gemfibrozil is a clofibrate congener. Both act mainly by increasing lipoprotein lipase activity to promote catabolism of VLDL. They may also decrease hepatic synthesis and secretion of VLDL. They decrease plasma triglycerides by lowering VLDL concentration and reduce plasma cholesterol by inhibiting hepatic cholesterogenesis.

- **Clinical use** These drugs are effective in familial dysbetaliproteinemia and hypertriglyceridemia. They are ineffective in primary chylomicronemia and familial hypercholesterolemia.

- **Adverse effects** Typical adverse effects include nausea and abdominal discomfort, myalgia with elevated plasma creatine phosphokinase, and an increased incidence of cholelithiasis or gallstones. Clofibrate and gemfibrozil also potentiate the anticoagulant action of indanedione and coumarin.

■ Bile Acid-Binding Resins: Colestipol and Cholestyramine

- **Basic pharmacology** Colestipol and cholestyramine are large cationic exchange resins that are insoluble in water. They have an unpleasant sandy or gritty quality. They act by binding bile acids to prevent their intestinal absorption. The reduction in bile acids increases hepatic LDL receptors, increasing the uptake of plasma LDL. The reduced LDL levels lower plasma cholesterol.

- **Clinical use** Fibric acid derivatives are effective whenever LDL is elevated as in heterozygous familial hypercholesterolemia and combined hyperlipoproteinemia.

- **Adverse effects** The bile acid-binding resins are the safest hypolipidemics because they are not absorbed. Their most common adverse effects are constipation and bloating. Steatorrhea may occur in patients with cholestasis, and enhanced gallstone formation may occur in obese patients. Bile acid-binding resins may also cause hypoprothrombinemia from vitamin K malabsorption, and they may impair absorption of some drugs, including digitalis, thiazide diuretics, tetracycline, thyroxine, and aspirin.

■ Neomycin

- **Basic pharmacology** Neomycin is an aminoglycoside antibiotic that lowers plasma LDL by inhibiting intestinal absorption of cholesterol and bile acids. It has variable effects on VLDL.

- **Clinical use** Neomycin is most effective for treating primary hypercholesterolemias when used in combination with other drugs.

- **Adverse effects** The use of neomycin is limited by severe adverse effects, including nausea, abdominal cramps, diarrhea, and malabsorption. It may produce enterocolitis from overgrowth of resistant microorgainisms. It impairs the absorption of digitalis glycosides.

HMG-CoA Reductase Inhibitors: Lovastatin, Pravastatin, and Simvastatin

HMG-CoA Reductase Inhibitors

Lovastatin
Pravastatin
Simvastatin

- **Basic pharmacology** These drugs are prodrugs that are hydrolyzed in the gut to form β-hydroxyl derivatives, the active medication. The active forms are structural analogs of the HMG-CoA intermediate formed in the synthesis of mevalonate. They reduce plasma LDL by inhibiting the reductase to increase high-affinity LDL receptors. They also decrease plasma triglycerides and increase HDL cholesterol.

- **Clinical use** The HMG-CoA reductase inhibitors are most effective when plasma LDL is elevated, as in heterozygous familial hypercholesterolemia or combined hyperlipoproteinemia.

- **Adverse effects** Adverse effects include elevations in serum transaminase, indicating hepatic toxicity, and an increase in creatine kinase with skeletal muscle pain.

■ Probucol
Probucol differs structurally from other hypolipidemic drugs. It may inhibit sterol synthesis and improve cholesterol transport. Probucol lowers HDL cholesterol, with minimal effects of LDL. It is effective in homozygous familial hypercholesterolemia.

■ Drug Combinations
Drug combinations are useful whenever treatment of hypercholesterolemia with a binding resin elevates VLDL levels significantly. LDL and VLDL levels are both elevated initially and LDL levels cannot be normalized using a single agent.

MULTIPLE CHOICE REVIEW QUESTIONS

1. A 48-year-old male with significant essential hypertension and a history of coronary vascular disease was prescribed minoxidil. Shortly after administration, the subject began to gain weight and experienced an exacerbation of his angina. Which of the following explanations is most likely correct?

    a. Minoxodil directly stimulates cardiac alpha receptors, resulting in decreased coronary blood flow (angina), and blocks the renal counter-current mechanisms (edema).

    b. Minoxidil would have lowered his blood pressure, decreasing myocardial after-load. Since the drug has no direct effect on the kidney, the angina and weight gain must be due to factors unrelated to the drug.

    c. Minoxidil causes salt and water retention because it increases proximal tubule reabsorption (edema) and because of its hypotensive action triggers a significant reflex tachycardia (angina).

    d. Minoxidil directly activates cardiac beta-1 receptors, increasing heart rate and myocardial oxygen demand, which in this patient produes angina. Fluid retention is secondary to congestive heart failure.

    e. Minoxidil is a beta-blocker that decreases myocardial inotropism. Angina and fluid retention is due to the congestive heart failure that ensues.

2. The above patient also developed pericardial effusion in addition to weight gain (10 kg) and an exacerbation of his angina. These adverse effects could probably have been avoided by use of drugs given along with minoxidil. Which combination would have been most appropriate?

    a. Minoxidil, chlorothiazide, phenoxybenzamine
    b. Minoxidil, furosemide, propranolol
    c. Minoxidil, acetazolamide, prazosin
    d. Minoxidil, mannitol, atropine
    e. Minoxidil, verapamil, tetrazosin

3. Which of the following agents could significantly reduce the tachycardia that is clinically observed after minoxidil administration?

    a. Hexamethonium
    b. Propranolol
    c. Trimethaphan
    d. Metoprolol
    e. All of the above

4. A 59-year-old female has a blood pressure of 160/109 mm. Blood pressure taken at home or in the physician's office confirms this systolic-diastolic relationship. The patient has a history of coronary vascular disease, which results in angina but has no evidence of congestive heart failure. The patient also has asthma, which is treated using terbutaline by aerosol inhalation. The physician prescribes propranolol to treat essential hypertension. Do you agree? Consider the following responses and explanations and choose the best answer.

    a. Propranolol is appropriate for this patient because it will reduce heart rate and cardiac output. It has a negative inotropic effect that will ameliorate her angina. It is a well-known, effective antihypertensive.

    b. Propranolol is inappropriate because it is useful in only mild hypertension. It would not be likely to reduce significantly at blood pressure of 160/109. A better drug for this patient would be minoxidil or hydralazine, either of which will produce a greater lowering of blood pressure.

    c. Propranolol is appropriate because it is an effective, low-cost antihypertensive. It will augment the effects of terbutaline and be of benefit in the treatment of the patient's asthma.

    d. Propranolol is inappropriate because it is contraindicated in a patient with asthma. A more appropriate drug would be diltiazem.

    e. None of the above.

5. A patient presents with episodic chest pain that may be due to angina or esophageal spasm. He is told, if the pain recurs, to take a sublingual nitroglycerin tablet and report what happens. When the pain recurs, the patient takes the "nitro" and notes that the pain goes away in about a minute. Which of the following conclusions is appropriate?

   a. The nitroglycerin test proves that the pain is due to myocardial oxygen insufficiency, which is relieved by the coronary vasodilatory activity of nitroglycerin.

   b. The pain is most likely due to esophageal spasm, because if it were due to the heart, relief would have taken longer to occur.

   c. The test is by itself not conclusive since the nitrates tend to relax almost all smooth muscle. Therefore it would effectively terminate pain from esophageal spasm.

   d. The nitroglycerin test proves that the pain is due to a relative myocardial oxygen insufficiency which is relieved by reduction in ventricular wall tension as preload is reduced.

   e. None of the above.

6. A 67-year-old male has multi-vessel coronary vascular disease confirmed by angiography. He also has severe COAD (chronic obstructive airway disease) and exertional angina. He is prescribed nifedipine to treat his angina. Shortly thereafter he begins his medication and complains of increased angina. Which explanation is most appropriate?

   a. Nifedipine is generally not appropriate for use in the treatment of angina.

   b. Nifedipine is a calcium channel blocker that has signifiant vasodilatory effects. The resultant hypotension and reflex cardiac stimulation are responsible for increased anginal episodes.

   c. Nifedipine in combination with propranolol would be appropriate, since the propranolol would block the reflex tachycardia that occurs with nifedipine.

   d. All of the above.

   e. None of the above.

7. Drugs that may be useful in treating congestive heart failure include:

   a. prazosin.
   b. captopril.
   c. hydralazine.
   d. sodium nitroprusside.
   e. all of the above.

8. Which of the following agents are classified as inotropic drugs that act by inhibiting phosphodiesterase Isozyme-III?

   a. Digoxin
   b. Dobutamine
   c. Amrinone
   d. Isoproterenol
   e. Hydralazine

9. Intravenous lidocaine is employed to treat:

   a. supraventricular tachycardia.
   b. angina pectoris.
   c. congestive heart failure.
   d. atrial flutter.
   e. ventricular arrhythmias.

10. Which of the following drugs used in treatment of hyperlipiemias can cause hyperglycemia, hyperuricemia, and facial flushing?

   a. Cholestyramine
   b. Colestipol
   c. Niacin
   d. Probucol
   e. Clofibrate

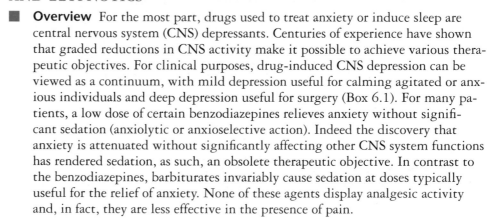

Chapter 6

Central Nervous System Drugs

SECTION 6.1 ANXIOLYTICS, SEDATIVES, AND HYPNOTICS

 Overview For the most part, drugs used to treat anxiety or induce sleep are central nervous system (CNS) depressants. Centuries of experience have shown that graded reductions in CNS activity make it possible to achieve various therapeutic objectives. For clinical purposes, drug-induced CNS depression can be viewed as a continuum, with mild depression useful for calming agitated or anxious individuals and deep depression useful for surgery (Box 6.1). For many patients, a low dose of certain benzodiazepines relieves anxiety without significant sedation (anxiolytic or anxioselective action). Indeed the discovery that anxiety is attenuated without significantly affecting other CNS system functions has rendered sedation, as such, an obsolete therapeutic objective. In contrast to the benzodiazepines, barbiturates invariably cause sedation at doses typically useful for the relief of anxiety. None of these agents display analgesic activity and, in fact, they are less effective in the presence of pain.

Box 6.1

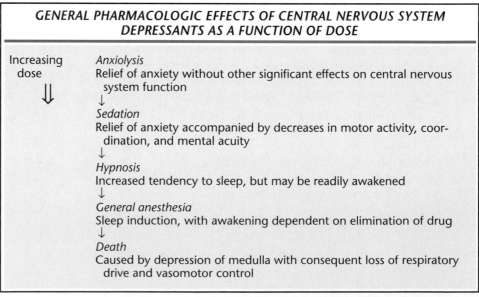

GENERAL PHARMACOLOGIC EFFECTS OF CENTRAL NERVOUS SYSTEM DEPRESSANTS AS A FUNCTION OF DOSE

Increasing dose ⇓

Anxiolysis
Relief of anxiety without other significant effects on central nervous system function
↓
Sedation
Relief of anxiety accompanied by decreases in motor activity, coordination, and mental acuity
↓
Hypnosis
Increased tendency to sleep, but may be readily awakened
↓
General anesthesia
Sleep induction, with awakening dependent on elimination of drug
↓
Death
Caused by depression of medulla with consequent loss of respiratory drive and vasomotor control

Although sedation and hypnosis are induced by increasing the dose of benzodiazepines, by themselves these drugs are not useful as general anesthetics, which suggests that they are incomplete CNS depressants. The barbiturates, on the other hand, and other members of this general class, such as **ethyl alcohol, chloral hydrate,** and **paraldehyde,** are complete CNS depressants that, depending on dose, induce sedation, hypnosis, general anesthesia, and death. The fact that the benzodiazepines by themselves are less likely to cause a fatal depression of CNS function while being capable of relieving anxiety with minimal or no sedation accounts for their popularity. Over the past three decades the benzodiazepines have largely replaced the barbiturates as the drugs of choice for treating anxiety and for inducing sleep.

From a pharmacologic standpoint there is nothing absolute about the various stages of CNS depression. Rather, the extent to which any stage is apparent depends solely on the dose of depressant administered.

Current research is aimed at developing anxiolytics that are not CNS depressants. **Buspirone** is an example of such an agent.

■ **Benzodiazepines** For the past 30 years the benzodiazepines have consistently ranked among the most prescribed medications in the United States. These drugs are used most often to relieve anxiety (anxiolytic), induce sleep (hypnotic), alleviate seizures (anticonvulsant), and reduce muscle tone (muscle relaxant).

● **Basic pharmacology** All benzodiazepines are highly lipophilic. As such they are readily absorbed after oral administration (within 30 minutes to 3 hours), with a significant fraction (80% to 95%) bound to plasma proteins. Few drugs dislodge benzodiazepines from plasma proteins because the binding sites are specific for this chemical class. This unique characteristic lessens the chance for drug interactions, contributing to the safety of the benzodiazepines.

Although these drugs are administered orally for most indications, preparations are available for sublingual, intramuscular (IM), and intravenous (IV) injections.

The benzodiazepines are extensively metabolized by liver microsomal enzymes, with the vast majority of the water-soluble metabolites excreted in urine. Induction of microsomal enzymes appears to be less of a problem with the benzodiazepines than with other CNS depressants. Some benzodiazepines are converted to active metabolites that extend their pharmacologic half-life. For example, both chlordiazepoxide and diazepam are converted to dimethyldiazepam and oxazepam, two of the several pharmacologically active metabolites of the parent compounds. Some metabolites, such as oxazepam and temazepam, were developed as pharmaceuticals in their own right. Given the importance of metabolism in terminating (and in some cases prolonging) the pharmacologic actions of the benzodiazepines, the response to these agents varies with changes in hepatic function. In the elderly, for example, elimination half-lives are increased up to three-fold because of compromised metabolism. This can lead to more severe and prolonged adverse effects if doses are not adjusted accordingly.

The benzodiazepines exert their effects by enhancing the response to the neurotransmitter γ-aminobutyric acid (GABA) (Fig. 6.1). Specific benzodiazepine receptors have been identified in the brain. These sites are located on a component of the GABA receptor such that activation of the benzodiazepine receptor increases the affinity of the GABA binding site for the neurotransmitter, increasing the sensitivity of the system to GABA. Because GABA is a major inhibitory neurotransmitter in the brain, augmentation of GABAergic transmission decreases neuronal excitability. Because only certain GABA receptors possess a benzodiazepine component, these

Benzodiazepines

Anxiolytic
Hypnotic
Anticonvulsant
Muscle relaxant

Benzodiazepines

Diazepam
Flurazepam
Chlorazepate
Clonazepam
Chlordiazepoxide
Alprazolam
Triazolam
Midazolam
Temazepam

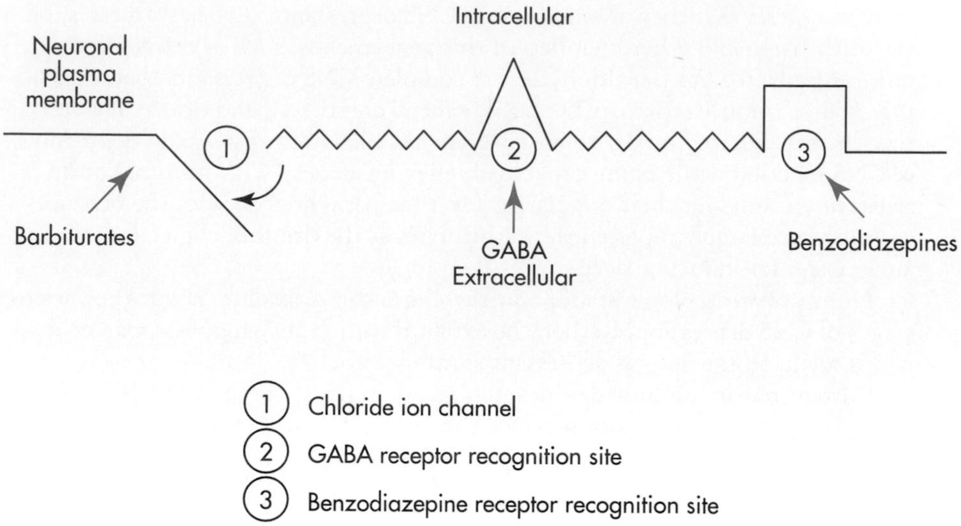

Intracellular

Neuronal
plasma
membrane

① ② ③

Barbiturates

GABA
Extracellular

Benzodiazepines

① Chloride ion channel

② GABA receptor recognition site

③ Benzodiazepine receptor recognition site

Fig. 6.1 Schematic representation of the GABA/benzodiazepine receptor complex.

Benzodiazepine Antagonist

Flumazenil

drugs are more selective than other CNS depressants, which tend to influence neuronal activity in a more generalized manner.

Benzodiazepine receptor antagonists attach to benzodiazepine sites in the brain but fail to enhance the response to GABA. Such agents are useful for blocking or reversing the effects of active benzodiazepines. **Flumazenil** is a benzodiazepine marketed for this purpose.

Other compounds, such as the beta-carbolines, attach to the benzodiazepine receptor but induce effects, such as anxiety and seizures, opposite to those observed after administration of a conventional benzodiazepine. These agents are considered inverse agonists because they evoke a response, which is typical of an agonist, but the effect is the inverse of that obtained with, for example, diazepam, which is, by convention, considered a pure agonist for this site. No inverse agonists are yet available for clinical use.

Work has also progressed in identifying partial agonists for the benzodiazepine receptor (Fig. 6.2). Such agents induce a response similar to benzodiazepine agonists, but they are somewhat less efficacious. In theory, the partial agonists would be safer than traditional benzodiazepines because they would be more limited as CNS depressants. Partial agonists reduce the response to a full agonist because they occupy the same receptor site. Moreover, partial agonists are less likely to induce physical dependence than full agonists. As yet, no partial agonist benzodiazepines have been approved for use in the United States.

Like all CNS depressants, the benzodiazepines produce tolerance and physical dependence. Tolerance develops especially to their sedative, hypnotic, and anticonvulsant effects. Less tolerance is observed to the anxiolytic action. The degree of dependence and the severity of withdrawal is a function of dose and duration of treatment. In general, benzodiazepines must be administered at high doses for months or years before observing an abstinence syndrome that could include seizures. There have been reports of minor withdrawal symptoms (insomnia, anxiety) after brief periods of administration of anxiolytic or hypnotic doses of these drugs. Withdrawal symptoms may be mitigated by the long half-life of some benzodiazepines. Because there is cross-tolerance among CNS depressants, the benzo-

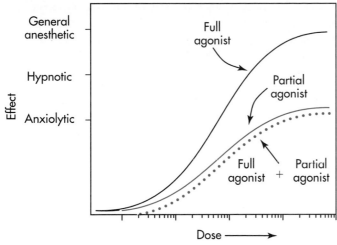

Fig. 6.2 Representative of the comparative effects of full and partial agonists at the benzodiazepine receptor.

diazepines are used to treat withdrawal symptoms associated with ethyl alcohol and the barbiturates.

- **Adverse effects** The most common adverse effects associated with the benzodiazepines are an extension of their primary pharmacologic actions. These include sedation, ataxia, and motor incoordination. Other troublesome CNS effects occasionally encountered are retrograde amnesia and paradoxic excitement. The benzodiazepines display no notable toxicities to individual organ systems.

- **Clinical use** As anxiolytics, longer-acting benzodiazepines such as diazepam and chlordiazepoxide are preferred. Table 6.1 lists the primary uses of some benzodiazepines.

    Benzodiazepines are also widely used as hypnotics. Although flurazepam, a longer-acting drug, was one of the first employed for this purpose,

Table 6.1 *Some Representative Benzodiazepines*

DRUG	MAXIMUM HALF-LIFE (HR)*	PRIMARY USE
Diazepam	150	Anxiolytic, anticonvulsant, muscle relaxant
Flurazepam	100	Hypnotic
Clorazepate	100	Anticonvulsant
Clonazepam	50	Anticonvulsant
Chlordiazepoxide	30	Anxiolytic
Alprazolam	15	Hypnotic
Triazolam	5	Hypnotic
Flumazenil	1	Benzodiazepine receptor antagonist

*Includes active metabolites.

short-acting benzodiazepines are preferred to minimize the risk of morning hangover. Alprazolam and triazolam are popular for this purpose.

The benzodiazepines have anticonvulsant activity, but their use is limited because tolerance develops to this effect. Diazepam, however, is a drug of choice for treating status epilepticus, an acute medical emergency, clonazepam is available for the treatment of petit mal (absence) epilepsy and myoclonic seizures, and clorazepate is used as adjunctive therapy for complex partial seizures.

Benzodiazepines, particularly diazepam, are also commonly used as skeletal muscle relaxants.

Benzodiazepines are often employed as preanesthetic medications to reduce the amount of general anesthetic necessary for surgery. They are also administered to suppress withdrawal symptoms in individuals addicted to other CNS depressants, and some, particularly alprazolam, are reported to be effective in treating panic disorder.

Panic Disorder

Alprazolam

- **Other clinical considerations** Although remarkably safe when used appropriately, benzodiazepines are a contributing factor in many accidental deaths and suicides because their effects are additive with other CNS depressants. Most troublesome is the mixture of benzodiazepines and ethyl alcohol.

■ **Barbiturates** Thousands of barbiturates were synthesized and tested during the first half of the twentieth century, but only a few are used today because of the superiority of the benzodiazepines as anxiolytics and hypnotics.

- **Basic pharmacology** The barbiturates are lipid-soluble, weak acids that are readily absorbed from the stomach. Barbiturates are available for oral, parenteral, rectal, and IV administration. Because of their lipid solubility barbiturates cross all membrane barriers, including the placenta. A significant fraction (80% or more) of an administered dose of barbiturate is bound to plasma proteins where it competes with other organic acids for these sites. The barbiturates are metabolized by liver microsomal enzymes. Although most members of this class are extensively metabolized, a significant fraction (up to 50%) of phenobarbital is excreted unchanged. The barbiturates are notorious for their ability to induce microsomal enzyme activity, which enhances their own metabolism and the metabolism of other agents. Parent compounds and metabolites are eliminated primarily in the urine.

    Barbiturates have historically been classified on the basis of their duration of action. Long-acting drugs, such as phenobarbital, were at one time the drugs of choice to relieve anxiety (sedatives), whereas intermediate-acting or short-acting agents, such as pentobarbital, were prescribed as hypnotics. Ultra short-acting barbiturates, as exemplified by thiopental, are typically administered IV as fixed general anesthetics.

    The relative duration of action of a barbiturate is a function of its lipid solubility and the time it takes to distribute throughout the body rather than a function of its rate of metabolism or excretion (Table 6.2). Thus, a thiopental-induced state of general anesthesia is terminated by the physical redistribution of thiopental from the brain, a highly vascularized, lipid-rich region, to other organs in the body. Because the concentration of less lipid-soluble long- and intermediate-acting drugs tends to rise more evenly throughout the body, the onset and termination of their effects on CNS functions are more gradual and of longer duration than for the more lipophilic thiopental.

Table 6.2 *General Classification of Barbiturates*

Duration	Drug	Primary Use
Long	Phenobarbital	Anticonvulsant
Intermediate	Pentobarbital	Hypnotic
Ultrashort	Thiopental	Fixed anesthetic

All barbiturates are complete CNS depressants, provoking responses from sedation to general anesthesia and death, depending on the dose administered.

The barbiturates enhance GABAergic transmission in the brain by interacting with a site on the GABA receptor different from that activated by the benzodiazepines. Thus the barbiturates appear to attach to a component of the GABA receptor coupled chloride ion channel, prolonging the amount of time the channel is open when the receptor is exposed to GABA. Because all GABA receptors of this type are associated with chloride channels, but only some have a benzodiazepine component, the barbiturates tend to have a more generalized effect on CNS function than the benzodiazepines, which may explain why the former are complete CNS depressants and the latter are not.

Tolerance and physical dependence develop to all members of this class. To some extent tolerance is due to the barbiturate-induced increase in microsomal enzyme activity (metabolic tolerance). Long-term administration of increasing doses of barbiturates leads to physical dependence. Withdrawal from barbiturates is more life threatening than opioid withdrawal and must be undertaken with care. Typically a benzodiazepine is substituted for the barbiturate and the dose of benzodiazepine is slowly reduced to prevent withdrawal symptoms (agitation, psychosis, nausea, vomiting, and seizures) as the patient is weaned off the drug.

● **Adverse effects** Sedation, ataxia, and motor incoordination are the most common adverse effects associated with the barbiturates. Up to and including hypnotic doses, the barbiturates have no adverse effects on any organ systems. At anesthetic doses and above there is a progressive decrease in respiration and, for some barbiturates, effects on cardiovascular tone are noted. Death from barbiturate overdose is due to paralysis of the respiratory and vasomotor centers in the brain.

● **Clinical use** Although a number of barbiturates are available for the treatment of anxiety and as hypnotics, these have been supplanted by the benzodiazepines. Two barbiturates that are still widely used are phenobarbital and thiopental. Phenobarbital remains a drug of choice for the treatment of grand mal seizures, whereas thiopental is employed as a fixed, or IV, general anesthetic.

Barbiturates
Phenobarbital
Thiopental

● **Other clinical considerations** When administered chronically there is a potential for drug interactions with the barbiturates. Thus weak organic acids, such as salicylates or certain antiepileptic medications, compete with phenobarbital for binding sites on plasma proteins. Moreover, because barbiturates induce microsomal enzyme activity, the response to drugs metabolized by these enzymes may be attenuated in patients taking phenobarbital. Coadministration of other CNS depressants, such as ethyl alcohol, can have deadly consequences in individuals taking barbiturates. Because barbiturates increase porphyrin synthesis, they are absolutely contraindicated in individuals suffering from intermittent porphyria.

■ **Other Central Nervous System Depressants** Dozens of drugs have been used as hypnotics or sedatives. None has any distinct advantages over the benzodiazepines or barbiturates (Box 6.2). As such, they could be discarded without compromising patient care. Nonetheless, some are still prescribed. One, ethyl alcohol, while having no distinctive clinical value, is one of the most commonly used drugs in our society.

Except for meprobamate, all of these agents are complete CNS depressants and are therefore capable of producing general anesthesia. None is used for this purpose, however, because the amount necessary to induce anesthesia is too near the lethal dose. All are readily absorbed from the gastrointestinal tract, are metabolized by the liver, and (except for paraldehyde, a portion of which is exhaled) are excreted primarily in urine. As with other CNS depressants, tolerance and physical dependence are noted with these agents.

● **Chloral hydrate** Used primarily as a hypnotic, chloral hydrate has a rapid onset but a short duration of action. In the body, chloral hydrate is reduced to trichloroethanol, an active metabolite. Chloral hydrate is irritating to the gastrointestinal tract. It is sometimes a preferred hypnotic for children.

● **Paraldehyde** Like chloral hydrate, paraldehyde has a rapid onset and a short duration of action. It is typically used only with institutionalized patients, although in the past it was employed in relieving the symptoms of alcoholic withdrawal. Paraldehyde is irritating to the gastrointestinal tract. One advantage over other hypnotics is that it can be administered in a retention enema when IV or oral administration is difficult.

● **Meprobamate** Meprobamate was introduced a few years before the benzodiazepines and rapidly gained wide acceptance as an antianxiety agent. Currently it is prescribed as a muscle relaxant, anxiolytic, or hypnotic, especially for the elderly. Although it appears to be an incomplete CNS depressant, its adverse effects are similar to those of the barbiturates.

● **Ethyl alcohol** Ethyl alcohol has no unique medicinal value, but it is widely used and abused for its sedative property, which imparts a feeling of well-being. Ethyl alcohol is oxidized in the liver to acetaldehyde by alcohol dehydrogenase, which is in turn converted to acetyl CoA. **Disulfiram** inhibits the conversion of acetaldehyde to acetyl CoA, raising the blood levels of the aldehyde, which induces dizziness, nausea, increased heart rate, and in some cases unconsciousness. For this reason disulfiram is sometimes used to help recovering alcoholics resist the temptation to indulge. Because of its CNS depressant properties, ethyl alcohol reduces muscular coordination, lengthens reaction time, impairs vision, and decreases anxiety. It is directly irritating to the gastrointestinal tract, and it decreases intestinal motility.

Ethyl alcohol has little effect on the respiratory system at subanesthetic doses, although it does cause vasodilation in moderate amounts. Ethyl alcohol increases urine flow and volume by inhibiting the release of antidiuretic hormone. When taken chronically it increases liver microsomal enzyme activity. The incidence of cirrhosis is higher in chronic alcoholics than in the general population. Ethyl alcohol is contraindicated in individuals suffering from hepatic or renal disorders, ulcers, or epilepsy. It should also be avoided by those taking other CNS depressants. Acute and chronic tox-

Box 6.2

CENTRAL NERVOUS SYSTEM DEPRESSANTS
Chloral hydrate
Paraldehyde
Meprobamate
Ethyl alcohol

icities, including addiction, are similar to those observed with the barbiturates.

■ **Non-Central Nervous System Depressant Sedatives and Hypnotics** Sedation is an effect common to a number of therapeutic agents. Although normally it is considered undesirable, in some cases it is a beneficial adjunct to the primary therapeutic indication. Most antipsychotics and many antidepressants display anticholinergic and antihistaminic activities, which are sedating. This effect can be beneficial for agitated psychotic or depressed patients. Examples are haloperidol, an antipsychotic, and imipramine, an antidepressant (Box 6.3). The hypnotic properties of trazodone, another antidepressant, are often used to help elderly depressed patients sleep.

Box 6.3

SEDATIVES AND HYPNOTICS THAT ARE NOT GENERAL CENTRAL NERVOUS SYSTEM DEPRESSANTS

Antipsychotics
Haloperidol
Chlorpromazine

Antidepressants
Imipramine
Trazodone

Anticholinergics
Atropine
Scopolamine

Antihistamines
Diphenhydramine
Pyrilamine

β-Adrenoceptor Antagonists
Propranolol

Buspirone

Antihistamines, such as diphenhydramine and pyrilamine, and anticholinergics, such as scopolamine and atropine, are found in over-the-counter hypnotics.

In some cases β-adrenoceptor antagonists (β-blockers), such as propranolol, are helpful in relieving anxiety. This effect is due to a decrease in the somatic symptoms (palpitations, sweaty palms) that reinforce anxiety.

Buspirone was developed as an anxiolytic devoid of CNS depressant properties. Unlike conventional anxiolytics, which are effective in a matter of minutes or hours, buspirone must be taken continuously for several days or weeks before its anxiolytic properties are apparent. Its mechanism of action is not completely understood, but it is thought to act as a partial agonist at serotonin$_{1A}$ receptors in brain. High doses of buspirone are dysphoric rather than euphoric. Tolerance and physical dependence are not observed with buspirone. Although it is not a CNS depressant, buspirone can cause confusion and drowsiness. It is prudent not to combine buspirone with ethyl alcohol or other CNS depressants, although buspirone is safer in this regard than other anxiolytics and hypnotics (Box 6.4).

Box 6.4

ANXIOLYTICS, SEDATIVES, AND HYPNOTICS
Drug Summary

Benzodiazepines
Alprazolam
Chlordiazepoxide
Clonazepam
Clorazepate
Flumazenil
Flurazepam
Triazolam

Barbiturates
Phenobarbital
Pentobarbital

**Miscellaneous Central
Nervous System
Depressants**
Chloral hydrate
Paraldehyde
Meprobamate
Ethyl alcohol

**Non–Central Nervous
System Depressants**
Haloperidol
Chlorpromazine
Imipramine
Trazodone
Atropine
Scopolamine
Diphenhydramine
Pyrilamine
Propranolol
Buspirone

SECTION 6.2 ANTIEPILEPTICS

 Overview Seizures are characterized by an excessive random discharge of neurons in the brain, with the type of seizure dependent on the location and extent of a brain lesion, or focus (Box 6.5). Whereas seizures are caused by head injury, stroke, or cancer, most forms of epilepsy are idiopathic.

Box 6.5

GENERAL CLASSIFICATION AND CHARACTERISTICS
OF SEIZURES

Partial Seizures
Usually no loss of consciousness, localized to specific
   area of the brain
Examples:
   Elementary symptomatology, such as cortical focal
      and jacksonian march
   Complex symptomatology, such as psychomotor

Generalized Seizures
Always loss of consciousness, all areas of the brain in-
   volved
Examples:
   Absence (petit mal)
   Tonic-clonic (grand mal)

Although there are numerous drugs available for treating seizures, most are effective in only certain types of epilepsy. Indeed, some antiepileptic medications may precipitate seizures in certain patients. It is important, therefore, to accurately diagnose the type of epilepsy before initiating therapy.

From a pharmacologic standpoint, seizures are categorized broadly into partial and generalized. With partial seizures the abnormal discharge is limited to a discrete brain region, whereas with generalized seizures neuronal excitability spreads from the focus throughout the entire CNS. Examples of partial seizures are jacksonian march and psychomotor epilepsy. Petit mal (absence) and grand mal (tonic-clonic) are examples of generalized seizures. Although the vast majority of seizures are self-limiting and, in themselves, not life threatening, status epilepticus, which is characterized by a rapid succession of seizures, is a major medical emergency.

Certain principles have been established in the pharmacologic management of epilepsy (Box 6.6). These include care in selecting the medication most appropriate for the type of seizures being treated. In addition, although monotherapy is most desirable, it is sometimes necessary to combine drugs for adequate seizure control. Given the chronic nature of the disorder, the potential for drug interactions and chronic toxicities is increased. Finally, care must be taken in terminating therapy or changing medications because abrupt withdrawal of an antiepileptic may precipitate a seizure.

Box 6.6

SOME GENERAL PRINCIPLES OF ANTIEPILEPTIC THERAPY

Drug selection determined by type of seizure
Monotherapy is preferred, but multiple drugs must
   sometimes be employed
Must be alert for drug interactions and chronic toxicities
Dosages should be gradually reduced when terminat-
   ing therapy to avoid inducing seizures

Of the antiepileptic medications available in the United States, only a few are used routinely in the treatment of this disorder. The others are less efficacious, more toxic, or limited in their use because tolerance develops to their antiepileptic effects.

Current research is aimed at developing medications having a broad spectrum of antiepileptic activity to simplify therapy and minimize the need for multiple medications. It is likely that several new antiepileptic drugs will soon be approved for use in the United States.

■ **Treatment of Grand Mal and Partial Seizures** Grand mal (tonic-clonic) epilepsy is characterized by a massive discharge of the CNS causing a loss of consciousness, intermittent contractions of the skeletal muscles (clonic phase), and muscular rigidity (tonic phase). Partial seizures are due to a random but localized discharge in a discrete brain region, which may be expressed as a tremor in a limb or digit or as a loss of emotional control. Although some medications are effective in controlling grand mal epilepsy, partial seizures are more resistant to therapy (Box 6.7).

● Hydantoins

— *Basic pharmacology* The absorption of **phenytoin,** the most important member of this chemical class, is slow and incomplete. A significant percentage is bound to plasma proteins, making it vulnerable to displacement by other medications. Phenytoin is metabolized by microsomal enzymes and, like the barbiturates, induces liver enzyme

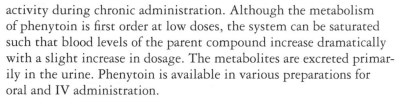

Box 6.7

PRIMARY DRUGS FOR THE TREATMENT OF GRAND MAL AND PARTIAL SEIZURES

Hydantoins
Phenytoin

Barbiturates
Phenobarbital
Primidone

Iminostilbene
Carbamazepine

activity during chronic administration. Although the metabolism of phenytoin is first order at low doses, the system can be saturated such that blood levels of the parent compound increase dramatically with a slight increase in dosage. The metabolites are excreted primarily in the urine. Phenytoin is available in various preparations for oral and IV administration.

Like all drugs effective against grand mal and partial seizures, phenytoin inhibits the spread of the discharge rather than depressing the focus itself. The primary mechanism of action of phenytoin is blockade of neuronal sodium channels, which stabilizes the membrane and increases the seizure threshold.

— *Adverse effects* The major adverse effects associated with phenytoin are diplopia, ataxia, sedation, nausea, and vomiting. Hyperplasia of the gums is effectively controlled with good oral hygiene. Hirsutism is encountered with most patients. Blood dyscrasias, such as agranulocytosis, are rare but possible.

— *Clinical use* Phenytoin is a drug of choice for the treatment of grand mal epilepsy and partial seizures. In general, it is less sedating than phenobarbital. There are some phenytoin congeners available for use, but they are either less effective (mephenytoin and ethotoin) or more toxic (phenacemide).

— *Drug interactions* Phenytoin competes for plasma protein binding sites with a variety of drugs, including antiinflammatory agents and some hypnotics. When coadministered with such agents there is a possibility that the blood levels of free phenytoin will increase, leading to adverse effects and toxicities not previously observed at that dose. Conversely, blood levels of phenytoin may drop if it is administered with drugs, such as phenobarbital and carbamazepine, that induce microsomal enzyme activity.

● **Barbiturates**

— *Basic pharmacology* **Phenobarbital** is the most important antiepileptic drug in this chemical class. Although there are other barbiturates available for treating seizure disorders (metharbital and mephobarbital), they are generally less effective than phenobarbital. The pharmacologic properties of phenobarbital are detailed earlier in this chapter. It is noteworthy that tolerance and physical dependence are not major problems with phenobarbital at the doses typically used to treat seizures. Phenobarbital appears to have a selective antiepileptic effect against certain types of seizures independent of its sedative and hypnotic actions.

Primidone is the other major antiepileptic in this chemical class. Although primidone itself has antiepileptic properties, much of its effectiveness is due to its metabolism to phenobarbital and phenylethylmalonamide (PEMA). Primidone is slowly absorbed after oral administration and a significant fraction (25% to 30%) is not bound to plasma proteins. The mechanism of action of the unmetabolized primidone is unknown, although it is believed to be similar to phenytoin.

— *Adverse effects* Sedation is the chief adverse effect of phenobarbital and primidone, although tolerance develops over time. Other adverse effects associated with primidone include nausea and vomiting, and, less commonly, skin rash, blood dyscrasias, and psychotic reactions.

— *Clinical use* Both phenobarbital and primidone are used for the treatment of grand mal and partial epilepsies. For many years phenobarbital was the drug of choice for these conditions, and it remains popular because of its safety, efficacy, and cost. Primidone is more often used when other medications fail to satisfactorily control the seizures, and it is sometimes administered in conjunction with phenytoin. There is little logic to combining primidone and phenobarbital because blood levels of the barbiturate are elevated in patients receiving primidone alone. Extreme caution must be exercised when withdrawing patients from phenobarbital or primidone because of the possibility of precipitating seizures, including status epilepticus.

— *Drug interactions* The potential for drug interactions is similar for phenobarbital and primidone. These include modifying the metabolism and thereby altering the blood levels of other drugs, particularly antiepileptic agents. Blood levels of phenobarbital and primidone, or the adjunctive therapy, may be increased or decreased depending on the level of competition for plasma protein binding sites and microsomal enzymes. Adjustment in dosage may be required to maintain seizure control when combining these agents with other drugs.

● Iminostilbene

— *Basic pharmacology* Carbamazepine is the only member of this chemical class used routinely for the treatment of seizures. Carbamazepine has a broad spectrum of therapeutic activities, also being effective in the treatment of bipolar depression and trigeminal and glossopharyngeal neuralgias. Its mechanism of action as an antiepileptic is unknown, although it is thought to be similar to phenytoin.

Carbamazepine is available only for oral administration. Its absorption is slow and erratic, with 70% of the absorbed dose bound to plasma proteins. Although a metabolite, carbamazepine-10,11-epoxide, displays antiepileptic activity, carbamazepine itself is primarily responsible for the theraputic response. Over 90% of the drug is metabolized before excretion in the urine.

— *Adverse effects* Sedation, ataxia, diplopia, nausea, and vomiting are the most common adverse effects associated with carbamazepine therapy. The drug has been associated with blood dyscrasias, but this is an infrequent occurrence.

— *Clinical use* Carbamazepine is considered by many the drug of choice for the treatment of grand mal epilepsy and partial seizures. It is thought to be less sedating than phenobarbital or phenytoin while being at least as efficacious.

— *Drug interactions* Although there appears to be little competition between other drugs and carbamazepine for plasma protein binding sites, carbamazepine is potent in inducing liver microsomal enzymes. Coadministration of carbamazepine with phenobarbital or phenytoin can reduce blood levels of these medications below that observed when they are used alone.

■ **Treatment of Petit Mal Seizures** Petit mal, or absence, epilepsy is characterized by loss of consciousness with some symmetric clonic activity, although it is much less dramatic than that associated with grand mal seizures. On occasion there is no obvious change in motor activity associated with a petit mal attack. Drugs typically used to treat grand mal or partial seizures are ineffective in controlling petit mal epilepsy (Box 6.8). Nonetheless, patients are sometimes administered phenobarbital or phenytoin along with the primary medication for treating petit mal since grand mal seizures are sometimes encountered with these individuals.

Box 6.8

PRIMARY DRUGS FOR THE TREATMENT OF PETIT MAL SEIZURES
Succinimides   Ethosuximide
Carboxylic Acids   Valproic acid
Benzodiazepines   Clonazepam
Oxazolidinediones   Trimethadione

● Succinimides

— *Basic pharmacology* Of the three succinimides approved for the treatment of epilepsy, **ethosuximide** is the most important member of this class. It is a drug of choice for the treatment of petit mal seizures.

Ethosuximide is rapidly and completely absorbed from the gastrointestinal tract, with little binding to plasma proteins. The majority of ethosuximide is metabolized and excreted in the urine, but a significant portion (24%) is eliminated as the parent compound. Ethosuximide is available only for oral administration.

There are several theories concerning the mechanism of action of the succinimides. Most evidence suggests that they reduce the current at T-type neuronal calcium channels.

— *Adverse effects* Anorexia, nausea, and vomiting are the chief adverse effects associated with ethosuximide. Adverse CNS effects include sedation, lethargy, and dizziness. Less frequently encountered are parkinsonian-like symptoms, skin reactions, and blood dyscrasias.

— *Clinical use* Ethosuximide is used only for the treatment of petit mal epilepsy. Because of its efficacy and safety relative to other agents, it is one of the most widely used drugs for treating this condition.

— *Drug interactions* When administered with valproic acid, the clearance of ethosuximide is slowed. Beyond this, ethosuximide has no significant interaction with other agents.

● Carboxylic acids

— *Basic pharmacology* **Valproic acid** is the only member of this class approved for use in the United States. It is the first example of a broad-spectrum antiepileptic because it displays efficacy against both grand mal and petit mal seizures, although it has been authorized for use only in the latter condition.

Valproic acid is rapidly and completely absorbed from the gastrointestinal tract, with 90% of the absorbed drug bound to plasma proteins. The vast majority of valproic acid is metabolized, with both the parent compound and metabolites excreted in the urine and feces. Valproic acid is available only for oral administration.

The mechanism of action of valproic acid remains unclear. Although there is evidence that it enhances GABAergic activity in the brain, perhaps by decreasing the metabolism of this amino acid transmitter, there is some question as to whether a sufficient concentration of the drug is attained in the brain to inhibit the breakdown of GABA. The possibility remains that valproic acid is capable of inhibiting GABA metabolism in discrete brain regions important for controlling seizure activity. The antiepileptic effect of valproic acid outlasts its sojourn in the body, suggesting an active metabolite or a long-lasting modification in neuronal excitability.

— *Adverse effects* Gastrointestinal disturbances, including anorexia, nausea, and vomiting, are the most frequent adverse effects encountered with valproic acid. Less frequently reported are sedation, ataxia, tremor, rash, and alopecia. Most troubling is the rare complication of fulminant hepatitis, which is most often encountered in young children and can be fatal.

— *Clinical use* Valproic acid has challenged ethosuximide as the drug of choice for the treatment of petit mal epilepsy. A major advantage of valproic acid is its effectiveness in controlling grand mal seizures as well, making it especially useful in those experiencing both types of seizures. However, although valproic acid has been used in millions of patients without serious incident, its potential to induce fatal hepatitis has made physicians more cautious in its use. Nonetheless, it is the only drug currently available that has been used for treating grand mal, myoclonic, and partial seizures, as well as petit mal epilepsy.

— *Drug interactions* Valproic acid modifies the blood levels of phenobarbital, phenytoin, and carbamazepine by altering the metabolism of these agents. In particular, valproic acid dramatically increases the likelihood of adverse effects to the barbiturates.

● **Benzodiazepines** Of the benzodiazepines, only **clonazepam** is specifically approved for the treatment of petit mal epilepsy. Its basic pharmacology, adverse effects, and drug interactions are similar to those described for this drug class earlier in the chapter (see p. 187). Although clonazepam is an outstanding antiepileptic agent, tolerance develops to this effect within a few months, rendering it inappropriate for long-term therapy. It is available only in tablet form for oral administration.

● **Oxazolidinediones**

— *Basic pharmacology* One of the earliest drugs developed for treating petit mal epilepsy, **trimethadione,** is now used only if other, safer medications fail to adequately control seizures.

Trimethadione is rapidly absorbed from the gastrointestinal tract and is not appreciably bound to plasma proteins. It is converted in the liver to dimethadione, an active metabolite, which is excreted in the urine. Several preparations are available for oral administration.

The mechanism of action of trimethadione is unknown, although it appears to be similar to ethosuximide in reducing T-type currents through calcium channels.

— *Adverse effects* Sedation and hemeralopia are the most common adverse effects associated with trimethadione. It is also known to cause blood dyscrasias, and it is sometimes toxic to the kidney and liver. These potential toxicities have relegated trimethadione to a backup role in the treatment of petit mal seizures.

— *Clinical use* Trimethadione is used for treating petit mal epilepsy only when other medications are found to be unsatisfactory. It must be used with caution because of the potential for fatal toxicities.

— *Drug interactions* There are no significant interactions between trimethadione and other medications.

■ **Treatment of Status Epilepticus** Status epilepticus is a repetitive series of seizures that, if uncontrolled, can lead to death. Because it is an acute, life-threatening condition, IV medications are administered to terminate the seizure as quickly as possible. If all else fails, inhalational anesthetics are used. Drugs most often used to treat status epilepticus are the benzodiazepines, **diazepam** or **lorazepam,** or the barbiturate **phenobarbital** (Box 6.9). An IV preparation of **phenytoin** is also available for this purpose. Care must be taken when administering any of these agents IV because they can cause fatal respiratory depression.

Box 6.9

PRIMARY DRUGS FOR THE TREATMENT OF STATUS EPILEPTICUS
Benzodiazepines   Diazepam   Lorazepam
Barbiturates   Phenobarbital

The basic pharmacology and other relevant properties of these drugs are detailed elsewhere in this chapter.

■ **Other Agents** The carbonic anhydrase inhibitor **acetazolamide** is a safe and effective treatment for petit mal epilepsy. However, tolerance develops to its antiepileptic effect within a few weeks. Its antiepileptic action is thought to be due to the increase in brain CO_2 that results from inhibition of carbonic anhydrase.

Vigabatrin is a new drug available in some European countries and awaiting approval in the United States. It is used primarily for control of partial seizures. Its mechanism of action is inhibition of GABA transaminase, the enzyme responsible for the metabolism of this amino acid. The increase in CNS GABA levels presumably enhances inhibitory neurotransmission in the brain. Vigabatrin is claimed to have a broader spectrum of activity than most antiepileptic agents.

■ **Drugs of Choice (Box 6.10 lists antiepileptic drugs)**

● **Grand mal epilepsy**
Phenytoin
Phenobarbital
Carbamazepine
Primidone

● **Petit mal epilepsy**
Ethosuximide
Valproic acid
Trimethadione

● **Partial seizures**
Carbamazepine
Phenytoin
Primidone

● **Status epilepticus**
Diazepam
Lorazepam
Phenobarbital

Phenytoin, phenobarbital, or primidone are sometimes administered with petit mal agents to control grand mal seizures in certain patients.

Box 6.10

ANTIEPILEPTIC DRUGS
Acetazolamide
Carbamazepine
Clonazepam
Diazepam
Ethosuximide
Lorazepam
Phenobarbital
Phenytoin
Primidone
Trimethadione
Valproic acid
Vigabatrin

Table 6.3	*Stages of General Anesthesia*
I. Analgesia stage	From administration to loss of consciousness
II. Delirium stage	From loss of consciousness to return of regular respiration
III. Surgical stage	From return of regular respiration to respiratory arrest
IV. Medullary paralysis stage	From respiratory arrest to death

SECTION 6.3 GENERAL ANESTHETICS

Inhalation Agents

Nitrous oxide
Halothane
Enflurane
Isoflurane
Methoxyflurane

Characteristics of General Anesthesia

Unconsciousness
Amnesia
Analgesia
Muscle relaxation

■ **Overview** General anesthesia was introduced to medicine in 1846 by William Morton, a second-year medical student at Harvard. Up to that time surgery was avoided but, when necessary, was generally conducted on conscious patients who were restrained by three or four large men. Given these circumstances, surgeons were admired more for their speed than for their skill or neatness. Although ethyl alcohol and opioids had been used to control patients, the doses necessary for major surgery are toxic and potentially fatal (Table 6.3). Thus Morton's demonstration revolutionized medical practice.

General anesthetics are divided into two categories: inhalational and fixed, or IV, agents. Inhalational anesthetics are administered as a gas or vapor, whereas fixed anesthetics are injected at a fixed dose, usually IV. Inhalational agents are subdivided further into gases and volatile liquids, depending on their physical characteristics at room temperature. The first general anesthetics were inhalational, including chloroform, ether, cyclopropane, and ethylene. None is currently used because of toxicities, flammability, or explosiveness. Only one gaseous anesthetic, nitrous oxide, and a few volatile agents, such as halothane, enflurane, isoflurane, and methoxyflurane, are used today. Likewise, only a few fixed anesthetics are employed routinely, including thiopental, ketamine, innovar, and propofol.

General anesthetics are seldom used alone for a major surgical procedure. The patient is normally treated with a preanesthetic medication, such as an anxiolytic or anticholinergic, to facilitate anesthesia and reduce adverse effects associated with the general anesthetic. In some cases a combination of anesthetics is used, such as nitrous oxide and halothane, to take advantage of the properties of the two agents. Other drugs, such as muscle relaxants, are administered during the operation to facilitate surgical procedures or to maintain vital functions.

Current research is directed toward developing general anesthetics that possess a wide margin of safety, are easily administered and readily terminated, and possess a range of useful pharmacologic properties, including analgesia and muscle relaxation. Although the ideal general anesthetic has yet to be discovered, the judicious use of preanesthetic medications and combinations of general anesthetics (balanced anesthesia) has made it possible to approach this objective.

■ **Inhalational Agents** For major surgical procedures general anesthetics are used to render the patient unconscious, to eliminate reflex motor responses to noxious stimuli, and to induce amnesia, analgesia, and muscle relaxation (Box 6.11). Most of these objectives are attained only by significantly depressing CNS activity. Thus all general anesthetics, whether administered by inhalation or injection, are CNS depressants.

Box 6.11

BASIC PRINCIPLES OF ANESTHESIA INDUCED BY INHALATIONAL AGENTS

Depth of anesthesia is directly related to the partial pressure or tension of anesthetic in the brain.

The time necessary to attain equilibrium between the partial pressure of an anesthetic in the brain, blood, and lungs (rate of induction) is directly related to the lipid solubility of the anesthetic, as is the time necessary to eliminate the anesthetic (rate of emergence).

Potency and efficacy are directly related to the lipid solubility (Ostwald coefficient, λ) of the anesthetic.

To gauge the depth of anesthesia, vital signs and other physiologic parameters are monitored during surgery. This makes it possible to maintain the minimum level of anesthesia for a particular procedure and provides warning if the depth of CNS depression becomes life threatening. The physiologic signs monitored vary with the general anesthetic and preanesthetic medications.

The responses to inhalational agents are generally divided into broad categories or stages representing different levels of anesthesia and CNS depression (see Table 6.3). The earliest stage (stage I) is characterized by analgesia but no loss of consciousness. This allows for procedures not requiring muscle relaxation, such as dental work and change of burn dressing. Nitrous oxide may be used alone for these purposes. Indeed, given its lack of efficacy, nitrous oxide alone cannot be used for anything other than stage I anesthesia.

An increase in the amount of anesthetic administered results in a loss of consciousness and entry into stage II. This stage is characterized by loss of bowel and bladder control, delirium, and excitement. With preanesthetic medications and appropriate combinations of general anesthetics it is possible to traverse stage II so quickly that these responses are avoided.

Major surgery is typically performed in stage III, the onset of which is signaled by the return of regular respiration after loss of consciousness. It is during this stage that skeletal muscle relaxation is most evident.

As the amount of anesthetic administered increases and CNS depression deepens, the patient enters stage IV, which is characterized by respiratory arrest caused by paralysis of the medullary respiratory center in brain. Stage IV represents a medical emergency and will end in death if anesthetic administration is not terminated.

- **Basic pharmacology** All inhalational anesthetics are highly lipophilic, some more so than others. As such they are readily absorbed from the lungs into the blood and are transferred from the blood to the brain and other organs.

     The degree of CNS depression, and therefore the depth of anesthesia, is directly related to the partial pressure or tension of the anesthetic in the brain. Inasmuch as the time necessary to attain the partial pressure required for anesthesia is proportional to the lipid solubility of the anesthetic, the rate of induction is slower for more lipophilic agents. Likewise, because the rate of elimination is related to lipophilicity, it takes longer for the more lipid-soluble agents to be cleared from the body.

     A measure of lipid solubility is the amount of anesthetic in blood compared with the amount in lungs at equilibrium. Equilibrium is attained when the partial pressure of the anesthetic in the blood is equal to the partial pressure of the gas in the lungs. The ratio of anesthetic in the blood

Increased Lipophilicity

Slow induction
Slow recovery

as compared with the amount in lungs at equilibrium is the blood:gas partition coefficient, or Ostwald coefficient (λ). The greater the Ostwald coefficient, the more lipid soluble the anesthetic and the slower the rates of induction and elimination. Ostwald coefficients vary from 0.47 (relatively less lipid soluble) for nitrous oxide to 12.0 (relatively more lipid soluble) for methoxyflurane.

Increased Lipophilicity
More potent

Anesthetic potency and efficacy are also related to lipid solubility. Thus at equilibrium much smaller quantities of more lipid-soluble agents are needed to maintain a given depth of anesthesia than are needed for less lipid-soluble substances. For example, up to 70% of the inhaled gases may be nitrous oxide, a less lipid-soluble agent, whereas only 1% to 3% is required for enflurane or isoflurane, more lipid-soluble anesthetics. Moreover, whereas enflurane or isoflurane alone can provide any stage of general anesthesia, nitrous oxide alone, even when administered at a concentration of 90% of the inspired gases, will barely attain stage II, indicating that it is a much less efficacious agent.

Anesthetic potency is expressed as the minimum alveolar concentration (MAC) in the inspired air at equilibrium when there is no response to a skin incision in 50% of the patients (Box 6.12). Inasmuch as more lipid-soluble anesthetics (higher Ostwald coefficient) are more potent, they have a lower MAC value than less lipid-soluble agents. Thus nitrous oxide (Ostwald coefficient = 0.47) has a MAC value >100, meaning that over 100% of the inspired air would have to be nitrous oxide to eliminate the response to a skin incision in 50% of patients. In contrast, the more lipid soluble methoxyflurane (Ostwald coefficient = 12.0) has a MAC of only 0.16, meaning the inspired air need contain only 0.16% methoxyflurane at equilibrium to eliminate the response to incision in half the population. Table 6.4 lists the major effects of general anesthetics.

Box 6.12

MINIMUM ALVEOLAR CONCENTRATION

The relative potency of an inhalational anesthetic (MAC value) is the concentration in the inspir ed air at equilibrium (when the partial pressure is identical in the lungs, blood, and brain) at which there is no response to a skin incision in 50% of patients. The numerical value of MAC is inversely related to the lipid solubility of an inhalational anesthetic.

MAC, minimum alveolar concentration.

Nitrous oxide, the gaseous agent, is excreted unchanged by the lungs, whereas the more commonly used volatile anesthetics are metabolized to some extent. Thus up to 70% of inspired methoxyflurane is metabolized in the liver, releasing fluoride ions and organic acids. Although much smaller quantities (2% to 5%) of halothane and enflurane are metabolized, halogen ions are the chief by-products, with fluoride being liberated in both cases. Because only about 0.2% of isoflurane is metabolized, it releases the least amount of fluoride of any of the volatile agents. This may account in part for the fact that isoflurane is less toxic to the liver and kidney than are the other volatile agents. In all cases the vast majority of unmetabolized drug is exhaled.

The precise mechanism of action of inhalational anesthetics is unknown.

		MAC AND **OSTWALD** **COEFFICIENT**	**RATE OF** **INDUCTION AND** **EMERGENCE**	**MUSCLE** **RELAXATION**	**EFFECT ON CARDIOVASCULAR SYSTEM**	**TOTAL** **EFFECT ON** **LIVER AND KIDNEY**
AGENT	**TYPE**					
Nitrous oxide	Gaseous	>100 0.47	Rapid	None	↓ No arrhythmias	None
Halothane	Volatile	0.8 2.3	Slow	Very good	↓ Sensitizes heart to catechol- amines	Hepatotoxic
Enflurane	Volatile	1.7 1.8	Slow	Very good	↓ No arrhythmias, does not sensi- tize heart to catecholamines	Hepatotoxic
Isoflurane	Volatile	1.40 1.40	Slow	Very good	↓ No arrhythmias, does not sensi- tize heart to catecholamines	None
Methoxy- flurane	Volatile	0.16 12.0	Very slow	Excellent	↓ Sensitizes heart to catechol- amines	Hepatotoxic and nephrotoxic

Table 6.4 *Classification and Characteristics of Some Inhalational General Anesthetics*

MAC, minimum alveolar concentration.

Given the diversity of chemical structures, it is unlikely that they inter-act at a common receptor in the brain. Current theories hold that these substances reversibly modify neuronal elements, thereby disrupting neurotransmission. This action is thought to be related to the lipid solubility of the anesthetic because the more lipid-soluble substances are more potent.

● **Adverse effects** Postoperative nausea and vomiting are frequently associ-ated with volatile anesthetics. All four volatile agents reduce arterial blood pressure and respiration in a dose-dependent manner. All but isoflurane decrease cardiac output. Nitrous oxide, the gaseous anesthetic, has less ef-fect on blood pressure, cardiac output, and respiration than the volatile agents, possibly reflecting that nitrous oxide is much less potent than the others.

● **Clinical use** By itself nitrous oxide is employed only for surgical proce-dures not requiring unconsciousness or skeletal muscle relaxation, reflecting the fact that it is the weakest of the inhalational anesthetics. In contrast, halothane, enflurane, isoflurane, and methoxyflurane induce all levels of general anesthesia and therefore may be used alone for most surgical proce-dures. In practice these agents are seldom, if ever, used alone. They are typically administered after initial induction with nitrous oxide or a fixed anesthetic.

The skeletal muscle relaxation attained with the volatile anesthetics ranges from good to excellent, depending on the efficacy of the agent. Often a skeletal muscle relaxant is administered during surgery to reduce the amount of anesthetic necessary to achieve the necessary reduction in muscle tone.

General anesthetics are used to terminate status epilepticus when con-ventional therapy (e.g., diazepam) fails.

● **Other clinical considerations** Halothane, enflurane, and methoxyflurane sensitize the heart to catecholamines, thereby increasing the possibility of ventricular arrhythmias. Of the three, halothane is most likely to cause arrhythmias. Isoflurane and nitrous oxide are devoid of this property.

Likewise, neither nitrous oxide nor isoflurane are hepatotoxic or nephrotoxic, unlike the other three agents. Hepatic necrosis and renal failure associated with volatile anesthetics, although rare, can be fatal. The precise cause is unknown but is thought to be related to the formation of toxic metabolites, particularly the fluoride ion.

Given these considerations, isoflurane has overtaken halothane as the preferred volatile anesthetic. Nitrous oxide is also widely used, both alone and in combination with the volatile agents.

■ **Fixed (IV) Anesthetics** In some circumstances fixed anesthetics are preferred over inhalational agents. Box 6.13 lists some commonly used fixed anesthetics. The chief advantages of the fixed anesthetics over the inhalational agents are ease of administration, rapid and smooth induction, and lack of adverse effects on the heart (no arrhythmias), liver, and kidneys. The chief disadvantage of the fixed anesthetics as compared with the inhalational agents is the inability to rapidly terminate anesthesia. Thus fixed anesthetics must be metabolized and excreted, whereas the majority of inhalational anesthetics are rapidly eliminated.

Box 6.13

COMMONLY USED FIXED, OR INTRAVENOUS, GENERAL ANESTHETICS

Innovar
Combination of droperidol and fentanyl
Neuroleptanalgesia

Ketamine
Dissociative anesthesia
Hallucinations

Thiopental
Barbiturate
No analgesia

Propofol
Similar to barbiturates, but more rapid recovery

Midazolam
A benzodiazepine

● **Basic pharmacology** Five of the more popular fixed anesthetics are **innovar,** a combination of the neuroleptic droperidol and the opiate fentanyl; **ketamine,** a structural analog of the hallucinogen phencyclidine; **thiopental,** a barbiturate; **midazolam,** a benzodiazepine; and **propofol.** All are available in IV formulations, with midazolam and ketamine also provided for IM administration.

For thiopental, propofol, and midazolam in particular, their brief duration of action is due to redistribution from the brain to other organs and tissues. All five of the listed anesthetics are extensively metabolized by the liver and excreted in the urine or bile. Durations of action are variable (a few minutes to a few hours) depending on the dose.

Droperidol acts primarily by blocking dopamine receptors in the brain, fentanyl stimulates opiate receptors, ketamine is a glutamic acid receptor antagonist, and midazolam stimulates the benzodiazepine component of GABA receptors in the brain. Both thiopental and propofol enhance GABAergic transmission in the brain by acting at the GABA receptor-associated ion channel.

Innovar and ketamine are potent analgesics, whereas thiopental, propofol, and midazolam are not and in fact may increase the awareness of pain. The latter three are sometimes administered with nitrous oxide, a powerful analgesic.

- **Adverse effects** Respiratory depression is commonly associated with innovar, thiopental, and propofol. Whereas thiopental and propofol are CNS depressants, innovar-induced respiratory depression, and nausea are caused by fentanyl, an opioid. Prominent adverse effects associated with ketamine are hallucinations and nightmares. Children are less susceptible to these actions of ketamine. Ketamine also stimulates heart rate and increases blood pressure, limiting its use in patients with cardiovascular disorders. Midazolam is relatively free of adverse effects when used as a fixed anesthetic or as a preanesthetic medication.

- **Clinical uses** Fixed anesthetics are typically used for brief and minor surgical procedures, changing burn dressings, and certain diagnostic procedures. Innovar and ketamine are particularly useful if there is a need for the patient to respond to suggestions while being left with little memory of the procedure. Fixed anesthetics are frequently used in combination with inhalational agents. In some cases they are administered with nitrous oxide to take advantage of the analgesic activity of the gaseous agent. Commonly, propofol, thiopental, or midazolam are injected before administration of a volatile anesthetic. This speeds the rate of induction and attainment of stage III anesthesia while reducing the amount of inhalational agent required to maintain the desired level of CNS depression.

- **Other clinical considerations** Fentanyl, a short-acting opioid analgesic, causes significant respiratory depression, nausea, and vomiting. These effects can be reversed by naloxone, an opioid receptor antagonist. Like all neuroleptics, droperidol can induce extrapyramidal muscle movements.

Because of its effects on blood pressure, ketamine should be used with caution in hypertensive patients. Moreover, care should be taken in administering this anesthetic to individuals with psychiatric disorders because of its tendency to induce hallucinations.

Although the benzodiazepines, such as midazolam, have little effect on respiration and the cardiovascular system, significant depression of both may be noted when they are used in combination with opioids.

Thiopental and propofol cause significant respiratory depression in a dose-dependent manner. Because there are no antagonists for these substances, the respiratory depressant effect cannot be easily reversed. Propofol also causes a significant decrease in systemic blood pressure. Nonetheless, it is now one of the most widely used fixed anesthetics because recovery is more rapid after propofol than with other agents.

■ **Preanesthetic Medications** A number of drugs are used as preanesthetic medications (Table 6.5). Fixed anesthetics such as **midazolam, thiopental,** and **propofol** are administered to speed the induction of anesthesia with the inhalational agents and to reduce the amount of volatile anesthetic necessary to maintain the desired level of anesthesia.

Anxiolytics, such as **diazepam,** are sometimes administered preoperatively

Table 6.5 *Preanesthetic Medications*

PURPOSE	AGENTS
Speed induction and reduce amount of general anesthetic needed to maintain desired level of anesthesia	Midazolam Thiopental Propofol
Reduce preoperative anxiety	Diazepam
Reduce preoperative and postoperative pain	Morphine
Reduce adverse effects of inhalational anesthetics	Scopolamine Glycopyrrolate

to reduce anxiety because an anxious patient requires more anesthetic than a calm individual.

When pain is present before surgery or is anticipated postsurgically, opioids, such as **morphine,** may be administered preoperatively. This also helps calm the patient and ease induction, especially if the pain is severe.

Some preanesthetic medications are administered to counter anticipated adverse effects of the general anesthetics. Anticholinergics, such as **scopolamine** and **glycopyrrolate,** are used for this purpose. These agents counteract the bradycardia associated with some general anesthetics and inhibit secretions induced by inhalational agents that are irritating to the respiratory tract. Scopolamine also has antiemetic properties.

Other drugs sometimes used as preanesthetic medications are antihistamines, such as **hydroxyzine,** and antiemetics, such as **cyclizine** (Box 6.14).

Box 6.14

AGENTS USED IN GENERAL ANESTHESIA

Inhalational Anesthetics

Nitrous oxide
Halothane
Enflurane
Isoflurane
Methoxyflurane

Fixed Anesthetics

Innovar
Ketamine
Thiopental
Propofol
Midazolam

Preanesthetic Medications

Diazepam
Morphine
Scopolamine
Glycopyrrolate
Hydroxyzine
Cyclizine

Section 6.4 Local Anesthetics

■ **Overview** Nerve conduction is blocked by a variety of drugs, some of which are used as local anesthetics. These agents are classified on the basis of their chemical structures into two types: esters, such as **procaine,** and amides, such as **lidocaine** (Box 6.15).

> ### Box 6.15
>
> | **LOCAL ANESTHETICS** |
> |---|
> | **Esters** |
> | Cocaine |
> | Procaine |
> | Tetracaine |
> | Benzocaine |
> | **Amides** |
> | Lidocaine |
> | Mepivacaine |
> | Bupivacaine |

Local anesthetics must penetrate to the membrane of axons of peripheral nerves without causing irritation, must stabilize nerve membranes at physiologic pH, and must bind reversibly to nerves. An ideal local anesthetic should act promptly, predictably, and reversibly to interrupt conduction of nerve impulses. It should have a reasonably rapid onset of activity, and the effect should last for the time necessary to complete the procedure with minimal adverse effects. Procaine, lidocaine, and **tetracaine** come closest to this ideal.

■ **Basic Pharmacology** Local anesthetics are applied topically or injected near the nerve to be blocked. To prolong anesthesia, vasoconstrictors, such as epinephrine, may be added to the preparation. Because less local anesthetic is required in this case, there is a lower systemic toxicity. Local anesthetics can penetrate all tissues, including the brain and the placenta.

Local anesthetics stabilize nerve membranes by depressing sodium and potassium conductance, thereby slowing the propagation of the action potential. Duration of action of different local anesthetics varies significantly.

Local anesthetics are destroyed either by esterases (serum or liver) or amidases (liver). Therefore the metabolism of local anesthetics takes place after the drugs have reached the circulatory system. Because esters are hydrolyzed more readily, they are shorter-acting than amides.

■ **Pharmacotherapeutics**

● **Clinical use** Some local anesthetics, such as **cocaine** and **benzocaine,** are effective topically because they penetrate mucous membranes. Procaine is an example of an agent useful only for infiltration anesthesia or spinal block. Some agents such as lidocaine, **mepivacaine,** or **bupivacaine,** are used for infiltration, peripheral nerve block, or epidural block.

Local anesthetics are useful in surgical procedures that are not extensive. They are of greatest use for outpatient surgery. Their use eliminates the need for the extensive postanesthesia care required with general anesthetics.

Hemorrhoidectomy and transurethral resection of the prostate are examples of procedures that lend themselves to regional local anesthetic block.

■ Adverse Effects

- **Central nervous system** Esters have a greater stimulatory effect than amides on the CNS. Convulsive seizures are therefore more common with the ester-type local anesthetics.

- **Cardiovascular** Both the amide and ester local anesthetics are depressants for both the myocardial conduction system and the peripheral vascular tone. Hypotension is a common adverse effect for all local anesthetics.

SECTION 6.5 ANTIDEPRESSANTS

■ **Overview** Antidepressants have several therapeutic applications. Their primary use is in the treatment of affective illness. Antidepressants are used most frequently in endogenous depression, a serious depression not correlated with life events. Other depressive states include reactive depression and bipolar disease. Reactive depression is related to life events, such as a personal loss or physical illness. Bipolar disease, or manic-depressive disorder, is least common.

Endogenous depression is a life-threatening disorder. Symptoms include profound sadness, pessimism, loss of interest, sleep disturbances, change in appetite, diminished libido, and difficulty in concentration. About 15% of endogenously depressed individuals commit suicide.

Several chemical classes of drugs display antidepressant properties. Included are the first-generation tricyclic antidepressants, second-generation agents, and monoamine oxidase (MAO) inhibitors. Although these drugs cause numerous well-defined neurochemical changes, their precise mechanism of action as antidepressants remains unclear.

■ **Basic Pharmacology** Many antidepressants block norepinephrine and serotonin reuptake into neurons. Fluoxetine, a second-generation agent, is more effective and selective at serotonin neurons than first-generation agents. Desipramine, a first-generation compound, blocks norepinephrine and serotonin uptake. Bupropion and trimipramine are weak inhibitors of norepinephrine and serotonin uptake. It is unclear whether the effectiveness of antidepressants is related to their selectivity for either norepinephrine or serotonin uptake sites. However, serotonin uptake inhibition is required for effective treatment of certain anxiety disorders and obsessive compulsive disorder.

First-generation antidepressants are also potent antagonists at various receptor systems. Of particular note is the inhibition of histamine H_1 and muscarinic cholinergic receptors by the tricyclic antidepressants. Many tricyclics also block α-adrenoceptor and dopamine D2 receptor sites (Box 6.16).

Box 6.16

FIRST-GENERATION TRICYCLICS
Receptor Blockade
Histamine
α-Adrenergic
Muscarinic cholinergic

■ **First-Generation Antidepressants** Because of their chemical structure, many first-generation antidepressants are referred to as tricyclics. These drugs are absorbed orally and undergo significant first-pass metabolism. High lipid solubility and protein binding yields a large volume of distribution. The tricyclics are extensively metabolized.

Examples of first-generation tricyclic antidepressants are imipramine, amitriptyline, desipramine, doxepin, nortriptyline, and protriptyline (Box 6.17).

The prototypes of the first-generation tricyclic antidepressants are imipramine and amitriptyline. These drugs are highly effective antidepressants, although they require several weeks of continuous administration before clinical improvement is noted.

- **Adverse effects** The anticholinergic effects associated with first-generation tricyclics include dry mouth (xerostomia), decreased near vision (mydriasis), urinary retention, constipation, sinus tachycardia, and anticholinergic psychosis (Box 6.18). Antihistaminic effects of these agents include sedation, weight gain, and possibly hypotension, whereas the α_1-adrenergic blockade (α_1-adrenoceptor) is responsible for orthostatic hypotension.

Box 6.17

> ### FIRST-GENERATION AGENTS—TRICYCLICS
>
> Imipramine
> Amitriptyline
> Doxepin
> Desipramine
> Nortriptyline
> Protriptyline
> Clomipramine

Box 6.18

> ### ADVERSE EFFECTS ASSOCIATED WITH FIRST-GENERATION TRICYCLICS
>
> Dry mouth
> Orthostatic hypotension
> Blurred vision
> Urinary retention
> Sedation

■ **Monoamine Oxidase Inhibitors** The MAO inhibitors display significant antidepressant activity. These agents are well absorbed orally and require several weeks of treatment for antidepressant activity to be clinically meaningful. Drugs included in this group are **tranylcypromine, phenelzine** and **isocarboxazid.** The therapeutic effects of MAO inhibitors require monoamine oxidase to be inhibited to a significant extent.

The cardiovascular side effects can be serious and result from their anticholinergic effects, reuptake blockade of monoamines, and a direct myocardial depressant. Sexual dysfunctions include loss of libido, impaired erection or erectile function, impaired ejaculation, and priapism. The tricyclic antidepressants are epileptogenic, although the frequency of this effect is low.

- **Adverse effects** The MAO inhibitors can cause myoclonus. Autonomic nervous system-related adverse effects include dry mouth, blurred vision, constipation, and urinary hesitancy. Sexual dysfunction or hypertension may occur with MAO inhibitors. Hypertension is a risk with the MAO inhibitors.

The combination of MAO inhibition and ingestion of foods containing tyramine (primarily fermented foods and beverages) can result in hypertensive crisis. This reaction is due to the inhibition of the metabolism of tyramine, an indirect-acting sympathomimetic agent.

■ **Second-Generation Antidepressants**

- **Basic pharmacology** The second-generation agents have significantly fewer adverse effects than the first-generation antidepressants. They are less cardiotoxic and have fewer anticholinergic effects. Second-generation

Monoamine Oxidase Inhibitors
Phenelzine
Isocarboxazid
Tranylcypromine

Second-Generation Agents
Fewer side effects

agents have similar pharmacokinetics to those described for first-generation antidepressants.

Second-Generation

Amoxapine
Maprotiline
Trazodone
Bupropion

**Second-Generation
Selective Serotonin
Reuptake Inhibitors (SSRI)**

Fluoxetine
Paroxetine
Sertraline
Fluvoxamine

Fluoxetine is one of the most popular second-generation antidepressants. Fluoxetine is well absorbed after oral administration and is metabolized by the liver to an active metabolite. Fluoxetine has been found to be at least as effective as imipramine or amitriptyline for the treatment of endogenous depression. Like the tricyclics, the onset of the therapeutic response to fluoxetine is delayed one to three weeks. Fluoxetine is a highly selective and potent inhibitor of serotonin reuptake.

Amoxapine resembles two effective antipsychotic drugs, loxapine and clozapine, and may exhibit some antipsychotic side effects.

Maprotiline has almost no effect on the serotonergic system.

Trazodone is a serotonin uptake inhibitor with few anticholinergic or cardiovascular side effects.

● **Adverse effects** Nausea, nervousness, headache, and insomnia are adverse effects associated with fluoxetine (Box 6.19). Fluoxetine may cause mania or hypomania.

Box 6.19

SIDE EFFECTS ASSOCIATED WITH FLUOXETINE ADMINISTRATION
Nausea Nervousness Insomnia Headache

Extrapyramidal symptoms are associated with the use of amoxapine, and maprotiline displays some anticholinergic effects, although less so than the tricyclic agents.

■ **Pharmacotherapeutics: The Treatment of Depression**

● **Clinical use** Antidepressants are used in the treatment of major endogenous depressive disorders (Box 6.20). The tricyclics and second-generation drugs are typically the drugs of choice. The MAO inhibitors are used in individuals who have atypical depression, which is characterized by anxiety, phobic features, and hypochondriasis. The MAO inhibitors are also effective in endogenous depression, but their use is limited because of the potential for adverse cardiovascular effects associated with the ingestion of tyramine.

Box 6.20

CLINICAL USES FOR ANTIDEPRESSANTS
Major endogenous depression Atypical depression Obsessive compulsive disorder Chronic pain treatment Posttraumatic stress syndrome

The elderly population has a higher incidence of suicide than any other group in the United States. First-generation agents used for treating depression in geriatric patients include **nortriptyline** and **desipramine**. Desipramine has less anticholinergic and hypotensive effects and is relatively nonsedating as compared with other tricyclics. Other first-generation agents are avoided because they are more likely to induce orthostatic hypotension. The MAO inhibitors are effective in treating depression in the elderly. These drugs are less sedating and more stimulating than the tricyclics. The second-generation agents **fluoxetine, trazodone,** and **fluvoxamine** are routinely prescribed for treating depression in the elderly.

Obsessive Compulsive Disorders
Clomipramine

    Clomipramine is an imipramine derivative effective in treating obsessive compulsive disorder. Like fluoxetine and fluvoxamine, which are also effective in this condition, clomipramine is a selective serotonin reuptake inhibitor.

● **Other clinical considerations** Physiologic effects of posttraumatic stress include autonomic hyperreactivity, nightmares, and flashbacks. All of these symptoms are effectively treated with tricyclic antidepressants. Some of the autonomic effects may be lessened by propranolol, a β-adrenoceptor antagonist, and persistent flashbacks may be diminished by carbamazepine.

    Alprazolam, a benzodiazepine, has been found useful in the treatment of mild to moderate endogenous depression. In some cases alprazolam is as effective as imipramine, amitriptyline, or doxepin and displays fewer adverse effects.

    Tricyclic antidepressants are also useful in the treatment of some types of chronic pain.

SECTION 6.6 OPIOID ANALGESICS AND ANTAGONISTS

■ **Overview** The opioid analgesics are primarily used for the treatment of severe pain. These analgesics are effective for both acute, sharp, and continuous visceral pain. Opioid agonists alter the psychologic perception of pain rather than reducing the pain itself. The classical prototype drug in this class is **morphine,** a naturally occurring opiate (Box 6.21).

Box 6.21

OPIOID ANALGESICS
Morphine
Hydromorphone
Oxymorphone
Methadone
Meperidine
Fentanyl
Sufentanyl
Oxycodone
Codeine
Pentazocine
Propoxyphene

■ **Opioid Analgesics** The opioid agonists may also be used in treatment of acute pulmonary edema, renal and biliary colic, and for cough suppression. The use of these agents is limited somewhat by the development of physical dependence and tolerance. Depending on the duration of treatment and response, withdrawal symptoms may occur after discontinuation of medication. Opioid agonists can produce severe, life-threatening respiratory depression and are drugs of abuse.

- **Basic pharmacology** Opioid analgesics are well absorbed from IM and subcutaneous (SQ) sites and from the gastrointestinal tract and nasal mucosa. They rapidly leave the blood and distribute to major organs, with most localized in muscle. **Fentanyl,** a highly lipophilic opioid agonist, accumulates in fat. Some agents, including heroin and codeine, readily cross the blood-brain barrier. Opioid agonists easily pass the placental barrier and readily gain access to the fetal brain. This can result in respiratory depression in the newborn.

    Opioid analgesics are metabolized primarily to more polar compounds that are excreted by the kidney. Small quantities of parent compound may also be excreted in the urine. Some agents, such as morphine, are conjugated with glucuronic acid. Others, such as **meperidine,** are hydrolyzed by tissue esterases.

    Opioid agonists combine with specific opioid receptor subtypes to produce pharmacologic effects (Box 6.22). The activation of mu opioid receptors produces respiratory depression, euphoria, physical dependency, and supraspinal analgesia.

Box 6.22

SPECIFIC OPIOID RECEPTORS
Mu
Respiratory depression
Physical dependency
Euphoria
Kappa
Miosis
Sedation
Sigma
Dysphoria
Cardiac stimulation
Hallucinations

Stimulation of kappa opioid receptors causes miosis, sedation, and spinal cord analgesia.

Endogenous opioid peptides (endorphins) interact with these receptors. Several different classes of endorphins have been isolated, one of which is the enkephalins.

Physical dependence to opioids occurs after repeated administration. Abrupt discontinuation of opioids may precipitate withdrawal symptoms, which are often physiologic effects exactly opposite to those observed after administration of the opioid. For example, although opioid agonists cause constipation, diarrhea is a characteristic of withdrawal. Although CNS hyperactivity accompanies withdrawal, convulsions are rarely observed. In those with compromised cardiovascular function, withdrawal from opioid agonists may be life threatening. Overall, the signs and symptoms of withdrawal include apprehension, tremor, headache, irritability, sweating, muscular weakness, diarrhea, increased heart rate, muscle spasm, ketosis, vomiting, and anorexia.

Symptoms of Withdrawal

Apprehension
Tremor
Headache
↑ Heart rate
Muscle spasm
Ketosis
Vomiting
Anorexia

- **Central nervous system effects** The effects of opioid analgesics on the CNS are among the most significant. These include analgesia, euphoria, sedation, cough suppression, and respiratory depression. The analgesia results primarily from an altered perception and reaction to painful stimuli. Opioid agonists also raise the pain threshold, although this effect is of secondary importance. The analgesic response to morphine is especially prominent in anxious patients.

  Opioid agonists reduce anxiety and induce euphoria. The potential for opioid abuse is a result of these properties. However, pain relief should not be denied solely because opioids have abuse potential. Moreover, individuals who are not in pain may experience dysphoria and restlessness at analgesic doses.

- **Gastrointestinal** The major effect of opioid agonists on the gastrointestinal tract is constipation.

- **Genitourinary** Opioid agonists depress renal function by decreasing renal plasma flow. They also increase urethral and bladder tone, which can cause urinary retention in the postoperative state.

- **Uterine** Opioid analgesics prolong labor. This is due to effects on the CNS and to direct relaxation of smooth muscle.

- **Neuroendocrine** Opioid analgesics stimulate the release of prolactin, somatropin, and antidiuretic hormone, and inhibit the release of luteinizing hormone.

- **Adverse effects** Major adverse effects of the opioid analgesics include miosis, sedation, constipation, respiratory depression, euphoria, dysphoria, nausea, emesis, mental clouding, and biliary spasm. The most important organ system toxicity is respiratory depression secondary to an action of the opioid on the medulla. These opioids lessen sensitivity of the respiratory control center to carbon dioxide. Most deaths associated with opioid analgesics are due to respiratory failure.

- **Pharmacology** Meperidine is a synthetic morphine-like drug. It is less potent and shorter-acting than morphine and has significant anticholinergic properties. As a result it should be used with caution in the presence of tachycardia.

  Methadone is another synthetic morphine-like drug. Longer-lasting and more effective orally than morphine, methadone is used for maintenance therapy in heroin dependency. Methadone withdrawal is milder than morphine withdrawal. Methadone also blocks the euphoriant effects of IV heroin.

  Fentanyl is a synthetic opioid analgesic that is administered IV. Considerably more potent than morphine, fentanyl is used both as an analgesic and as a fixed anesthetic. Sufentanyl, which is ten times more potent than fentanyl, is used for anesthesia. The combination of fentanyl and droperidol is used as a fixed general anesthetic.

  Pentazocine is a partial agonist at opioid receptors. Its general properties are similar to morphine when it is used as an analgesic. If given after morphine, pentazocine can precipitate withdrawal because, as a partial agonist, it blocks the response to a full agonist.

  Codeine and d-propoxyphene are used to treat mild pain. Codeine is also an effective antitussive agent, although it has been largely replaced by dextromethorphan.

  Several drugs chemically related to the opioids are used as antitussives,

Opioid Agonists
Respiratory depression

Adverse Effects
Miosis
Sedation
Constipation
Respiratory depression
Euphoria
Dysphoria
Nausea
Emesis
Mental clouding
Biliary spasm

Antitussives

Codeine
Dihydrocodeine
l-propoxyphene
Dextromethorphan
Noscapine

Opioid Antagonists

Naloxone
Naltrexone

Antidiarrheals

Diphenoxylate
Loperamide

Hyperpyretic Coma

Opioids
+
MAO inhibitors

including codeine, dihydrocodeine, l-propoxyphene, dextromethorphan, and noscapine. Dextromethorphan is commonly used in cough syrups. It is not addictive unless taken in large quantities.

Opioid receptor antagonists are useful because they reverse the potentially lethal respiratory depressant response to opioids. The principal drugs in this class are **naloxone** and **naltrexone**. Naloxone has a duration of action of only 1 to 4 hours and must be given by injection because it is poorly absorbed orally. Naltrexone is given orally and has a half-life of about 10 hours. Naloxone is mainly used to treat acute overdosage of opioid agonists.

● **Pharmacotherapeutics**

— *Clinical use* The primary use of opioid agonists is for the relief of pain, especially sharp pain. The severe pain associated with renal and biliary colic is effectively managed with opioid agonists. These drugs increase smooth muscle tone and as a result increase the spasm around the stone. Because this effect increases pain, higher doses of opioids are required for effective analgesia in this condition.

Opioid agonists are used in the treatment of acute pulmonary edema. A decrease in myocardial preload, afterload, perception of shortness of breath, and anxiety contribute to relief of dyspnea.

Opioid analgesics are used to treat diarrhea. Agents with selective gastrointestinal effects, such as **diphenoxylate** and **loperamide,** are particularly useful.

— *Other clinical considerations* Cancer pain must be treated without regard to tolerance and dependence. Thus the dosage of opioid analgesics should be individualized. The preferred route of administration is oral because of convenience and because tolerance develops at a slower rate when drugs are given orally. Continuous administration of the analgesic is important if cancer pain is constant. Frequent administration will result in sedation, constipation, nausea, vomiting, and respiratory depression. The sedation may be reduced if the frequency of dosing is increased and the dosage is decreased. Constipation may be relieved by stool softeners and laxatives. Nausea and vomiting are controlled by **hydroxyzine.**

Opioid agonists are sometimes combined with other drugs in treating cancer pain. Anticonvulsants such as **carbamazepine** are useful in management of neuralgias that complicate tumor progression. Phenothiazines may help in the opioid tolerant patient, and tricyclic antidepressants are suggested for terminal use in posttherapy neuralgia, vincristine- and cisplatin-induced neuropathy, and postthoracotomy incisional pain.

Some opioids should not be used for treating chronic cancer pain. For example, meperidine is too short-acting and yields a metabolite, normeperidine, which can produce anxiety, tremor, and seizures.

● **Prominent drug interactions** Concomitant use of sedative-hypnotics with opioid analgesics enhances the likelihood of respiratory depression. The combination of opioids and antipsychotics results in greater sedation and enhances the anticholinergic and α-adrenoceptor antagonist effects on the cardiovascular system. Opioid agonists should not be administered with MAO inhibitors because this combination can produce hyperpyretic coma and hypertension.

SECTION 6.7 CENTRAL NERVOUS SYSTEM STIMULANTS/DRUGS OF ABUSE

■ **Overview** CNS stimulants include methylxanthines, which are found in coffee, tea, cocoa, and colas, nicotine, which is found in tobacco products, amphetamines, and cocaine (Box 6.23).

> **Box 6.23**
>
> ### MAJOR CENTRAL NERVOUS SYSTEM STIMULANTS
>
> Methylxanthines
> Nicotine
> Amphetamines and cocaine

■ **Methylxanthines** Methylxanthines affect many organ systems, including the CNS, heart, and kidney. The CNS effects induce enhanced mental acuity and reduced mental fatigue.

  ● **Basic pharmacology** Methylxanthines are readily absorbed after oral administration and distribute throughout the body. These agents, which include **caffeine, theobromine,** and **theophylline,** cross the placenta. Methylxanthines are metabolized by the liver and are excreted in the urine.

  Methylxanthines stimulate the CNS and increase heart rate and cardiac output. Cardiac arrhythmias may be produced by these drugs. Caffeine has a mild diuretic action.

  Although caffeine is the most widely consumed methylxanthine, theophylline is more important therapeutically. Theophylline is a primary therapy for the treatment of asthma because it relaxes the bronchiolar smooth muscle.

  Mechanisms of action of methylxanthines include blockade of adenosine receptors, increases in cyclic nucleotides, and effects on calcium distribution.

■ **Nicotine** Nicotine is an addictive drug that is very lipid soluble, easily entering and stimulating the brain. It acts as a CNS depressant at higher doses.

  ● **Basic pharmacology** Nicotine from tobacco is absorbed by the mucosa and rapidly enters the circulation, affecting many organ systems. In addition to CNS stimulation, nicotine increases blood pressure and heart rate. Peripheral vasoconstriction in the fingers and toes is prominent. Coronary blood flow may also be decreased because of vasoconstriction. Mechanisms of action of nicotine include ganglionic stimulation followed by blockade, and activation of CNS nicotine receptors.

■ **Amphetamines** Amphetamines are potent stimulants of the CNS and produce many of the same effects observed with methylxanthines. They are well absorbed from the gastrointestinal tract and are metabolized by the liver and excreted by the kidney.

  ● **Basic pharmacology** The CNS effects of the amphetamines produce feelings of increased energy, self-confidence, and euphoria and are accompanied by increases in motor activity, appetite suppression, and insomnia. Amphetamines act by promoting release of CNS neurotransmitters, especially dopamine.

Use

Narcolepsy
Hyperkinetic syndrome

Anorexiants

Diethylpropion
Fenfluramine
Phendimetrazine
Phentermine

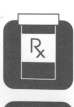

● Pharmacotherapeutics

— *Clinical use* The clinical uses of the amphetamines (dl-amphetamine, d-amphetamine, methamphetamine) include treatment of narcolepsy and of hyperkinetic syndrome in children. In some hyperactive children, amphetamine increases the ability to concentrate and to perform tasks. Methylphenidate is a CNS stimulant used to treat hyperactivity.

Some CNS stimulants are used as anorexiants. These drugs should be used only as a temporary adjunct to an overall weight-reduction program. The development of adverse effects and loss of effectiveness occur rapidly with these agents. Many are available as over-the-counter drugs. Included are diethylpropion, fenfluramine, phendimetrazine, and phentermine.

● **Adverse effects** Adverse effects associated with the use of stimulants include tachycardia, hypertension, increased reflex vagal tone, and cardiac arrhythmias. The signs and symptoms of acute overdosage can be characterized as mild, moderate, and severe. Mild effects are restlessness, tremors, talkativeness, anorexia, irritability, tachycardia, flushing, sweating, analgesia, and hyperactive reflexes. Moderate effects include confusion, delirium, hallucinations (visual), profuse sweating, fever, hypertension, cardiac irregularities, and panic states. Severe effects include convulsions, circulatory collapse, hyperpyrexia, coma, and death. Severe intoxication occurs rarely in the healthy adult.

■ **Chemical Abuse and Dependence**

● **Overview** Alcohol, opioids, and other CNS-active agents may be drugs of abuse.

● **Alcohol** Alcohol is a drug for which self-induced intoxication is widely accepted. Suicides, accidental deaths, and homicides result from alcohol abuse. With the possible exception of cigarette smoking, alcoholism is the most serious medical problem associated with nonprescription drugs in the United States.

— *Basic pharmacology* The development of tolerance accompanies the chronic abuse of alcohol and permits consumption of larger amounts without the individual exhibiting many of the signs of drunkenness. Although tolerance to many of the effects of alcohol is increased about twofold or threefold, the lethal dose is not significantly altered. The major cause of tolerance in alcoholics is adaptive changes in the CNS and other organ systems, rather than a more rapid metabolization of the drug.

— *Pharmacotherapeutics*
Clinical considerations. The main objective in treating acute alcohol overdosage is the prevention of severe respiratory depression and aspiration of vomitus. Successful management of alcohol intoxication requires support of the cardiovascular and respiratory systems. In addition, metabolic abnormalities and dehydration may require treatment.

With chronic alcoholics, initial withdrawal symptoms include an increase in blood pressure, respiratory rate, temperature, and pulse and a slight tremor. Vomiting, anxiety, nausea, sweating, hyperreflexia, and seizures can occur. Grand mal seizures are a dangerous complication of withdrawal. A severe withdrawal syndrome, delirium tremens, occurs within 2 days after the last dose of alcohol. Characteristics of this syndrome include hypertension, hyperthermia, tremor, hallucinations, and tachycardia. The major objective in the treatment of alcohol withdrawal is prevention of delirium, seizures, and arrhythmias.

Alcohol detoxification may require the temporary use of another sedative-hypnotic as an alcohol substitute. The drug of choice for this purpose is diazepam. For alcoholics who have confirmed liver disease, oxazepam may be preferred. Oxazepam is metabolized to a water-soluble, inactive metabolite that does not accumulate in the body.

— *Drug interactions* Alcohol can influence the response to many drugs because of its effect on microsomal enzyme activity. Many drugs, especially other CNS depressants, augment alcohol-enhanced CNS depression.

— *Other sedatives* Treatment of withdrawal from barbiturates and other sedative-hypnotic agents is the same as for alcohol. Convulsions associated with withdrawal are the most serious problem in the clinical management of withdrawal. As with alcohol, the addict is treated with a substitute agent, such as diazepam, and the dose is tapered over time.

● **Opioids** The most frequently abused opioids are morphine, oxycodone, and heroin. The user must increase the dose of these drugs over time to continue to obtain the desired effect.

— *Pharmacotherapeutics*

Clinical considerations. Special medical problems are associated with opioid abuse. Many of these relate to the fact that these drugs are administered IV; hepatitis B viral infections occur frequently because of shared use of contaminated hypodermic syringes, IV drug abuse is a risk category for HIV infection, and bacterial infections from IV drug use can lead to meningitis and osteomyelitis.

— *Treatment of opioid dependency* Substitution of a long-acting, orally active opioid is the preferred method to wean an addict from the opioid. **Methadone** has been used for this purpose and more recently **clonidine**, an α-adrenoceptor agonist, has been found useful. Clonidine, a nonaddicting, nonopioid compound, probably works by reducing sympathetic outflow, decreasing the physiologic components of withdrawal.

● **Stimulants** Abused stimulants include amphetamines and cocaine. Amphetamine abuse is characterized by repeated IV injections to produce feelings of euphoria and alertness. Following days of use, a paranoid schizophrenic-like syndrome may appear. Intense periods of abuse end when the individual is exhausted from sleeplessness. Withdrawal characteristics include mental depression, exhaustion, hunger, and sleepiness. Overdose with amphetamines is seldom fatal. With chronic amphetamine abuse, necrotizing arteritis can lead to fatal brain hemorrhages or renal failure.

● **Cocaine** Cocaine has been characterized as a highly potent amphetamine. It is far more likely to lead to dependence than amphetamines. Sniffing and freebasing are two popular methods of administration. IV injection is not as common, in part because of the high risk of overdosage. Overdoses of cocaine may be rapidly fatal, with the individual dying within a few minutes. Death is caused by respiratory depression and convulsions. CNS actions of cocaine are probably due to inhibition of CNS neurotransmitter re-uptake. Effects on dopamine levels may be responsible for euphoric effects noted with cocaine.

Hallucinogens

Mescaline
LSD
Psilocybin
Phencyclidine (PCP)
"Designer drugs"

● **Hallucinogens** Mescaline, LSD, psilocybin, phencyclidine (PCP), and the increasingly popular "designer drugs" are hallucinogens. Hallucinogenic effects include distortions of perspective, less discriminate hearing, visual illusions, and distortion of time perception. There are also memory impairments, altered moods, and poor judgment. Pupillary dilation, hyperactivity of the sympathetic system, tremor, and increased heart rate are some physiologic signs. These hallucinogens may be acting through 5-HT and 5-HT receptor subtypes.

     Scopolamine, an antimuscarinic agent, can produce delirium disorientation, memory loss, and delusions. **Phencyclidine** produces feelings of detachment and disorientation. Physiologic effects include nystagmus, tachycardia, and hypertension. Overdosage has been lethal.

● **Marijuana** The most common route of administration of marijuana in western countries is by smoking. The very high lipid solubility of the primary active component, tetrahydrocannabinol (THC), results in trapping on the surfactant lining of the lungs. As a result, smoking is similar, pharmacokinetically, to IV administration. Early stages of marijuana intoxication include euphoria, laughter, time distortion, and sharpened vision. Heightened pulse rate and reddening of the conjunctiva are two prominent signs of marijuana use. Heavy marijuana smoking can cause respiratory problems similar to those of cigarette smoking. This includes chronic bronchitis, airway obstruction, and squamous cell metaplasia.

     Some samples of marijuana contain pathogenic aspergillus, which can cause invasive pulmonary and allergic aspergillosis. This problem has been noted when marijuana is used as an antiemetic drug in immunodeficient patients with cancer receiving chemotherapy.

Inhalants

Nitrous oxide
Industrial solvents
Aerosols
Propellants
Organic nitrites

● **Inhalants** Abused inhalants include nitrous oxide, industrial solvents, aerosol propellants, and organic nitrites. These agents nonspecifically alter CNS function.

Box 6.24

NEUROMUSCULAR BLOCKING AGENTS
Competitive
Tubocurarine
Metocurine
Atracurium
Doxacurium
Mivacurium
Pancuronium
Pipercuronium
Rocuronium
Vecuronium
Depolarizing
Succinylcholine
Decamethonium

SECTION 6.8 SKELETAL MUSCLE RELAXANTS

■ **Overview** Skeletal muscle relaxants interact with nicotinic receptors at the neuromuscular junction and to some extent on postganglionic neurons to produce paralysis. Peripherally acting neuromuscular blocking agents fall into two categories: competitive and depolarizing (Box 6.24). The actions of these drugs are modified by other drugs and physiologic states.

■ **Clinical Uses** Skeletal muscle relaxants are used primarily as an adjunct to anesthesia. The muscle relaxation they produce facilitates intubation and incision. This decreases the amount of general anesthetic required.

     In addition to surgery, these drugs are used in electroconvulsant therapy (succinylcholine), in the diagnosis of multiple sclerosis (D-tubocurarine), and in the diagnosis of pain caused by nerve root compression masked by muscle spasm.

■ **Competitive Neuromuscular Blocking Agents** Competitive neuromuscular blocking agents act as competitive antagonists at the neuromuscular nicotinic receptor, thus blocking the actions of acetylcholine. Examples of competitive neuromuscular blocking agents are D-tubocurarine, metocurine, and pancuronium.

Competitive Agents

D-tubocurarine
Metocurine
Pancuronium

  ● **Pharmacologic effects** Competitive neuromuscular blocking agents produce muscle weakness and flaccidity. Small muscles are affected first, and respiratory muscles are affected last.

■ **Depolarizing Agents** Depolarizing agents are nicotinic receptor agonists used at high doses to produce depolarization blockade. Under these circumstances sodium channels are inactivated. Depolarizing agents include succinylcholine, which is the most commonly used drug in this class, and decamethonium.

Depolarizing Agents

Succinylcholine
Decamethonium

  ● **Pharmacologic effects** Because they are agonists, the initial effects of depolarizing agents are muscle fasciculation or contraction followed by relaxation. Limbs are affected first, and respiratory muscles are affected last.

  ● **Pharmacokinetics** Skeletal muscle relaxants are almost always administered IV. They have a short duration of action. Metabolism varies with the drug.

  ● **Drug interactions** The actions of neuromuscular blocking agents are modified by many other drugs and physiologic states. Accordingly, care must be taken in the use of these agents. For example, general anesthetics depress motor centers in the brain and decrease the sensitivity of the motor end plate to acetylcholine by interfering with opening of Na^+-K^+ channels. Halothane is particularly potent in this regard. The aminoglycosides and tetracycline antibiotics inhibit neuromuscular transmission by decreasing acetylcholine release. The calcium channel blockers potentiate the effects of both competitive and depolarizing neuromuscular blockers. The potency of D-tubocurarine increases in acidosis and decreases with alkalosis. Body temperature alters the rate of excretion and metabolism of the muscle relaxants as well as the rate of muscle membranes.

     The response to skeletal muscle relaxants varies greatly among patients, depending on the status of their renal function and the activity of nonspecific cholinesterase. Numerous other drugs, including certain opioids, local anesthetics, anticonvulsants, and cardiovascular drugs, also interact with neuromuscular blocking agents to enhance or reduce their effectiveness (Table 6.6).

  ● **Adverse effects** D-Tubocurarine causes histamine release which can result in hypotension and bronchospasm. Other neuromuscular blocking agents release histamine, but they do so to a lesser extent. This effect can be dangerous in patients with asthma or ulcers. Cardiovascular effects vary with individual agents, as shown in Table 6.7. Blockade of ganglionic transmission can result in decreased gastrointestinal motility.

SECTION 6.9 PARKINSONISM AND OTHER MOVEMENT DISORDERS

■ **Overview** Parkinson's disease is an idiopathic disorder resulting from the degeneration of the nigrostriatal dopamine pathway (Fig. 6.3). Symptoms include tremor, rigidity, and bradykinesia. Similar symptoms can occur with viral infection, certain medications such as antipsychotics, and other neurologic disorders

Table 6.6   *Comparison of Competitive and Depolarizing Neuromuscular Blocking Agents*

EFFECTS	COMPETITIVE	DEPOLARIZING
Action at receptor	Antagonist	Agonist
Effect on motor end plate depolarization	None	Partial persistent depolarization
Initial effect on striated muscle	None	Fasciculation
Muscles affected first	Small muscles	Skeletal muscle
Muscles affected last	Respiratory	Respiratory
Effect of AchE inhibitors	Reversal	No effect or increased duration
Effect of Ach agonists	Reversal	No effect
Effect on previously administered D-tubocurarine	Additive	Antagonism
Effect on previously administered succinylcholine	No effect of antagonism	Tachyphylaxis or no effect
Effect of halothane	Increase potency	Decrease potency
Effect of antibiotics	Increase potency	Decrease potency
Effect of Ca^{++} channel blockers	Increase potency	Increase potency

Table 6.7   *Attributes of Neuromuscular Blocking Agents*

	D-TUBOCURARINE	METOCURINE	PANCURONIUM	SUCCINYLCHOLINE
Type	Competitive	Competitive	Competitive	Depolarizing
Site of action junction	N-M junction and ganglion	N-M junction and ganglion	N-M junction	N-M junction and ganglion
Enters CNS	No	No	No	No
Crosses placenta	Negligible	—	—	—
Effect on				
Histamine release	+++	++	+	++
Heart rate	Decrease	Decrease	Increase	Decrease
Blood pressure	Decrease	Decrease	Increase	Increase or decrease
Potency altered by pH	Yes	No	No	No
Other effects				1. Increase intraocular pressure 2. K$^+$ release from muscle leading to electrolyte imbalance
Duration of action	20 min Residual effects 2-4 hours	20 min	20 min	20 min
Metabolism and excretion	1. urinary 2. bile Some metabolism	1. urinary 2. bile Some metabolism	Hepatic metab	Hydrolyzed by plasma and liver cholinesterases
Uses	Surgery MS diagnosis	Surgery More potent than D-tubocurarine	Surgery	Surgery Electroconvulsive therapy

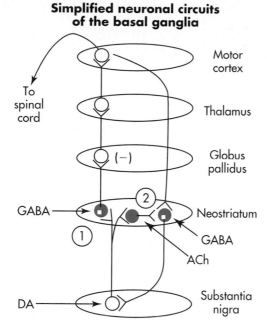

**Simplified neuronal circuits
of the basal ganglia**

Motor cortex

To spinal cord

Thalamus

Globus pallidus   (−)

GABA   Neostriatum

GABA

ACh

DA   Substantia nigra

Site of action for:
1. Levodopa, Bromocriptine, Selegiline
2. Anticholinergics

Fig. 6.3 Site of action within the neuronal circuits of the basal ganglia from drugs used to treat parkinsonian disorders. *DA,* dopamine; *GABA,* γ-amino-butyric acid; *ACh,* acetylcholine.

such as carbon monoxide poisoning, progressive supranuclear palsy, and Creutzfeldt-Jakob disease. The primary therapeutic approach (Box 6.25) to treat this condition is to increase the availability of dopamine in the brain. Anticholinergic drugs are also beneficial.

■ **Levodopa (L-dopa)** L-Dopa is a dopamine precursor that is able to cross the blood-brain barrier. After entering the brain, it is metabolized to dopamine (Fig. 6.4).

● **Pharmacokinetics** L-Dopa is administered orally. Absorption depends on gastrointestinal transit time. Peak activity is usually observed in ½ to 2 hours with a plasma half-life of 1 to 3 hours.

— *Biotransformation and excretion* More than 95% of L-dopa is decarboxylated in the periphery by aromatic amino acid decarboxylase and excreted in the urine.

● **Pharmacologic effects** Simulation of dopamine receptors in the brain reverses the rigidity, tremor, and bradykinesia associated with Parkinson's disease, improves mental function, and enhances a sense of wellness.

● **Adverse effects** The most prominent adverse effects associated with L-dopa therapy are due to the stimulation of central and peripheral dopamine receptors. These effects are dose dependent and reversible. Included are nausea and vomiting, postural hypotension, arrhythmias, tachycardia, and inhibition of prolactin secretion.

Box 6.25

DRUGS USED IN THE TREATMENT OF MOVEMENT DISORDERS

Parkinsonism
Levodopa
Carbidopa
Bromocriptine
Pergolide
Amantidine
Seligeline
Anticholinergics
    Trihexyphenidyl
    Antihistamines
    Diphenhydramine

Spasticity
Baclofen
Diazepam
Dantrolene

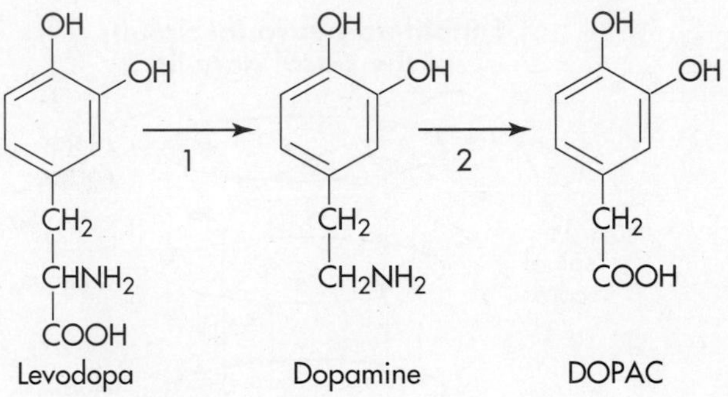

1. Aromatic amino acid decarboxylase (AADC)
   inhibited by carbidopa
2. MAO-B
   inhibited by selegiline

Fig. 6.4 Carbidopa inhibits dopamine formation in the periphery, whereas selegiline inhibits dopamine metabolism in the brain.

Adverse effects occurring after prolonged L-dopa administration include fluctuations in efficacy, such as the *on-off effect,* in which symptoms reappear periodically, and *wearing off,* in which drug effects do not last as long. A general loss of efficacy can also occur with L-dopa over time. Abnormal movements such as dystonia, dyskinesias, and chorea are common. Psychic effects can also occur, including hallucinations, paranoia, mania, anxiety, and depression. Renewed sexual interest and behavior can result from the actions of L-dopa on the neuroendocrine system.

■ **Carbidopa** Carbidopa blocks amino acid decarboxylase in the periphery, thereby increasing the amount of L-dopa entering the brain (Fig. 6.5). This permits the use of lower doses of L-dopa, yielding fewer adverse effects. Carbidopa has no pharmacologic effects when administered alone.

■ **Bromocriptine** Bromocriptine and related agents such as **pergolide** and **lisuride** are ergoline dopamine D_2 receptor agonists. Bromocriptine is used as an adjunct to L-dopa treatment in patients who are not adequately controlled with L-dopa.

● **Pharmacokinetics** Bromocriptine is rapidly absorbed from the gastrointestinal tract after oral administration. Extensive first-pass metabolism occurs. The plasma half-life is about 3 hours.

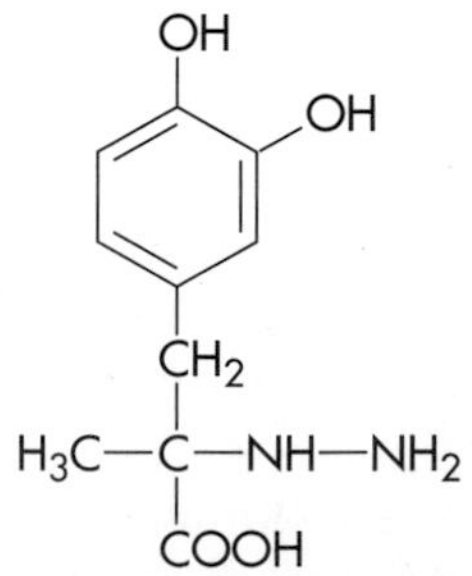

Fig. 6.5 Structure of carbidopa.

- **Adverse effects** As with L-dopa, adverse effects of bromocriptine are primarily due to its dopamine receptor agonist activity. Principal among these are nausea, vomiting, postural hypotension, and hallucinations.

■ **Amantadine** Amantadine is an antiviral agent that has been shown to have some efficacy in treating Parkinson's disease. Although its precise mechanism is unknown, it may release dopamine or have anticholinergic properties. Amantadine in usually used as an adjunct to L-dopa therapy to improve motor symptoms.

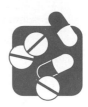

- **Pharmacokinetics** Amantadine is administered orally. The plasma half-life is relatively long, allowing for twice-daily dosing. It is excreted unchanged in the urine.

- **Adverse effects** This drug produces numerous CNS side effects. It can also cause livido recticularis (i.e., discolored spots on the skin).

- **Other** Tachyphylaxis may occur in patients treated with amantadine.

■ **Selegiline** Selegiline is an irreversible inhibitor of a subtype of monoamine oxidase, MAO-B. It decreases degradation of dopamine, thereby prolonging the action of L-dopa. This allows the dose of L-dopa to be decreased, minimizing its adverse effects. The use of selegiline also decreases the on-off effect.

■ **Drug Interactions** A variety of drugs interact with those used in the treatment of Parkinson's disease. Included are MAO inhibitors, which inhibit the catabolism of dopamine, enhancing the response to L-dopa. Dopamine receptor antagonists and dopamine depleting agents (antipsychotics, reserpine) block the effects of L-dopa. Because they decrease gastrointestinal motility, anticholinergics delay and decrease absorption of L-dopa. Pyridoxine increases the metabolism of L-dopa (see Fig. 6.4).

■ **Other Treatments**

- **Anticholinergics** Anticholinergics are used in the treatment of parkinsonism to block the action of striatal cholinergic interneurons, which are disinhibited in the absence of dopaminergic innervation. Drugs used for this purpose include **trihexyphenydyl, benztropine,** and **procyclidine.**

Anticholinergics
Trihexyphenydyl
Benztropine
Procyclidine

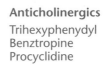

  — *Pharmacokinetics* The centrally active anticholinergics are administered orally, with the extent of absorption being dependent on gastrointestinal transit time. Peak plasma levels are obtained 1 to 2 hours after administration. The plasma half-life is 10 to 12 hours.

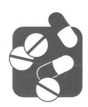

  — *Pharmacologic effects* Centrally active anticholinergics decrease the tremor associated with Parkinson's disease but are generally less effective than L-dopa. They are usually used in L-dopa-resistant patients.

  — *Adverse effects* Adverse effects are those typically encountered with anticholinergic agents. These include cycloplegia, constipation, urinary retention, mental confusion, and hallucinations.

- **Antihistamines** Antihistamines, such as **diphenhydramine,** are used in the treatment of Parkinson's disease because some are also potent anticholinergics. In general, these drugs are well tolerated but less efficacious than other anticholinergics.

Table 6.8   *Attributes of Drugs for the Treatment of Spasticity*

	BACLOFEN	DIAZEPAM	DANTROLENE
Mechanism	$GABA_B$ agonist: inhibits release of excitatory transmitters, increases threshold for excitation	Augments GABAergic transmission	Inhibits release of Ca^{2+} from sarcoplasmic reticulum
Site of action	Spinal cord	Spinal and supraspinal	Muscle
Adverse effects	Drowsiness, insomnia, weakness, dizziness, ataxia, confusion	Sedation Ataxia	Generalized muscle weakness Hepatotoxicity
Uses	Spinal cord injury Multiple sclerosis	All types of spasticity Spinal cord injury Cerebral palsy	Paralysis Cerebral palsy Multiple sclerosis

■ **Spasticity**

● **Overview** Spasticity results from a dysfunction of descending motor input resulting in violent, painful, involuntary muscle contractions. This condition can result from trauma or inflammation and is associated with disorders such as multiple sclerosis and cerebral palsy. Therapeutic strategies are directed toward modifying skeletal muscle tension (Table 6.8).

● **Baclofen** Baclofen is an agonist at a subclass of GABA receptors, the $GABA_B$ site. As such it inhibits release of excitatory transmitters and hyperpolarizes central neurons, increasing their threshold for excitability. It decreases monosynaptic and polysynaptic spinal reflexes. The gamma-motor system is most affected by baclofen. It is used primarily to treat diseases and injuries affecting the spinal cord as well as in multiple sclerosis.

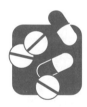

— *Pharmacokinetics* Baclofen is rapidly absorbed after oral administration. The plasma half-life is 3 to 4 hours. It is excreted unchanged in the urine.

— *Adverse effects* Adverse effects include drowsiness, insomnia, dizziness, weakness, ataxia, and mental confusion.

● **Diazepam** Diazepam exerts it antispastic actions by enhancing GABAergic transmission at spinal and supraspinal levels. It is used in all types of spasticity, but especially to treat spasticity associated with spinal cord lesions. It is also sometimes used for cerebral palsy.

— *Adverse effects* Adverse effects include sedation and ataxia.

● **Dantrolene** Dantrolene reduces muscle contraction by decreasing Ca^{++} release from sarcoplasmic reticulum. It is used in the treatment of paralysis and hemiparalysis, cerebral palsy, and multiple sclerosis. It is also used in the treatment of malignant hyperthermia.

— *Pharmacokinetics* Dantrolene is administered orally. The plasma half-life is 9 hours. It undergoes hepatic metabolism and is excreted in urine.

— *Adverse effects* Adverse effects of dantrolene include generalized muscle weakness and hepatotoxicity.

SECTION 6.10 ANTIPSYCHOTICS
AND LITHIUM

■ **Overview** Antipsychotic drugs (Box 6.26), also called neuroleptics or major
tranquilizers, are used in the treatment of schizophrenia, a disorder thought to
be related to hyperactivity of one or more of the dopamine systems in the brain.
This condition is characterized by positive symptoms, such as paranoia, hallucinations, and delusions, and negative symptoms, such as flat or inappropriate
affect and social withdrawal.

Box 6.26

ANTIPSYCHOTIC DRUGS
Phenothiazines
Chlorpromazine
Thioridazine
Trifluoperazine
Perfenazine
Fluphenazine
Butyrophenones
Haloperidol
Thioxanthines
Chlorprothixene
Thiothixene
Miscellaneous
Pimozide
Loxapine
Molindone
Clozapine
Risperidone
Remoxipride

■ **Mechanism of Action** Although the precise mechanism of action of antipsychotics is unclear, all drugs of this class are antagonists of the dopamine D_2 receptor subtype in the brain. Because the clinical potency of these drugs correlates with their affinity for this receptor, it is believed that the blockade of the
dopamine D_2 site is the primary mechanism of action. The potency of these
drugs at D_2 receptors also correlates with their propensity to produce adverse
neurologic effects. These drugs also interact with a number of other receptors,
including dopamine D_1, α-adrenoceptors, histamine, cholinergic, and serotonin
receptors. In addition, there are suggestions that other dopamine receptor
subtypes, such as the D_3 and D_4 receptors, may play a role in the therapeutic
effects of these drugs.

Antipsychotics
D_2 receptor blockers

■ **Pharmacologic Effects** The initial effect of antipsychotics is sedation. In
healthy volunteers, these drugs produce disinterest, limited range of emotion,
and dysphoria. In schizophrenics, the antipsychotic effects develop after a week
or more of continuous treatment. In general, positive symptoms are improved
significantly with little effect on negative symptoms. Antipsychotics are also antiemetics, an effect mediated by an action on the chemoreceptor trigger zone
in the brain. Accordingly, these drugs are not effective in the treatment of
motion sickness.

Parkinsonian-like Symptoms

Tremor
Bradykinesia
Akathisia
Dystonia
Perioral tremor

■ **Adverse Effects** Although antipsychotic drugs have a relatively high therapeutic index, they produce numerous adverse effects. These include orthostatic hypotension from blockade of α-adrenoceptors, anticholinergic effects, such as xerostomia, and antihistaminergic effects, such as sedation.

Extrapyramidal effects are characterized by parkinsonian-like symptoms, including tremor, bradykinesia, akathisia, dystonia, and perioral tremor. These typically occur early in therapy and can be attenuated with anticholinergic or antihistaminergic drugs.

Additional adverse effects include delirium, agitation, cardiovascular effects, and alterations in the endocrine system resulting in increased prolactin release, gynecomastia, and ammenorhea. The antipsychotics can also induce ocular abnormalities such as blurred vision and retinitis pigmentosa. They decrease seizure threshold and body temperature.

Neuroleptic malignant syndrome is a life-threatening condition that develops in patients with extreme sensitivity to the extrapyramidal effects of antipsychotics, especially when sweat production is inhibited by concomitant treatment with anticholinergics.

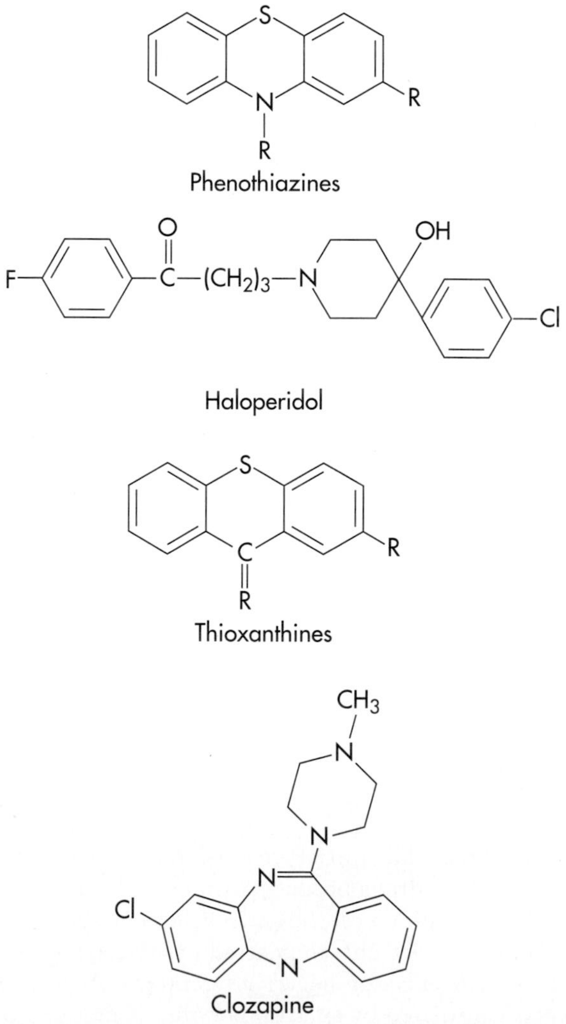

Phenothiazines

Haloperidol

Thioxanthines

Clozapine

Fig. 6.6 Structures of different classes of antipsychotic agents.

Tolerance develops to the hypotensive, sedative, and anticholinergic effects of the antipsychotics after continued treatment.

During long-term treatment, additional adverse effects may develop. The most notable is tardive dyskinesia. This condition is characterized by stereotyped abnormal movements and facial disfigurement. It is sometimes irreversible. Perioral tremor may also occur. Agranulocytosis may occur during treatment with clozapine and some phenothiazines.

■ **Classes of Antipsychotic Agents** Antipsychotics are classified according to their chemical structure. Structural classes include the phenothiazines, butyrophenones, and thioxanthines. Three types of phenothiazines display antipsychotic actions: aliphatic phenothiazines, such as chlorpromazine, which are the least potent; piperidine phenothiazines, such as thioridazine, which have the lowest incidence of extrapyramidal effects among the phenothiazines because of their intrinsic anticholinergic activity; and piperizine phenothiazines, such as trifluoperazine, perphenazine, and fluphenazine, which have the highest incidence of extrapyramidal effects of the phenothiazines (Fig. 6.6).

Included among the butyrophenones is haloperidol. The thioxanthine derivatives include chlorprothixene and thiothixene. A summary of the actions of antipsychotic agents are given in Table 6.9.

Table 6.9 *Summary of Actions of Antipsychotics*

	CHEMICAL CLASS	CLINICAL POTENCY	EPS LIABILITY	SEDATIVE EFFECT	HYPOTENSIVE ACTIONS	ANTICHOLINERGIC EFFECTS
Drug/Presumed Site of Action		**DA**	**DA**	**Histamine**	**α-Adrenergic**	**Ach**
Chlorpromazine	Aliphatic phenothiazine	low	moderate	high	high	moderate
Fluphenazine	Piperazine phenothiazine	high	high	low	v. low	moderate
Thiothixene	Thioxanthene	high	moderate	moderate	moderate	moderate
Haloperidol	Butyrophenone	high	v. high	low	v. low	low
Clozapine	Dibenzodiazepine	moderate	v. low	high	v. low	v. low
Risperidone	Benzisoxazole	high	low	low	v. low	low

EPS, extrapyramidal syndrome; DA, dopamine; Ach, acetylcholine; V, very.

Several antipsychotics do not fall into any of these classes. These miscellaneous drugs include loxapine, molidone, pimozide, risperidone, remoxipride, and clozapine. Among these, clozapine is most notable because it has been shown to be effective in patients who fail to respond to other antipsychotics. It is also relatively unique in that is has low affinity for dopamine receptors and higher affinity for serotonin receptors. Furthermore, there has been no reported incidence of extrapyramidal effects with clozapine. However, regular blood monitoring must be performed during clozapine treatment because of the high incidence of agranulocytosis associated with its use.

Clozapine
Agranulocytosis

■ **Pharmacokinetics** Antipsychotics may be administered by oral, IM, or IV routes. IM or IV administration affords rapid onset and are particularly useful in noncompliant patients. The onset of action is slow after oral administration.

These drugs are highly lipophilic. Accordingly, they accumulate in the brain, lungs, and other organs with rich blood supply.

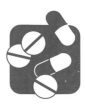

Antipsychotics undergo extensive hepatic metabolism. Metabolites, which are numerous and vary with each drug, accumulate in the body and may persist for months.

The action of a single dose usually persists for at least 24 hours, although there is considerable variation among patients.

■ **Clinical Uses** The primary use for antipsychotics is in the treatment of schizophrenia. Typically, 3 weeks or more of continuous administration are required before beneficial clinical effects are obtained.

Antipsychotics are sometimes used in the treatment of pruritis (itching) (trimeprazine), nausea and vomiting (chlorpromazine), intractable hiccoughs (chlorpromazine), Gilles de la Tourette's syndrome (haloperidol), Huntington's disease (haloperidol), alcohol-induced hallucinations, and mania.

■ **Lithium** Lithium salts are used in the treatment of manic-depressive illness because of their mood-stabilizing effects. Lithium may occasionally be used in addition to or in place of other antidepressants in nonbipolar, depressed patients.

● **Mechanism of action** The mechanism by which lithium stabilizes mood is unknown. It has been suggested that this ion affects membrane transport, synaptic neurotransmission, or second messenger systems, particularly phosphoinositol hydrolysis.

● **Pharmacokinetics** Lithium salts are rapidly absorbed after oral administration. Peak plasma levels are achieved within 2 to 4 hours. Because lithium accumulates slowly in the brain, therapeutic effects are usually noted only after 6 to 10 days of treatment. More than 95% of the administered dose is excreted in the urine.

● **Adverse effects** Because lithium salts have a low therapeutic index, adverse effects are quite common. Included are thyroid enlargement, polydipsia and polyuria, alterations in electrocardiogram, leukocytosis, edema, acne, and tremor. Tremor associated with lithium can be treated with propranolol.

Acute, mild lithium intoxication is characterized by nausea, vomiting, abdominal pain, diarrhea, sedation, and tremor. In severe cases, ataxic confusion, seizures, coma, and ultimately death occur. Symptoms of severe intoxication include cardiac arrhythmias, hypotension, and albuminuria.

There is no specific treatment for lithium toxicity. Efforts should be made to maintain proper hydration and electrolyte balance.

The use of lithium salts is contraindicated in patients with renal or cardiovascular disease. Lithium crosses the placenta and can be teratogenic.

Multiple Choice Review Questions

1. An antianxiety drug that binds to the $5\text{-}HT_{1a}$ receptor is:

   a. triazolam.
   b. buspirone.
   c. diazepam.
   d. paraldehyde.
   e. pentobarbital.

2. A 63-year-old male has problems with insomnia. For cost reasons, his physician decides against prescribing benzodiazepines to this patient. If a drug is to be used in the case, which agent would be most reasonable?

   a. Triazolam
   b. Diphenhydramine
   c. Trazodone
   d. Chlorpromazine
   e. Buspirone

3. A patient whose depression is being treated with tranylcypromine is admitted to the emergency room suffering from pounding occipital headache and palpitations. Both systolic and diastolic blood pressures are significantly elevated. Before becoming ill, the patient was having dinner consisting of a corned beef sandwich with a glass of a nice Chianti (red wine) with fava beans on the side. Suggest a probable cause of the patient's symptoms.

   a. In normal use tranylcypromine causes hypertension.
   b. Tranylcypromine is a beta blocker so that an underlying hypertensive condition can be unmasked.
   c. Tranylcypromine is a monoamine oxidase inhibitor. After ingestion of tyramine-containing foods, the tyramine can produce a hypertensive response.
   d. Tranylcypromine is a first-generation tricyclic antidepressant and can produce hypertensive responses as a side effect.
   e. None of the above.

4. Choose the correct statement concerning buspirone.

   a. Buspirone is a new benzodiazepine.
   b. Buspirone is advantageous as compared with other benzodiazepines in that it has a rapid onset of action.
   c. Buspirone does not produce sedation as seen with the benzodiazepines.
   d. Buspirone is one of the new antidepressants with few side effects.
   e. Buspirone shows cross-tolerance with the benzodiazepines.

5. Which of the following drugs has numerous side effects resulting from antiadrenergic and anticholinergic actions and may produce extrapyramidal syndromes?

   a. Chloral hydrate
   b. Haloperidol
   c. Meprobamate
   d. Tranylcypromine
   e. Lithium

6. A patient is admitted to the emergency room experiencing high fever and chills. A CBC was drawn and the report indicated a total WBC of 725 with 0% segmented neutrophils and bands, 95% lymphocytes, and 5% monocytes. The patient's daughter indicated that the patient was being treated for schizophrenia and recently had been switched to a new medication. She remembered that after this change in medication, her father had to go every Friday to get his blood checked. If the fever and chills were to be related to the patient's new medication, what was the drug?

   a. Loxapine
   b. Clozapine
   c. Hydralazine
   d. Chlorpromazine
   e. Doxepin

7. The primary drug used in the treatment of moderate to severe cases of Parkinson's disease is:

   a. amantadine.
   b. L-dopa.
   c. selegiline.
   d. pergolide.
   e. bromocriptine.

8. Which of the following is the first choice for treating absence seizures?

   a. Primidone
   b. Phenytoin
   c. Ethosuximide
   d. Thiopental
   e. I.V. diazepam

9. A 29-year-old schizophrenic female has been suffering from paranoid delusions despite being treated at various times with haloperidol, chlorpromazine, loxapine, thiothixene, and lithium. At this stage which antipsychotic might be appropriate to try?

    a. Trifluoperazine
    b. Amoxapine
    c. Clozapine
    d. Benztropine
    e. Molindone

10. The most common serious side effect of the narcotic agonists is:

    a. cardiac arrhythmia.
    b. endogenous depression.
    c. gastrointestinal hypermotility.
    d. respiratory depression.
    e. convulsion.

11. An example of a pure narcotic antagonist is:

    a. fentanyl.
    b. pentazocine.
    c. naloxone.
    d. droperidol.
    e. oxycodone.

PART 3

Toxicology and Selective Toxicity

Chapter 7

Chemotherapy Drugs

SECTION 7.1 INTRODUCTION TO CHEMOTHERAPY

 Overview Chemotherapy is an exercise in **selective toxicity**. Inasmuch as all chemotherapeutic agents are toxic, the goal in chemotherapy is to achieve a selective toxic effect against the pathogen, whether it be bacteria, fungi, viruses, protozoa, helminths, or tumor cells, while being minimally toxic to normal cells.

Toxicity to pathogens versus host is often relative. The difference in relative sensitivities between the patient (host) and the pathogen is quantified as the chemotherapeutic index (CTI). The CTI is defined as toxicity to pathogen divided by toxicity to patient, or LD_{50} for patients divided by the LD_{50} for pathogen. The higher the CTI, the more selective the drug for the pathogen.

Selective toxicity is related to the characteristics of the target organism or cell, the dose of the drug, and the specificity of drug action.

Selective toxicity can be achieved if there is a unique target present in the pathogen that is absent in the host. Alternatively, the target may be structurally different or more important in the pathogen than in the host (Box 7.1). Common targets for chemotherapeutic agents include cell wall synthesis, membrane integrity and function, protein synthesis, nucleic acid synthesis, nucleic acid integrity, cytoskeletal integrity, lipid (sterol) synthesis, and energy production (Box 7.2).

Box 7.1

SELECTIVE TOXICITY
Unique target must be present in pathogen, absent in host
Target must be structurally different in pathogen than in host
Target must be more important in pathogen than in host

Box 7.2

TARGETS FOR SELECTIVE TOXICITY
Cell wall synthesis
Membrane integrity and function
Protein synthesis
Nucleic acid synthesis
Nucleic acid integrity
Cytoskeletal integrity
Lipid (sterol) synthesis
Energy production

Sites of Exclusion

Cerebral spinal fluid
Ocular fluid
Synovial fluid
Pleural fluid cysts
Necrotic tissue

Sites of Concentration

Urine
Bile
Liver
Kidney
Bone
Fat
RBCs
Skin

When those targets are not unique to pathogens, structural and functional differences between species and cell types may enhance the selective toxicity of chemotherapeutics.

■ **Pharmacokinetics** Because the degree of selective toxicity is dose dependent, the pharmacokinetic properties of chemotherapeutic drugs are often critical factors for effective therapy.

Chemotherapeutic drugs are commonly excluded from the brain and cerebrospinal fluid, ocular fluid, synovial fluid, pleural fluid, cysts, and necrotic tissue. They are often concentrated in urine, bile, liver, kidney, bone, fat, red blood cells (RBCs), and skin.

Host metabolism is not important for many antimicrobial agents, but it is required for some antitumor drugs. Metabolism by pathogen is, in some cases, necessary for activity.

■ **Pharmacodynamics**

● **Mechanism of action** The mechanism of action for chemotherapeutics is typically defined by the target in the pathogen and the interactions between the drug and that target. Similarities between target sites in the pathogen and the host are often the reason for adverse effects.

● **Spectrum of activity** Chemotherapeutic agents are not selectively toxic toward a single organism; they destroy a range of related pathogens. Narrow-spectrum drugs are effective against a few species or classes of pathogens, whereas broad-spectrum agents attack many. Each type of drug displays certain advantages over the other. Thus narrow-spectrum drugs are employed when sensitivity of a particular pathogen is documented based on the results of culture and sensitivity tests. In this case the use of a narrow-spectrum agent yields maximal efficacy with fewer adverse effects because other cells are less likely to be influenced by the drug. This is an example of targeted selective toxicity. Broad-spectrum drugs, on the other hand, are used for mixed infections, such as when several pathogens are involved or when pathogen identities and sensitivities are unknown. The toxicity of a broad-spectrum agent on a wider range of pathogens maximizes the probability of it destroying unknown pathogens that may also be present.

● **Cytostatic versus cytocidal agents** Cytostatic agents inhibit growth and proliferation of susceptible target cells but do not kill them. Cytocidal agents, in contrast, kill susceptible cells. Antibacterials are classified further as bacteriostatic and bactericidal. Although not absolute, these classifications reflect the concentration of the chemotherapeutic agent, indicate the duration of the maintenance of an effective concentration, or vary with the strain of bacteria. For example, high doses of some bacteriostatic agents may be bactericidal. All other factors being equal, a cytocidal agent is preferable to a cytostatic drug because of its ability to decrease the pathogen population rather than merely preventing it from increasing.

An important concept in chemotherapy is the relationship between cytostatic and cytocidal agents. Cytostatic and cytocidal agents should *never* be mixed because many cytocidal drugs require that a pathogen population be actively growing for the drug to be effective. Cytostatic drugs block active growth and thus minimize the efficacy of cytocidal agents.

● **Development and incidence of resistance** Because only those pathogens sensitive to a given drug or combination of drugs are affected by it, resistant organisms enjoy a selective advantage for growth and proliferation. Thus chemotherapeutic agents select for resistant strains of the pathogen, which, by definition, will not respond to the drug over the long term. As a result, chemotherapeutic drugs are useful for only a period of time against a given population or in a particular patient. Ensuring that drugs are used only when they are appropriate and employing effective dosing regimens and duration of treatment maximize the usefulness of a drug by slowing the emergence of resistant strains. Box 7.3 lists some general mechanisms for resistance.

Box 7.3

MECHANISMS FOR RESISTANCE
1. Pathogen does not absorb drug
2. Pathogen pumps drug out
3. Pathogen metabolism inactivates drug
4. Modified target in pathogen not affected by drug
5. Increased production of target molecules
6. Development of altered metabolic pathways to bypass target

Nongenetic, or temporary, resistance is a reflection of the physiologic state of the target cells. Pathogens may be metabolically inactive, or dormant, either as a part of their life cycle or because of the actions of a cytostatic agent. Thus they will not be susceptible to agents that are effective only against metabolically active or proliferating cells. Genetic, or permanent, resistance arises either through chromosomal mutations or acquisition of new genes through plasmid transfer. Chromosomal mutations conferring drug resistance generally do not affect the function of the target molecule, but rather cause the loss of, or a significant decrease in, the ability of the molecule to interact with the drug. This normally results in resistance to a single drug or drug class. The acquisition of plasmids that mediate drug resistance is particularly important in the development of resistance. Such transfer of information does not require mitosis and therefore confers resistance to nonprogeny cell populations. Moreover, these plasmids often contain multiple genes, which may confer resistance to several classes of drugs. Such multidrug resistance is a major problem in chemotherapy.

To minimize the emergence of resistance, chemotherapeutic agents should only be used when clearly indicated. Narrow-spectrum drugs known to be effective against a specific pathogen minimize the selection of resistant organisms. The use of multiple drugs attacking different targets provides a therapeutic effect while blocking the proliferation of pathogens that may rapidly develop resistance to an individual agent.

● **Superinfections** A superinfection is a new, often more severe, infection as a result of chemotherapy. The primary chemotherapeutic agent often alters the normal flora of the gastrointestinal, genitourinary, or respiratory tracts. This can lead to an overgrowth of other microorganisms not affected by the primary agent. Most common are resistant bacterial or fungal overgrowths observed after antibacterial chemotherapy. Although oral and genitourinary superinfections are well known, gastrointestinal effects are more common. These appear as diarrhea or other types of gastrointestinal distress.

Symptoms of a gastrointestinal superinfection must be differentiated from direct irritation to the gastrointestinal system. These may be distinguished on the basis of the time course because direct irritant effects are noted frequently after the initial drug dose, whereas a superinfection usually requires 2 to 5 days of therapy to develop.

Three major classes of gastrointestinal superinfections are known. The first and most common is intestinal candidiasis. This fungal overgrowth does not necessitate alteration in antibacterial therapy, but it does require the addition of an antifungal drug.

The second type of superinfection is staphylococcal enterocolitis. This is a potentially life-threatening condition that requires not only the administration of an appropriate antibacterial, such as vancomycin, but also the cessation of the original therapy.

Pseudomembranous colitis, which is associated with *Clostridium difficile*, is another potentially fatal superinfection. As in the case of staphylococcal enterocolitis, the primary therapy should be terminated and the superinfection treated with either vancomycin or metronidazole.

Superinfections
Fungal
Staphylococcal enterocolitis
Pseudomembraneous colitis

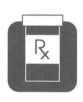

● **Role of host defenses** Chemotherapy itself seldom produces a cure. Instead, chemotherapy limits or decreases the size of the target cell population to enable the host immune system to provide the cure. This dependence on the immune response limits the effectiveness of chemotherapy in debilitated or otherwise immune-compromised individuals. In immune-compromised patients, bactericidal agents may be more effective than bacteriostatic agents.

● **Adverse effects** Adverse effects of certain classes of chemotherapeutic agents include hypersensitivity (allergic reactions) and idiosyncratic responses. Such effects are generally not related to the therapeutic mechanism of action of the drug. Dose-related toxicity is seen, however, with certain agents. This is often characterized as a loss of selectivity in the targeting of the desired effect. That is, the drug is exhibiting a toxic effect on host systems in addition to the target cell population. Such dose-related effects may be due to alterations in the pharmacokinetics of the drug.

■ **Pharmacotherapeutics** As with any drug, the goal of chemotherapy is to produce an effective concentration of the active drug where it is needed and to maintain that concentration for a sufficient length of time to elicit the desired response. These objectives are directly related to the pharmacokinetics of the individual drug. In the treatment of infections or malignancies, pharmacokinetics may be affected by inflammation, alteration or destruction of normal tissue architecture, changes in vascularization, and necrosis. The duration of therapy should be sufficient to ensure the eradication of the target cell population. Patient compliance in completing a full course of chemotherapy is sometimes difficult to achieve, is a common cause of failure, and is a contributing factor in the development of drug resistance.

Ideally, the choice of drug is based on the results of culture and sensitivity testing to identify the responsible organism. Without such information, the choice of a chemotherapeutic agent is based on conjecture, which may include consideration of a recent pattern of susceptibility and resistance observed with similar infections in that institution or geographic area. Although empiric chemotherapy is often effective, it does not obviate the need for precise identification and targeting of pathogens as provided by culture and sensitivity tests.

● Special uses

— *Combination chemotherapy* Frequently the use of multiple drugs against the same pathogens may provide distinct therapeutic advantages over single-drug therapy. Indications for combination chemotherapy include the following:

Synergism between the actions of two or more drugs. For example, an inhibitor of cell wall synthesis, such as a penicillin, with an inhibitor of protein synthesis, such as an aminoglycoside, enhances the therapeutic response to both agents. The increase in bacterial permeability caused by the action of the penicillin allows for the accumulation of higher concentrations of the aminoglycoside in the cell, promoting its bactericidal effect. Note that both of these agents are bactericidal.

To delay development of resistance. As indicated, a single drug selects for pathogens resistant to it. The emergence of resistance may occur rapidly with certain drugs or pathogens. One way to minimize this development is to combine two drugs that act by different mechanisms. The probability of a single cell becoming resistant to two different classes of drugs is low, unless the resistance is mediated by a plasmid encoding multiple drug-resistant gene product.

For the treatment of "mixed" infections. An infection involving multiple pathogens may exceed the capability of any single agent, no matter how broad the spectrum might be. In such a situation, multiple drugs are employed to ensure that all pathogens are targeted.

To initiate therapy in life-threatening situations when the pathogens are not known. When treating critically ill patients it may not always be prudent to withhold chemotherapy pending the results of culture and sensitivity tests. In such instances chemotherapy can be initiated on the basis of an empiric diagnosis and may include broad enough chemotherapeutic coverage to attack all likely pathogens that might be involved. The therapy is later modified based on the results of culture and sensitivity tests.

— *Chemoprophylaxis* Chemoprophylaxis is chemotherapeutic intervention in individuals who have been exposed to pathogens or who are otherwise at risk before the development of symptoms (Box 7.4).

Box 7.4

> ### INDICATIONS FOR CHEMOPROPHYLAXIS
>
> 1. Protect healthy individuals after exposure to specific pathogens
> 2. Prevent postsurgical infections
> 3. Prevent bacterial endocarditis in susceptible individuals

Successful chemoprophylaxis is associated with several factors. First, the specific pathogen and its sensitivity should be known. Second, chemoprophylaxis should be of short duration to minimize the development of resistant pathogens. Chemoprophylaxis is most successful when the pathogen is slow to develop resistance to the chosen drug. The doses employed should be equal to those used for chemotherapy, which will help slow the development of resistance. Finally, the efficacy of chemoprophylaxis for a given clinical setting should be established. This is not often the case because chemoprophylaxis has become standard practice in some situations despite a lack of documentation for its efficacy. For example, chemoprophylaxis against endocarditis for patients undergoing dental procedures is common practice despite the fact that its efficacy has not been established.

■ **Misuse and Overuse of Chemotherapeutic Drugs** As with all drugs, there are established rules for using chemotherapeutic agents. Because of the nature of selective toxicity, the complexity of the microbial and eukaryotic populations that may be affected, and the progressive emergence of resistance, the unnecessary or improper use of chemotherapeutics may have negative consequences. For example, there is needless risk of developing resistance or of exposing the patient to adverse effects. Moreover, inappropriate use of chemotherapeutic agents can alter microbial flora, facilitating the development of superinfections and increasing the cost of health care (Box 7.5).

Box 7.5

CONSEQUENCES OF IMPROPER USE OF CHEMOTHERAPEUTIC DRUGS
Needless exposure of patients to sensitization or adverse effects Provide opportunities for the development of resistance Alter normal microbial flora, facilitating development of superinfections Needless increases in health care costs

Section 7.2 Inhibitors of Cell Wall Synthesis

■ **Overview** The bacterial cell wall is an ideal target for selective toxicity. This proteoglycan layer (highly cross-linked polypeptides and polysaccharides) between the cytoplasmic membrane and the outer membrane is absolutely essential for the viability of most bacteria and has no parallel in structure in mammalian cells. This unique target is the site of action of two major classes of antibacterials. Because the cell wall is found only in bacteria, drugs acting on this structure have a low incidence of adverse effects on the host.

Inhibitors of cell wall synthesis (ICWS) block various biosynthetic steps in the production of the cell wall. The most widely used are the β-lactam antibiotics. These compounds, represented by the penicillins and cephalosporins, block enzymatic steps in cell wall synthesis that occur outside of the cell in the periplasmic space. Other ICWS act at intracellular sites.

■ **Penicillins** All penicillins are amide derivatives of 6-aminopenicillanic acid. The various congeners differ in the structure of the organic acid added to the 6-amino moiety. The penicillins are one of the most widely used classes of antibacterials primarily because of their highly selective toxicity (extremely high chemotherapeutic index). These bactericidal agents are particularly useful in treating infections caused by gram-positive organisms (Table 7.1).

● Pharmacokinetics

— *Absorption* Although some penicillins are acid labile (β-lactam is hydrolyzed), they still may be administered orally. The dose employed depends on the amount of drug destroyed by the gastric acid. Many synthetic penicillins are acid stable (e.g., phenoxymethyl penicillin,

**Cell Wall Synthesis
  Inhibitors**

Penicillins
Cephalosporins
Aztreonam
Imnipenem
Vancomycin
Bacitracin

Table 7.1   *Properties of Penicillin Congeners*

Congener	Acid Stability	B-Lactamase Resistance	Comment
Penicillin G (Benzylpenicillin)	No	No	Active against gram-positive organisms
Benzathine penicillin G	No	No	Depot preparation of Pen G
Phenoxymethyl penicillin (penicillin V)	Yes	No	Acid-resistant Pen G
Nafcillin	Yes	Yes	Biliary excretion
Oxacillin	Yes	Yes	Like Pen G
Cloxacillin	Yes	Yes	Like Pen G
Ampicillin	Yes	No	Increased gram-negative activity
Amoxacillin	Yes	No	Increased gram-negative activity
Carbenicillin	No	No	*Proteus* and *Pseudomonas*
Ticarcillin	No	No	*Proteus* and *Pseudomonas*
Piperacillin	No	No	*Pseudomonas* and *Klebsiella*

nafcillin, oxacillin, cloxacillin). Penicillins are also administered parenterally, with intravenous (IV) administration favored over intramuscular (IM) because of local irritation by the latter route. Benzathine penicillin G is a low-solubility salt that is administered in a relatively large IM dose. This serves as a "depot" that slowly releases penicillin into the circulation over a period of 3 to 4 weeks.

— *Distribution* The penicillins penetrate into most tissues and fluids, including pleural, pericardial, and synovial fluids. Little is found in the eye and central nervous system (CNS). The penicillins accumulate to a greater extent in the CNS during active meningitis because of disruption of the blood-brain barrier. However, the amount may be insufficient to be effective in this condition.

— *Metabolism* Host metabolism of penicillins is variable and usually not significant.

— *Excretion* Penicillins are rapidly excreted into the urine by the organic acid secretory system in renal tubules. This limits the plasma half-life of most penicillins to 1 hour or less. Probenecid, a competing substrate for the acid secretory system, is sometimes used to prolong the half-life of penicillins. Nafcillin is an exception in that it is primarily cleared by biliary secretion rather than through the kidney.

● Pharmacodynamics

— *Mechanism of action* Penicillins bind to penicillin-binding proteins in the periplasmic space. This blocks the transpeptidation reaction necessary for the cross-linking of the cell wall, thereby preventing synthesis of the structure. The requirement for continued cell wall synthesis is observed only with actively growing bacterial populations. Growth also requires murein hydrolases, enzymes that break down the cell wall, allowing for the insertion of new cell wall components. Penicillins not only block cell wall synthesis, but they also activate murein hydrolases, enhancing the degradation of the existing cell wall.

— *Resistance* Bacteria without cell walls are not susceptible to the penicillins or other inhibitors of cell wall synthesis. Similarly, resting (nonproliferating) bacteria have no need for cell wall synthesis and so are not affected by these agents. Although some bacteria are susceptible to the inhibitory effects on cell wall synthesis, their murein hydrolase is not affected, reducing the bactericidal effect of penicillins. If the permeability of the outer membrane is altered, access of penicillins to the binding proteins may be blocked, resulting in resistance. An inability to reach or bind to the penicillin-binding proteins appears to be the cause of methicillin resistance in *Staphylococcus aureus*. The major mechanism of resistance to penicillins, however, is derived from the plasmid-mediated expression of β-lactamases, enzymes that hydrolyze the β-lactam ring, abolishing antibacterial activity. Certain synthetic penicillins, such as nafcillin, oxacillin, and cloxacillin, are not substrates for β-lactamases and therefore are not influenced by this mode of resistance. Alternatively, a β-lactamase inhibitor such as Clavulanic acid or Sulbactam may be coadministered with a penicillin.

β-lactamase Inhibitors
Clavulanic acid
Sulbactam

● **Adverse effects** Penicillins are relatively nontoxic. The major adverse effects noted with these agents are immune mediated. Thus a self-limiting, nonrecurring rash occurs in about 10% of patients receiving ampicillin. The incidence of this effect is about 90% for mononucleosis patients receiving ampicillin. Allergic reactions to penicillins may be more serious. Such hypersensitivity reactions can result in potentially fatal anaphylactic shock. Between 5% and 10% of patients report a history of penicillin allergy, although the actual incidence is thought to be lower. Allergy is characterized by complete cross reactivity with all penicillins. Cross-reactivity with cephalosporins is estimated at 5% to 15% in these patients. Sensitization occurs with exposure to any penicillin or penicillin-containing product, with the incidence increasing as the exposure to penicillins increases. The sensitizing agent appears to be a breakdown product of penicillins, which becomes covalently bound to proteins. Skin tests with degraded penicillins or penicillanic acid-polypeptide conjugates have some predictive utility.

Classic dose-related CNS toxicity is seen with high levels of penicillins, usually after intrathecal administration. In addition, the penicillins are associated with the emergence of bacterial or fungal superinfections. This is particularly common with broad-spectrum agents such as ampicillin and amoxacillin.

● **Clinical use** Penicillins are widely used and effective antibacterials, with a minimal incidence of serious adverse effects. Their site of action on bacterial cell walls yields an exceedingly selective toxicity. Penicillin G and V are primarily useful against gram-positive bacteria. Ampicillin and amoxacillin exhibit increased activity against gram-negative bacteria and are considered broad-spectrum penicillins. Newer agents include carbenicillin, piperacillin, and ticarcillin. These "extended-spectrum" penicillins are effective against *Proteus* and *Pseudomonas*. Piperacillin is effective against *Klebsiella* as well. The rapid emergence of resistance to carbenicillin is seen with *Pseudomonas*, so chemotherapy usually includes an aminoglycoside. The extended-spectrum penicillins are powerful drugs that should be used only when indicated to conserve their therapeutic value.

■ **Cephalosporins** Cephalosporins are a class of antibacterials with a structure and function similar to penicillins (Box 7.6). These β-lactams possess a broader spectrum of activity than the penicillins, but they possess other pharmacokinetic and pharmacodynamic properties that generally render them less useful than the penicillins. Cephalosporins are described as first, second, or third generation compounds. In addition to referring to the order of their discovery, this designation also relates to greater gram-negative activity, often at the expense of lower gram-positive activity, higher incidence and severity of adverse effects,

Box 7.6

CEPHALOSPORINS
First Generation Cephalothin Cephalexin Cefadroxil
Second Generation Cefoxitin Cefaclor
Third Generation Ceftriaxone Ceftazidime Cefixime Moxalactam

higher resistance to β-lactamases, and better distribution to the CNS.

● **Pharmacokinetics**

— *Absorption* Some cephalosporins, such as cefadroxil, cephalexin, cefaclor, and cefixime, are administered orally. The others are administered IV.

— *Distribution* Cephalosporins are widely distributed to most fluids and tissues. Only the third generation agents, including cefoperazone and cefixime, penetrate into the CNS.

— *Excretion* Cephoperazone and ceftriaxone are cleared in the bile. All other cephalosporins are excreted in the urine.

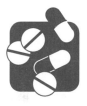

● **Pharmacodynamics**

— *Mechanism of action* The cephalosporins display a mechanism of action similar to the penicillins.

— *Altered response* Resistance to the cephalosporins is similar to penicillins. Often unique β-lactamases, referred to as cephalosporinases and penicillinases, are expressed that are specific for either cephalosporins or penicillins, but not for both.

● **Adverse effects** Hypersensitivity to cephalosporins occurs as described for penicillins. Between 6% and 18% cross-reactivity to penicillins is observed for those sensitive to β-lactam antibiotics. Renal toxicity is sometimes observed, but the incidence is low. Thrombophlebitis has been noted after IV administration. Superinfections can result from the overgrowth of gram-positive organisms subsequent to the use of second-generation and particularly third-generation cephalosporins, which are ineffective against these organisms.

● **Clinical use** Cephalosporins are considered secondary inhibitors of cell wall synthesis because of the need for parenteral administration, higher toxicity, and high cost. In general, the penicillins are preferred in most instances.

Other β-lactams
Aztreonam
Imipenem

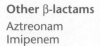

■ Other β-Lactams

● **Monobactams** Aztreonam is a monocyclic β-lactam (monobactam), whereas penicillins and cephalosporins are bicyclic. After IV administration, aztreonam is rapidly excreted in the urine. It is not inactivated by β-lactamases. Aztreonam is particularly effective against gram-negative organisms such as *Serratia* and *Pseudomonas*. It has little or no activity against gram-positive microbes or anaerobes.

● **Carbapenems** Imipenem is a bicyclic β-lactam that is administered IV. It is widely distributed throughout the body, including the CNS, and is readily excreted in the urine. Imipenem is not hydrolyzed by β-lactamases but is inactivated by renal tubule dihydropeptidases, necessitating the coadministration of **cilastatin,** a dihydropeptidase inhibitor. This is analogous to the use of clavulanate or sulbactam to inhibit β-lactamases, except that in this case, it is a host enzyme that must be blocked. Imipenem is a broad-spectrum antibacterial that affects many gram-negative and gram-positive organisms, as well as some anaerobes. *Pseudomonas* develops resistance rapidly, requiring that the drug be given with an aminoglycoside. Gastrointestinal disturbances have been noted, along with skin rashes and possible cross-reactivity in penicillin-sensitive patients.

■ Other Inhibitors of Cell Wall Synthesis

● **Vancomycin** Vancomycin inhibits the synthesis of the peptidoglycan, a cell wall component. Unlike the transpeptidation reaction inhibited by the β-lactams, the target for vancomycin is intracellular rather than in the periplasmic space. Vancomycin is administered orally for the treatment of gastrointestinal superinfections. Because it is not absorbed after oral administration, this represents a topical application. Previously it was thought that vancomycin was too toxic for systemic use. However, more effective purification of the drug removed contaminants responsible for most of the adverse effects. This allows for the parenteral (IV) use of vancomycin. After injection it is distributed to most fluids and tissues, but not to the brain. The plasma half-life is 5 to 10 hours, with renal excretion as the major clearance mechanism. Vancomycin is bactericidal for many gram-positive organisms. Resistance is becoming more common with increasing use. Because it is an irritant, local inflammation at the infusion site or systemic effects such as chills and fever can occur. Vancomycin also may trigger histamine release and diffuse flushing ("red man syndrome"). Decreasing the infusion rate or coadministration of antihistamines can minimize this effect.

● **Bacitracin** Like vancomycin, bacitracin inhibits early intracellular steps in cell wall synthesis. It is bactericidal for susceptible gram-positive organisms. It is used only as a topical antibacterial. Nephrotoxicity prevents its systemic use.

Membrane-Active
Polymixin B
Colistimethate

■ **Membrane-Active Antibacterials** Polymixin B and Colistimethate are cationic detergents that exert their antibacterial effect by permeabilizing the bacterial cell membrane.

Gram-negative organisms are most susceptible to these agents. Severe nephrotoxicity and neurotoxicity preclude their systemic use. Instead, they are applied as ointments for skin lesions, or they may be instilled into the pleural or joint cavities. Occasionally they are administered orally for the topical treatment of gram-negative bacterial overgrowth in the gastrointestinal tract.

SECTION 7.3 INHIBITORS OF PROTEIN SYNTHESIS

■ **Overview** Although both eukaryotes and prokaryotes must synthesize proteins, this process yields several sites for selective inhibition in prokaryotes, providing targets for selective toxicity. Unlike the inhibition of cell wall synthesis, inhibition of protein synthesis relies on a target that is somewhat different in the pathogen than in the host, rather than unique to the pathogen.

■ **Aminoglycosides** The aminoglycosides are irreversible inhibitors of bacterial ribosomal function and thus are bactericidal. Aminoglycosides are powerful agents, particularly against gram-negative organisms, but are limited in their usefulness by adverse effects and by the development of resistance.

● **Pharmacokinetics** Aminoglycosides are poorly absorbed from the gastrointestinal tract and therefore are usually administered IM. Occasionally they are given IV.

Being polar, aminoglycosides are rapidly absorbed from an IM injection site and distributed throughout the body. They do not enter the CNS, eye, or eukaryotic cells, except in the renal cortex.

Although host metabolism is negligible, microbial metabolism represents a major mechanism for resistance.

Aminoglycosides are rapidly excreted by glomerular filtration, yielding a serum half-life of 2 to 3 hours. Impairment of renal function must be considered when instituting aminoglycoside therapy.

● **Pharmacodynamics**

— *Mechanism of action* Aminoglycosides bind irreversibly to the small (30S) subunit of bacterial ribosomes. The association of aminoglycosides with the 30S subunit blocks the initial binding of mRNA to the ribosome, causes misreading of the mRNA, and destabilizes polysomes, resulting in a loss of functional synthetic complexes.

— *Resistance* The rapid development of resistance to aminoglycosides limits their use. They are administered alone for only relatively short periods of time. More commonly they are used in combination with a penicillin. Three mechanisms are known to confer resistance to aminoglycosides.

Alteration in bacterial uptake. To reach the bacterial ribosomes, aminoglycosides are taken up by an oxygen-dependent active transport. Alteration of this transport system retards accumulation of the drug, decreasing its effectiveness. Changes in the composition of the cell wall may also hinder the penetration of the aminoglycoside to the plasma membrane where the transporter is located. These alterations may be either chromosomal or plasmid derived. Temporary resistance caused by altered transport is seen in facultative anaerobes. Under anaerobic conditions the oxygen-dependent uptake of aminoglycosides does not occur, so strict anaerobes are not susceptible to these drugs.

Protein Synthesis Inhibitors
Aminoglycosides
Tetracyclines
Chloramphenicol
Macrolides
Spectinomycin
Clindamycin

Aminoglycosides
Streptomycin
Kanamycin
Neomycin
Gentamicin
Tobramycin
Amikacin
Netilmicin

Altered target (ribosomal protein). A structural change in the protein "receptor" for aminoglycosides may result in a ribosomal protein that no longer binds the drug.

Increased bacterial metabolism. Conjugation of aminoglycosides by adenylation, acetylation, or phosphorylation abolishes antibacterial activity. Plasmid-mediated induction of such conjugating enzymes is the most common mechanism of resistance.

Adverse Effects
Ototoxicity
Nephrotoxicity
Neuromuscular blockade

- **Adverse effects** Aminoglycosides display distinct adverse effects, including ototoxicity and nephrotoxicity. Ototoxicity may be auditory (hearing loss, often beginning with the loss of high-frequency sensation) or vestibular (loss of balance, vertigo). Nephrotoxicity results in a loss of function as demonstrated by increasing serum creatinine levels. Although nephrotoxicity is usually reversible, auditory ototoxicity is often irreversible.

  Both the ototoxicity and the nephrotoxicity are dose-dependent and time-dependent effects. The ototoxicity is related to the plasma concentration of aminoglycoside because the drug concentrates in the perilymph of the cochlea. When plasma levels fall, the drug diffuses out and cochlear damage does not ensue. Nephrotoxicity results from the high levels of aminoglycosides in the renal proximal tubular cells as the drug is cleared. Plasma concentrations are a critical factor in both types of toxicity and thus must be closely monitored. This is particularly critical in patients with renal impairment.

  Neuromuscular blockade is a rare adverse effect of aminoglycosides and is observed only with an extremely high concentration of the drug. This effect, similar to that of curare, can cause respiratory paralysis. It is most common in surgical patients in whom other neuromuscular blocking drugs may be present. There is also a higher incidence in patients with myasthenia gravis.

- **Clinical use** Aminoglycosides are used primarily for the treatment of nonresistant gram-negative infections. Combination chemotherapy with a penicillin is often used to enhance penetration of the aminoglycoside into the organism and to delay the emergence of resistance. The choice of a particular aminoglycoside is often based on the susceptibility of the organisms in a given institution or geographic area.

- **Congeners** Because **streptomycin** is an older aminoglycoside, wide-spread resistance is a limiting factor in its use. **Kanamycin** and **neomycin** were formerly used as systemic agents, but the frequency of adverse effects and the availability of newer, more selective aminoglycosides has limited them to use as topical agents. **Gentamicin** and **tobramycin** are popular aminoglycosides, with similar antibacterial spectra and toxicities. Tobramycin is slightly less nephrotoxic than gentamicin. **Amikacin** and **netilmicin** are newer aminoglycosides effective against bacterial strains resistant to the older aminoglycosides. This advantage will probably disappear with further exposure of pathogens to these drugs.

- **Tetracyclines** Tetracyclines are a group of bacteriostatic inhibitors of protein synthesis that display activity against a broad range of gram-negative and gram-positive organisms. A common feature of the tetracyclines is their high affinity for Ca^{++} and other divalent metal ions, a characteristic that in large part defines their pharmacokinetics and adverse effects.

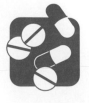

- **Pharmacokinetics** Despite the fact that their absorption is highly variable, tetracyclines are most commonly administered orally. Parenteral formulations are available for IV administration. All tetracyclines are potent chelators of divalent metal cations, primarily Ca^{++}, Mg^{++}, and Fe^{++}. Trivalent aluminum (Al^{+++}) is also chelated. This is of critical importance because the metal-associated forms of tetracyclines are not absorbed from the gut and do not possess antibacterial activity. Thus tetracyclines should not be administered orally with milk or milk products, iron supplements, or antacids (Table 7.2).

Absorbed tetracyclines are widely distributed to fluids and tissues, but they do not enter the cerebrospinal fluid in effective concentrations. Tetracyclines readily cross the placenta and are also found in breast milk. Calcium chelation yields high concentrations of tetracyclines in teeth and bones. This is particularly apparent in growing tissues.

The excretion of most tetracyclines occurs by both renal and hepatic clearance. The ratio of clearance in urine and feces varies with different tetracyclines, although the amount cleared by each route is at least 10%. Doxycycline is unique in that its clearance is entirely hepatic. Enterohepatic circulation of tetracyclines can yield concentrations in the bile tenfold higher than in the plasma.

- Pharmacodynamics

    — *Mechanism of action* Tetracyclines bind reversibly to the 30S ribosomal subunit, blocking the binding of aminoacyl-tRNAs required for peptide elongation. Reversibility renders this action bacteriostatic because the ribosomal binding sites are vacant when the drug concentration drops below the therapeutic level.

    — *Altered response* Plasmid-mediated alterations in the ability of bacterial cells to concentrate tetracyclines prevent the attainment of effective drug concentrations. This results either from changes in the active systems that transport tetracyclines or from a decrease in the passive transport of the drug. Resistance is especially common in strains of *Pseudomonas, proteus,* and in some coliform bacteria.

- Adverse effects Tetracyclines cause gastrointestinal distress in two different ways. First, the drugs may be direct irritants to the gastrointestinal mucosa, resulting in nausea, diarrhea, and anorexia. This must be distinguished from the potentially more serious gastrointestinal superinfection. Overgrowth of tetracycline-resistant bacteria or fungal organisms can produce similar initial complaints as seen with direct irritation, but with a delayed onset. Identification and proper intervention of superinfections is critical.

Tetracyclines may be hepatotoxic, especially those with a high hepatic clearance. Hepatotoxicity is usually a high-dose phenomenon that occurs most often if there is a preexisting impairment of hepatic function.

Renal toxicity may occur in individuals with diminished kidney func-

Table 7.2 *Extent of Absorption of Some Tetracyclines after Oral Administration*	
CONGENER	ABSORPTION OF ORAL DOSE
Chlortetracycline	Very incomplete (~30%)
Oxytetracycline	Incomplete (60%-80%)
Tetracycline	Incomplete
Doxycycline	Complete (90%-100%)
Minocycline	Complete

tion. This also appears to be concentration dependent, resulting from excessive accumulation of tetracycline because of reduced excretion. Outdated tetracycline preparations are particularly associated with renal toxicity. Photosensitization may also occur with tetracyclines.

Calcium chelation is the underlying cause of the most significant adverse effects of the tetracyclines. The ability of tetracyclines to follow calcium, and thus to deposit in teeth and bones, results in discoloration and dysplasia. These effects are particularly pronounced in the fetus, in infants, and in young children, when growth of teeth and bones is ongoing. Deposition in bone can result in deformity, growth inhibition, and structural weakness. These effects are common when tetracyclines have been administered during pregnancy but are also seen in infants and children undergoing long-term therapy.

- **Clinical use** The tetracyclines are broad-spectrum antibacterials exhibiting bacteriostatic effects against both gram-positive and gram-negative organisms. These agents are particularly popular for the treatment of infections involving *Mycoplasma, chlamydia,* and *rickettsiae.* Lyme disease is treated with tetracycline.

■ **Chloramphenicol** Chloramphenicol, like the tetracyclines, is a broad-spectrum bacteriostatic inhibitor of protein synthesis. Although chloramphenicol is an extremely effective drug, its use is severely limited by its toxicity.

- **Pharmacokinetics** Chloramphenicol is well absorbed after all modes of administration. It is widely distributed throughout the body, including the CNS.

   In contrast to most antibacterials, host metabolism of chloramphenicol is extensive and plays a major role in determining blood levels of the drug. Up to 90% of administered chloramphenicol is glucuronidated in the liver, a reaction that abolishes antibacterial activity.

   Chloramphenicol is excreted entirely in the urine. About 10% of the excreted substance is chloramphenicol itself, which is filtered, and about 90% is glucuronide secreted by the tubules. Because the glucuronidation of chloramphenicol in the liver is the rate-limiting step for its inactivation and clearance, a dose adjustment is indicated with changes in hepatic status, but not renal status.

- **Pharmacodynamics**

   — *Mechanism of action* Chloramphenicol binds reversibly to a specific site on the large (50S) bacterial ribosomal subunit. This prevents the addition of new amino acids to the growing peptide chain (peptidyl transferase reaction).

   — *Resistance* The major mechanism of resistance to chloramphenicol is plasmid-mediated acquisition of chloramphenicol acetyltransferase, an enzyme that acetylates the drug, abolishing its antibacterial activity. Such plasmids often contain genes coding for other products conferring drug resistance. Less common is resistance to chloramphenicol from permeability changes in the bacterium, which may diminish uptake of the drug. Such changes are slow to develop and usually result in only a twofold to fourfold decrease in drug potency.

- **Adverse effects** The gastrointestinal effects of oral chloramphenicol include nausea, vomiting, and diarrhea. More serious are gastrointestinal or genitourinary fungal superinfections caused by alterations in the endogenous flora. The major limiting factor for chloramphenicol use is the development of anemias. This includes a defect in red cell maturation, apparently from inhibition of mitochondrial protein synthesis in bone marrow cells. This anemia is dose related and usually reversible. Aplastic anemia can also result from chloramphenicol use. Its incidence does not correlate directly with dose or duration of therapy, but rather appears to be an idiosyncratic response. Chloramphenicol-induced aplastic anemia, although rare, is usually irreversible and fatal.

Because neonates are deficient in glucuronyl transferase, they are particularly prone to chloramphenicol toxicity. Excessive accumulation of chloramphenicol causes the gray baby syndrome, characterized by gray color, flaccidity, hypothermia, vomiting, and severe shock. Chloramphenicol is also an inhibitor of cytochrome P-450 and therefore will significantly potentiate the effects of phenytoin, warfarin, and tolbutamide, drugs metabolized by cytochrome P-450-dependent reactions.

- **Clinical use** Because of its adverse effects, chloramphenicol use is limited to the treatment of anaerobic and mixed CNS infections, sensitive *Salmonella* infections, such as typhoid fever, and *H. influenzae*.

■ **Macrolide Antibiotics** Erythromycin and various erythromycin esters and derivatives are macrocyclic lactones, or macrolides. These compounds may be either bacteriostatic or bactericidal, depending on the concentration of the drug and on the susceptibility of the organism.

- **Pharmacokinetics** Although erythromycin is absorbed from the gastrointestinal tract after oral administration, it is acid labile. Thus the drug is given in acid-resistant capsules or as an acid-stable ester. It may also be given IV.

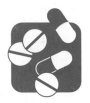

  Except for the CNS, erythromycins penetrate into all tissues and fluids. They readily cross the placental barrier.

  Clearance of erythromycins is primarily hepatic, with excretion in the bile. Biliary levels may be 50 times higher than the plasma concentrations. About 5% of the parent drug appears in the urine.

- **Pharmacodynamics**

  — *Mechanism of action* Macrolides bind reversibly to the rRNA component of the 50S bacterial ribosomal subunit, blocking peptide bond formation.

  — *Resistance* The primary mode of resistance to macrolides is a plasmid-mediated methylation of rRNA. This maintains ribosomal function while reducing the binding of the macrolide. A second plasmid-mediated resistance is seen in coliforms and is due to the expression of an esterase, which hydrolyzes and inactivates the macrolide, similar to the actions of a β-lactamase on a penicillin or cephalosporin.

- **Adverse effects** Gastrointestinal distress, including nausea, vomiting, and diarrhea, is common with oral administration of macrolides. Hepatotoxicity may also occur, particularly in response to erythromycin estolate. This may be due to a hypersensitivity reaction. Macrolides inhibit certain cytochrome P-450 isozymes, resulting in alterations in the pharmacokinetics of other drugs cleared by those pathways. Particularly affected are oral anticoagulants, oral digoxin, and terfenadine. Fatal cardiac arrhythmias have resulted from high levels of terfenadine in patients receiving macrolide antibiotics.

- **Clinical use** Erythromycins are frequently employed in penicillin-sensitive patients. They are also used in the treatment of corynebacterial infections, chlamydial infections, and for mycoplasma pneumonia and legionnaire's disease.

■ Other Inhibitors of Protein Synthesis

- **Spectinomycin** Spectinomycin is structurally related to the aminoglycosides but is a bacteriostatic inhibitor of protein synthesis. It is administered IM and is used for the treatment of penicillin-resistant gonorrhea.

- **Clindamycin** A bacteriostatic inhibitor of protein synthesis, clindamycin is administered either orally or IV. It distributes throughout the body, except for the CNS. Clearance is both hepatic and renal.

  Clindamycin binds to the rRNA of the 50S subunit, a site similar or identical to that targeted by erythromycin. Resistance appears to be chromosomal rather than plasmid mediated. Various cocci are resistant, and resistance is common in *C. difficile.* Gastrointestinal distress, skin rashes, and decreased liver function are adverse effects associated with clindamycin. The frequent resistance of *C. difficile* favors the development of pseudomembranous colitis, a life-threatening superinfection. Clinical use is limited mainly to treatment of mixed anaerobic infections.

Section 7.4 Inhibitors of Nucleic Acid Synthesis and Other Synthetic Antibacterials

Sulfonamides

Sulfisoxazole
Sulfacytine
Sulfamethaoxazole
Sulfasalazine
   (salicylazosulfapyridine)
Silver sulfadiazine
Sodium sulfacetamide
Co-trimoxazole
   (sulfamethoxazole-
   trimethoprim)

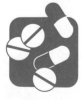

- ■ **Overview** Antibacterials of this class block the ability of bacteria to make (sulfonamides) or use (trimethoprim) folate derivatives required for the synthesis of purine bases. The quinolones and fluoroquinolones inhibit bacterial topoisomerase II, also called DNA gyrase. This enzyme catalyzes the unwinding of supercoiled DNA necessary for transcription and replication. The target for sulfonamides is unique to the bacterium, whereas trimethoprim and the quinolones attack a site present in both pathogen and host, although the bacterial enzyme has a higher affinity for these drugs. These agents are often used in the treatment of urinary tract infections. An additional drug used for this condition (nitrofurantoin) will also be considered in this chapter.

- ■ **Sulfonamides** All sulfonamides are structurally related to *p*-aminobenzenesulfonic acid amide, or sulfanilamide. Congeners possess different substituents on the amide or amine nitrogen. These substitutions alter the pharmacokinetics and, occasionally, the spectrum of activity of the sulfonamides.

  - **Pharmacokinetics** Sulfonamides are readily absorbed from the stomach or small intestine after oral administration, the preferred route. **Silver sulfadiazine** and **sodium sulfacetamide** are applied topically for treating burns and conjunctivitis, respectively. Sulfonamide preparations for IV administration are sometimes used with comatose patients. Once absorbed, sulfonamides are widely distributed through the body, including the CNS and across the placenta. Unlike most antibacterials, metabolism of sulfonamides by the patient is significant. They are acetylated, primarily in the liver, to an extent determined by both the chemical structure of the drug and the phenotype of the patient. Excretion is primarily by glomerular filtration, with urine concentrations of active drug being 10 to 20 times higher than plasma concentrations.

Sulfasalazine, a sulfonamide linked to 5-aminosalicylate, is not absorbed from the gastrointestinal tract and is split by bacteria into the free sulfonamide and amino salicylate. Amino salicylate is a potent antiinflammatory agent and is effective in the treatment of inflammatory bowel disease. If free amino salicylate is given, it is readily absorbed and shows little activity in the intestine where it is needed. By combining it with sulfonamide, it is possible to deliver more amino salicylate to the target tissue.

● **Pharmacodynamics** Sulfonamides are antimetabolites because they compete with the endogenous substrate *p*-aminobenzoic acid for binding to dihydropteroate synthase. This blocks the pathway synthesizing dihydrofolic acid, inhibiting folate-dependent reactions required for purine synthesis. The competitive inhibition of dihydropteroate synthase disappears when the sulfonamide concentration falls. Thus sulfonamides are bacteriostatic. Their effect can also be overcome by abnormally high concentrations of *p*-aminobenzoic acid.

Resistance to sulfonamides results from a mutation that causes the bacterium to produce greatly increased levels of *p*-aminobenzoic acid, displacing sulfonamide from the binding site. Changes in bacterial permeability to sulfonamides also afford resistance by preventing access to the enzyme target. Finally, mutations may occur in the target enzyme that maintain its function by increasing its ability to discriminate between the normal metabolite and the antimetabolite. The low cost and wide availability of sulfonamides has contributed to their extensive use and misuse, and as a result resistance is widespread. This is a major limitation to their use.

● **Adverse effects** are due to hypersensitivity or other immune-based phenomena. Rashes and related reactions occur in up to 5% of patients, and occasionally the more severe Stevens-Johnson syndrome, which includes fever, malaise, erythema multiforma, and mucous membrane ulceration in the mouth and genitalia, is seen. Hematopoietic effects occur in rare cases, and patients with glucose-6-phosphate dehydrogenase deficiency may develop hemolytic anemia. Finally, adequate hydration and renal function must be maintained to prevent the crystallization and precipitation of sulfonamides in the urinary tract.

● **Clinical Use** Sulfonamides are broad-spectrum, bacteriostatic agents. In addition to the uses noted, they are employed in the treatment, or chemoprophylaxis, of a wide range of gram-positive and gram-negative infections. They are particularly popular in the initial treatment of uncomplicated urinary tract infections because of the susceptibility of the offending organisms to these drugs and the pharmacokinetics of these agents. Infections involving chlamydia and various cocci may be treated with sulfonamides if resistance has not developed.

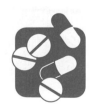

■ **Trimethoprim** Rather than inhibiting the synthesis of folates, trimethoprim blocks the reduction of dihydrofolate to tetrahydrofolate, a reaction catalyzed by dihydrofolate reductase. Tetrahydrofolate is required for the use of folate as a cofactor in purine and amino acid synthesis. Unlike dihydropteroate synthase, an enzyme unique to the target, dihydrofolate reductase is present in mammalian cells. The affinity of trimethoprim for the bacterial enzyme is about 50,000 times higher than for the mammalian enzyme, the basis for its selective toxicity. The pharmacokinetics of trimethoprim are similar to those of sulfamethoxazole, with rapid absorption of an oral dose, widespread distributions, and excretion in the urine. Trimethoprim is commonly used in combination with a sulfonamide because the use of agents that block two separate steps in the same metabolic pathway yields a significant synergism. A combined preparation, **co-trimoxazole,** is available and is used routinely.

Although the difference in affinity for trimethoprim between the bacterial and mammalian enzyme appears vast, adverse effects of trimethoprim are due to its action as an antimetabolite. Megaloblastic anemia, leukopenia, and granulocytopenia may all occur and may be treated with a folinic acid supplement because most pathogens do not accumulate folinic acid. Co-trimoxazole produces adverse effects attributable to both trimethoprim and sulfamethoxazole. Fever, rashes, nausea, vomiting, and diarrhea may also accompany the use of co-trimoxazole. The incidence of those effects is noted especially in AIDS patients receiving co-trimoxazole for the treatment of *pneumocystis* pneumonia.

DNA Gyrase Inhibitors
Quinolone—nalidixic acid
Fluoroquinolones—ciprofloxacin, norfloxacin

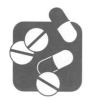

■ **DNA Gyrase Inhibitors** The prototype for this class of antibacterial is a quinolone, **nalidixic acid.** Nalidixic acid inhibits bacterial DNA replication by blocking DNA gyrase (topoisomerase II) activity. It is particularly effective against gram-negative organisms, with much lower activity against gram-positive organisms. The usefulness of nalidixic acid is limited by the fact that although it is readily absorbed after oral administration, its metabolism and excretion are too rapid to provide a prolonged systemic antibacterial effect. About 80% of the dose is glucuronidated in the liver, and both the parent compound and conjugate are excreted in the urine. The 20% of dose excreted in active form is toxic to gram-negative organisms in the urinary tract.

Use of nalidixic acid is also limited by the rapid emergence of resistance, particularly in *Pseudomonas*.

Nalidixic acid may cause gastrointestinal disturbances and superinfections, hyperglycemia, and glucosuria. Nalidixic acid treatment can also yield false-positive results for urinary glucose.

The fluoroquinolones **ciprofloxacin** and **norfloxacin** possess broader antibacterial spectra than nalidixic acid. These drugs are readily absorbed and widely distributed throughout the body after oral administration. Parenteral formulations of ciprofloxacin are also available. Less than 20% of the dose of fluoroquinolone is metabolized, and like nalidixic acid, it is cleared by the kidney. Its excretion can be slowed by administration of probenecid.

Fluoroquinolones are effective against both gram-negative and gram-positive organisms. They are used in the treatment of urinary tract infections, but also in the treatment of various respiratory, gynecologic, and soft tissue infections. Because this is the first new class of antibacterials introduced in decades, its use is still being defined. Despite their recent introduction, resistance to fluoroquinolones has already been observed. Resistance occurs from a mutation in DNA gyrase, diminishing the binding of the quinolone. *Pseudomonas, staphylococci,* and *Serratia* have all shown resistant strains.

Adverse effects of fluoroquinolones include nausea and vomiting, headaches, dizziness, and insomnia. Abnormal liver function and skin rashes have also been reported. Fluoroquinolones inhibit the clearance of theophylline, with the potential to cause theophylline toxicity, including seizures.

■ **Nitrofurantoin** Nitrofurantoin is used solely for the treatment of urinary tract infections caused by gram-negative or gram-positive organisms. Although the mechanism of action is unclear, it appears to involve reduction of the nitro group and generation of reactive oxygen species. Nitrofurantoin may be either bacteriostatic or bactericidal, depending on the pathogen. Although it is rapidly absorbed after oral administration, it is also rapidly metabolized and excreted into the urine. Clearance of nitrofurantoin is so efficient that even when administered IV it is not systemically active. This not only limits the use of this drug to treatment of urinary tract infections, it also lessens adverse effects. In patients with renal insufficiency nitrofurantoin accumulates systemically and is associated with anorexia, gastrointestinal disturbances, and occasionally oxidative hemolytic anemia, leukopenia, and hepatotoxicity.

Section 7.5 Antimycobacterial Agents

- ■ **Overview** Several characteristics of mycobacteria make effective chemotherapy a prolonged and complex effort. Mycobacteria do not have a peptidoglycan cell wall. Moreover, they are often intracellular pathogens, requiring that antimycobacterial agents be accumulated by the mammalian cells before they can be absorbed by the pathogen. In addition, mycobacteria often enter prolonged dormant periods between acute, active stages of infection. These resting pathogens are immune to the effects of antibacterial agents yet will enter active stages that can be fatal to the patient. Tuberculosis and leprosy are two of the best-known disorders of this type.

- ■ **Chemotherapy in Tuberculosis** Tuberculosis is a systemic mycobacterial infection characterized by long, asymptomatic dormant periods interrupted by acute, symptomatic active periods of bacterial growth and proliferation. Although the disease is apparent only during the active periods, chemotherapy continues until the pathogen is eradicated. Chemotherapy for simple cases of tuberculosis lasts 6 to 9 months, whereas treatment of tuberculosis meningitis or of miliary tuberculosis can take up to 2 years. Patient compliance is a major challenge in such cases because the individual will be asymptomatic much of the time. Resistance is also a problem, requiring combinations of three separate drugs.

    Antituberculosis drugs are generally classified as either first-line or second-line drugs (Box 7.7). The defining features are the frequency and severity of adverse effects. First-line drugs exhibit more selective toxicity than second-line drugs and thus are preferred unless the particular strain has acquired resistance to them. Such resistance was once rare, but within the last decade multidrug resistant tuberculosis has become a significant urban problem in the United States. This is coincident with a general rise in the number of reported cases of tuberculosis, and it parallels the spread of AIDS.

Box 7.7

ANTITUBERCULAR DRUGS
First-line Drugs Isoniazid (INH) Ethambutol Rifampin Pyrazinamide
Second-line Drugs Para-aminosalicylic acid Ethionamide Cycloserine

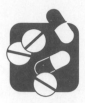

- **First-line antitubercular agents**

  — *Isoniazid* Isoniazid (INH) is the most frequently used antituberculosis drug. It is well absorbed after oral administration and is distributed through the body with brain levels about 20% of the serum level. It readily crosses mammalian cell membranes, as required for antimycobacterial therapy. The drug is primarily acetylated in the liver, which abolishes its antimycobacterial effect. The variation in acetylation activity is a well-described genetic polymorphism, dividing patients into slow and fast acetylator phenotypes. The African American and Caucasian populations in the United States are about 50% fast acetylators and 50% slow. Most Native Americans and Asian Americans are fast acetylators. The fast phenotype yields to a half-life of less than 90 minutes for INH, whereas slow acetylators clear the drug with a half-life in excess of 3 hours. Serum levels of INH in fast acetylators are between 30% and 50% of the levels in slow acetylators. Excretion of INH and its acetylated metabolite is in the urine. Acetylation is so important that dosing regimens are sometimes altered in response to changes in hepatic status, not to changes in renal status.

    Isoniazid blocks the synthesis of mycolic acids, key components of the mycobacterial cell wall. As with the inhibitors of peptidoglycan cell wall synthesis, this is a bactericidal effect in growing cells only. Resistance to INH results from the loss of genes coding for catalase and a peroxidase. Because resistance is widespread, INH is seldom used alone. Its use is limited to the treatment or chemoprophylaxis of tuberculosis. In the latter case, INH alone is given to individuals with documented tuberculosis exposure or positive tuberculin tests. For the treatment of tuberculosis, INH is used in combination with other antimycobacterial drugs, such as ethambutol, rifampin, or pyrazinamide.

    Adverse effects of INH are dose and time dependent. Hepatotoxicity occurs, particularly in elderly patients and in fast acetylators. Peripheral and central neuropathy result from an antipyridoxine effect. Because INH is structurally similar to pyridoxine, the neuropathy, but not the antimycobacterial effect, is reversed by supplementation with pyridoxine (vitamin B_6). Optic neuritis has been linked to INH. Finally, INH is contraindicated in seizure-prone patients.

  — *Ethambutol* The absorption and distribution of ethambutol closely resemble those of INH. Ethambutol is concentrated in erythrocytes, providing a depot for continuous release of drug. About 50% of the absorbed dose is excreted unchanged in the urine, with up to 15% excreted as urinary metabolites. The mechanism of action of ethambutol is unknown but may involve inhibition of polyamine synthesis. Because resistance to ethambutol can emerge rapidly, it is usually employed in combination with other agents. The primary adverse effect of ethambutol is a usually reversible optic neuritis with loss of visual acuity. This is a dose-dependent effect. Preliminary and periodic ophthalmologic examinations are recommended.

  — *Rifampin* Rifampin is a powerful bactericidal that is useful against gram-positive and gram-negative cocci and chlamydia in addition to mycobacterial infections. Like the other antimycobacterials, rifampin is readily absorbed and distributed after oral administration, reaching 40% of the serum level in the brain. Hepatic uptake, deacetylation, excretion into the bile, and enterohepatic circulation are noted with rifampin. The deacetylated metabolite retains antibacterial activity. Rifampin is an inhibitor of bacterial RNA synthesis, binding to the beta subunit of bacterial DNA-dependent RNA polymerase. Human polymerases are not affected. Resistance may result from permeability changes in the bacterium or from mutations that diminish drug binding by the polymerase. Resistance is common, so rifampin is used in combination chemotherapy for complete coverage of pathogens. It is a frequently used first-line antitubercular drug, with its relatively high cost being the major limiting factor for its use. Rifampin is present in tears, sweat, urine, and saliva, giving these fluids a distinct orange color. Occasional renal and hepatic impairment is seen, as is a flulike syndrome. Rifampin is a noted inducer of cytochrome P-450, enhancing the clearance of anticoagulants, contraceptive steroids, ketoconazole, cyclosporine, and chloramphenicol.

— *Pyrazinamide* This tuberculocidal drug is well absorbed and widely distributed after oral administration. Significant deamination and oxidation occur, followed by urinary excretion by glomerular filtration. Because resistance develops rapidly, combination chemotherapy is required. Up to 5% of patients receiving pyrazinamide develop dose-dependent and time-dependent hepatotoxicity, and all patients exhibit some measure of hyperuricemia. Pyrazinamide-induced gout does not respond to treatment with probenicid.

● **Second-line antitubercular drugs**

— *Para-aminosalicylic acid* Like all second-line drugs, the use of para-aminosalicylic acid (PAS) is limited by the frequency of serious adverse effects. It is well absorbed and widely distributed (except to the brain) after oral administration. Rapid urinary excretion of PAS and acetylated metabolites occurs. The drug blocks the dihydropteroate synthetase of tubercle bacilli, but not other bacteria. This is the opposite of sulfonamides. The use of PAS is frequently accompanied by severe gastrointestinal disturbances and pain. Hypersensitivity is relatively common after several weeks of PAS administration.

— *Ethionamide* This analogue of INH also inhibits mycolic acid synthesis. Ethionamide causes intense gastric pain, and it may be neurotoxic as well. Resistance develops rapidly.

— *Cycloserine* Cycloserine is effective after oral administration. It inhibits alanine racemase. Although it is an effective antitubercular agent, CNS toxicity and drug-induced psychosis limit its use.

■ **Chemotherapy of Leprosy** Although rifampin is effective in treating leprosy, **dapsone** is more widely used. Dapsone is widely distributed throughout the body with long-term use. Particularly high levels are found in skin, liver, kidney, and muscle. Dapsone and its acetylated metabolite are excreted in the urine. It is effective against *M. leprae*, the causative agent for leprosy, and *Pneumocystis carinii*. Dapsone frequently causes hemolytic anemia, particularly in glucose-6-phosphate dehydrogenase-deficient individuals, and it induces methemoglobinemia. Gastrointestinal disturbances and skin rashes are sometimes encountered with this agent.

Antileprosy Drugs
Dapsone

SECTION 7.6 ANTIFUNGAL CHEMOTHERAPY

■ **Overview** Selective toxicity against bacteria is aided by fundamental differences between them and the host. Even though prokaryotes and eukaryotes perform many of the same metabolic functions, the chemicals and pathways involved may differ. Protein synthesis uses different ribosomal structures in the two cell types, for example, with fungi, these differences are lost because they are composed of eukaryotic cells, as is the host. This makes selective toxicity more difficult to achieve and helps explain why the adverse effects of antifungals are more frequent and often more severe than with antibacterial drugs. Fungal infections are most common in debilitated or immunosuppressed patients, which limits their incidence. However, because normal defenses are weak or absent in the host, the course of chemotherapy is complicated and prolonged. Box 7.8 lists the antifungal agents discussed in this section.

■ **Polyenes**

● **Amphotericin B** A broad-spectrum fungicidal agent, amphotericin B is used systemically. Its high incidence of severe adverse effects limits its use.

— *Pharmacokinetics* Amphotericin B is not well absorbed from the gastrointestinal tract. Therefore oral administration is primarily a topical treatment for intestinal infections. When administered IV, amphotericin B is widely distributed throughout the body, except for the CNS. Intrathecal administration is required for the treatment of fungal meningitis. Circulating amphotericin B is extensively bound to plasma proteins and is slowly excreted in the urine.

— *Pharmacodynamics* Ergosterol is a key structural component in the fungal cell membrane, analogous to cholesterol in mammalian membranes. Amphotericin B binds to ergosterol, altering membrane structure, increasing its permeability. This loss of membrane integrity and the resultant inability to maintain internal homeostasis is fungicidal. Resistance occurs because there is a decrease in the uptake of amphotericin by the fungal membrane. This is due to either a decrease in ergosterol content or to structural changes in the membrane structure that inhibit the binding of amphotericin to ergosterol.

Box 7.8

ANTIFUNGAL AGENTS

Polyenes
Amphotericin B
Nystatin

Antimetabolite
Flucytosine
(5-fluorocytosine)

Antifungal Azoles
Clotrimazole
Miconazole
Ketoconazole
Fluconazole

Other
Griseofulvin

● **Adverse effects** associated with amphotericin B are frequent and many, giving rise to the expression "amphoterrible." Systemic administration of amphotericin is often accompanied by fever, chills, and nausea. Headache is common with this agent. Therapy may begin by titrating the dose on the basis of what the patient can tolerate, *not* on what is effective against the pathogen. Aspirin, acetaminophen, or antihistamines are given to treat fever and chills. More troublesome are the nephrotoxicity, hepatotoxicity, and anemia caused by standard doses of amphotericin B. The nephrotoxicity may be irreversible. Liposomal preparations of amphotericin B display a greatly decreased incidence of nephrotoxicity.

● **Pharmacotherapeutics** Amphotericin B is effective in the treatment of a wide range of systemic fungal infections. It is used in combination with flucytosine to delay the development of resistance. This combination allows for the use of lower doses of amphotericin B, diminishing the potential for adverse effects.

● **Nystatin** Like amphotericin B, nystatin is a polyene macrolide that binds to ergosterol in fungal membranes. Nystatin is even more toxic than amphotericin B, limiting its use to topical applications. This includes oral administration for the treatment of fungal infections and superinfections in the lumen of the gastrointestinal tract. The drug is not absorbed after oral administration.

■ Antimetabolite

● **Flucytosine** This pyrimidine, actually the cytosine analog 5-fluorocytosine, functions as a fungistatic antimetabolite.

— *Pharmacokinetics* Flucytosine is well absorbed after oral administration and distributes to all fluids and tissues, including the brain. Flucytosine is actively secreted in the urine, generating urinary concentrations of the drug up to tenfold higher than those found in serum. As an antimetabolite, the drug is metabolized most extensively by the metabolic pathways in the target cell.

— *Pharmacodynamics* Flucytosine is deaminated by a fungal-specific enzyme to form 5-fluorouracil, which is converted to the corresponding nucleotide. This form blocks thymidylate synthetase and ultimately DNA synthesis. Resistance develops rapidly, requiring the use of combination chemotherapy with amphotericin B. Flucytosine is relatively nontoxic to mammalian cells. With prolonged use occasional alopecia and bone marrow suppression have been seen.

■ Antifungal Azoles

Members of this newest class of fungistatic agents display a broad spectrum of activity. Although these agents are efficacious, the degree of selective toxicity is less than optimal. The drugs to be considered are the imidazoles **clotrimazole, miconazole, ketoconazole,** and the triazole **fluconazole.**

● **Pharmacokinetics** Clotrimazole and miconazole are applied topically with little absorption through the skin. In contrast, ketoconazole and fluconazole are readily absorbed after oral administration. Miconazole and fluconazole also are administered IV. Orally administered azoles are widely distributed through the body. Fluconazole readily enters the CNS. Antifungal azoles target fungal cytochrome P-450 enzymes, so it is not surprising that they also bind to and may be metabolized by mammalian cytochrome P-450 isozymes as well. This is observed with all three systemic agents, which are either extensively metabolized by liver microsomal enzymes (miconazole, ketoconazole) or classified as inhibitors of cytochrome P-450s (ketoconazole, fluconazole). (It must be appreciated that a *substrate* for a given enzyme, such as ketoconazole, will be a competitive inhibitor of the metabolism of another substrate for that same enzyme.) Miconazole and ketoconazole are excreted as inactive metabolites in the bile, whereas about 80% of fluconazole appears as the parent compound in the urine.

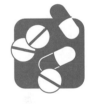

● **Pharmacodynamics** The primary action of the antifungal azoles is to inhibit the fungal cytochrome-450-dependent enzyme necessary for the synthesis of ergosterol. This results in a fungistatic effect. Resistance to these drugs is not yet apparent.

● **Adverse effects** are relatively common and can often be linked to inhibition of mammalian cytochrome P-450 enzymes. Hepatic effects, including increased levels of hepatic enzymes in the serum, may result from treatment with ketoconazole or fluconazole, and have even been attributed to the minute amounts of clotrimazole absorbed during topical administration.

This effect is usually reversible and causes no obvious symptoms. However, about 1 in 10,000 patients receiving ketoconazole may develop a progressive hepatotoxicity, which can be fatal. Competition with other substrates for cytochrome P-450 binding results in pronounced drug-drug interactions. Ketoconazole increases the serum levels and half-lives of cyclosporine and terfenadine similar to the macrolide antibiotics. An increase in the blood levels of terfenadine can lead to potentially fatal cardiac arrhythmias. Fluconazole administration also increases the blood levels of phenytoin and cyclosporine and of hypoglycemic and anticoagulant drugs. Because ketoconazole is effective as an inhibitor of the cytochromes involved in androgen formation, gynecomastia may occur. This antiandrogenic effect has been used in the treatment of prostatic carcinoma. Ketoconazole use also has been linked to thrombophlebitis at injection sites and on rare occasions with anaphylaxis and cardiotoxicity. Nausea and vomiting occur with significant frequency after systemic administration of these compounds and is particularly prominent with miconazole.

■ **Griseofulvin** This drug must be administered orally to be effective against topical mycotic infections. The absorption of oral griseofulvin is facilitated when taken with a high-fat meal. Once absorbed, it is concentrated in tissues containing keratin, which avidly binds griseofulvin. This characteristic makes it especially effective for the treatment of ringworm and athlete's foot. The mechanism of actions appears to involve either inhibition of nucleic acid synthesis or a disruption of microtubule structure in the fungus. Allergic reactions to griseofulvin have been noted. Headaches and gastrointestinal disturbances are also associated with this agent.

SECTION 7.7 ANTIPARASITIC CHEMOTHERAPY

■ **Overview** Although the argument could be made that all chemotherapy targets parasites, the definition of antiparasitic chemotherapy is limited to attacks on protozoans and helminths. Sites of attack may differ greatly from those targeted in chemotherapy of bacterial or fungal infections, but the basic principles of selective toxicity and the strategies for obtaining that selectivity are similar to these other classes of chemotherapeutics.

■ **Antiprotozoal Chemotherapy**

Antimalarial Agents

Chloroquine
Mefloquine
Primaquine
Pyrimethamine
Fansidar

● **Antimalarials** To understand the classification and use of antimalarials, the life cycle of the protozoans that cause the disease must be understood. Any of four species of *Plasmodium* may be transferred to the blood of a human bitten by an infected mosquito. The infectious agents, known as sporozoites, infect and reproduce in the liver. The progeny are termed *tissue schizonts*. Drugs that kill at this stage of the life cycle are termed *tissue schizonticides*. The progeny are released into the general circulation, where they infect red blood cells. During this erythrocytic phase the organisms are susceptible to the effect of blood schizonticides. These drugs are also called suppressive agents. Blood schizonts are converted to their reproductive forms, the gametocytes, and released into the blood. These are taken in by mosquitoes, which infect other individuals.

P. falciparum and *P. malariae* go through only one life cycle, resulting in an infection that completes its tissue stage in about 4 weeks. Treatment with blood schizonticides for at least 1 month generally eradicates infection.

P. vivax and *P. ovale*, in contrast, maintain dormant populations of tissue schizonts in the liver. These cells periodically reproduce and are released into the circulation, causing relapse. This is similar to the dormant populations of mycobacteria that complicate the chemotherapy of tuberculosis. This form of malaria requires the use of primaquine, the only known tissue schizonticide, to eradicate the infection.

● **Quinolines and aminoquinolines**

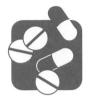

— *Chloroquine* Chloroquine is a 4-aminoquinoline. It is well absorbed from the gastrointestinal tract and widely distributed through the body. Parenteral formulations are available but are not commonly used. The pharmacokinetics of chloroquine are dominated by extensive tissue binding, resulting in an apparent volume of distribution of over 10,000 liters. Erythrocyte concentrations range from 10 to 20 times the plasma concentration in normal cells and to as much as 500 times in *Plasmodium*-infected erythrocytes. Such concentrations in infected erythrocytes facilitate the antimalarial activity of chloroquine. However, binding to other sites results in the sequestration of the drug and necessitates the use of a high loading dose for acute chemotherapeutic activity. Chloroquine is slowly released from tissue stores and excreted in the urine.

Although the mechanism of action of chloroquine is unclear, it is believed that disruption of the metabolism of hemoglobin by the parasite and other metabolic blocks may be involved. Resistance primarily arises by expression of a membrane P-glycoprotein pump, which expels chloroquine from the parasite. *P. falciparum* is the most likely species to exhibit resistance.

Chloroquine is the most widely used antimalarial for the chemosuppression and eradication of the parasitemia of all *Plasmodia*. It is used in combination chemotherapy with primaquine, a tissue schizonticide, for *P. vivax* and *P. ovale.* It is also administered prophylactically to travelers entering areas where there is a significant risk of malaria. Oral chloroquine is well tolerated, with gastrointestinal disturbances and headache being the most common complaints. Large cumulative doses may result in irreversible retinopathy, myopathy, and ototoxicity. Large IM and IV doses may trigger hypotension and cardiac arrest.

— *Mefloquine* Mefloquine is a quinoline derivative. It can be administered only orally, is well absorbed, and distributes throughout the body. It is cleared by the liver. Mefloquine is an effective blood schizonticide and is primarily used for prophylaxis or treatment of chloroquine-resistant *P. falciparum.* Adverse effects include vertigo, headache, gastrointestinal pain and disturbances, visual alterations, confusion, depression, hallucinations, and anxiety.

— *Primaquine* This 8-aminoquinoline is well absorbed and widely distributed after oral administration. It is extensively deaminated with the metabolite attaining much higher plasma concentrations than the parent compound. Both the parent and metabolite are excreted in the urine. The mechanism of action of primaquine is undefined. It is the only known tissue schizonticide. Primaquine is usually used in combination with chloroquine, for prophylaxis against or to cure *P. vivax* malaria. Primaquine can cause hemolytic anemia in patients with glucose-6-phosphate dehydrogenase deficiency. Prolonged use is often accompanied by gastrointestinal disturbances, headache, and pruritus.

- **Antifolates**

  — *Pyrimethamine* Pyrimethamine is a dihydrofolate reductase inhibitor with selectivity for the protozoal enzyme. The drug is well absorbed from the gastrointestinal tract and is cleared by the kidney. The half-life is 80 to 110 hours. Pyrimethamine is useful for prophylaxis against or treatment of infections by all susceptible strains of *Plasmodium*. This is particularly noted for chloroquine-resistant *falciparum*. Adverse effects include those associated with antifolates.

  — *Fansidar* This is a combination of pyrimethamine with the sulfonamide sulfadoxine. The utility of the combination is discussed on pp. 253-254.

■ Other Antiprotozoals

Metronidazole
Trichomoniasis
Giardiasis
Amebiasis

- **Metronidazole** This nitroimidazole is readily absorbed and widely distributed throughout the body after administration. Parenteral formulations are also available for IV administration. Effective concentrations are achieved in the brain. Intracellular concentrations are comparable to extracellular concentrations. The drug is cleared in the urine. Reduction of the nitro group of metronidazole by electron transport systems in protozoans leads to redox cycling and subsequent oxidative damage to the parasite. Metronidazole is used to treat a variety of intestinal, extraintestinal, and urogenital protozoal infections, including trichomoniasis, giardiasis, and amebiasis. It is also effective against various anaerobic bacteria. Adverse effects are common and include nausea, headache, and dry mouth. Metronidazole also has a pronounced disulfiram-like effect.

- **Pentamidine** Because this diamidine is not absorbed from the gastrointestinal tract, it is administered either IM or by aerosol inhalation. Absorbed pentamidine is concentrated in several tissues, including the liver, spleen, and kidneys. It does not cross the blood-brain barrier, but it does cross the placenta. The precise mechanism of action is not known, but it may involve inhibition of synthesis of protein, nucleic acids, or phospholipids. Pentamidine is an alternative drug for several protozoal infections. It is the primary drug for prophylaxis or treatment of *Pneumocystis* infections in AIDS patients. Pentamidine triggers the release of histamine from mast cells, causing pronounced and even life-threatening hypotension. Selective toxicity to the β-cells of the pancreatic islets is also noted, which may cause an initial hypoglycemia because of inappropriate insulin release. Hepatotoxicity and nephrotoxicity may also be noted. Serious adverse effects are seen in about 50% of AIDS patients receiving pentamidine.

Anthelmintic Drugs
Mebendazole
Thiabendazole
Praziquantel
Pyrantel pamoate

■ Anthelmintic Chemotherapy
The targets for anthelmintics are generally adult multicellular organisms. Described in this section are drugs most widely used in the United States, where the range of helmintic infections is narrow. It should be noted that a much larger number of parasites and drugs are of importance in other parts of the world.

- **Mebendazole** Although this benzimidazole compound is given orally, only about 10% is absorbed. When used for nonintestinal infections the drug should be taken with a fatty meal, which will enhance its absorption. The absorbed drug is excreted primarily in the urine. Mebendazole inhibits the synthesis of microtubules in nematodes, decreasing their ability to transport secretory vesicles and other cellular organelles, resulting in the death of the nematodes. Mebendazole is effective against pinworms, hookworms, and ascariasis. Normal doses of mebendazole elicit few adverse effects, mostly gastrointestinal disturbances.

- **Thiabendazole** Unlike mebendazole, thiabendazole is rapidly and efficiently absorbed from the gastrointestinal tract. Thiabendazole is almost quantitatively hydroxylated in the liver, with the metabolite and its conjugates excreted in the urine. Like mebendazole, thiabendazole blocks microtubule synthesis, but it also may inhibit fumarate reductase in the parasite. Adverse effects of thiabendazole are generally moderate, but their incidence is higher (up to 50%) than for mebendazole. These include nausea, vomiting, anorexia, and dizziness. Less common adverse effects include hepatotoxicity.

- **Praziquantel** Oral administration of praziquantel results in about 80% bioavailability. The drug is rapidly and extensively hydroxylated in the liver, and the metabolites are excreted primarily in the urine. The parent compound is the active form. Praziquantel increases the permeability of the helminth cell membrane to calcium, resulting in contraction, paralysis, and death. Praziquantel is used for the treatment of schistosomiasis and other helmintic infections. Headache, dizziness, and drowsiness are common adverse effects. Gastrointestinal disturbances and elevations in serum levels of liver enzymes may also occur.

- **Pyrantel pamoate** Pyrantel pamoate is poorly absorbed from the gastrointestinal tract and is therefore useful for the treatment of luminal helmintic infestations. Pyrantel triggers the release of acetylcholine in susceptible helminths, causing depolarizing neuromuscular blockade and paralysis of the helminth. Pyrantel pamoate has a broad spectrum of activity and is used primarily for the treatment of *Ascaris* and pinworm infections. Adverse effects include gastrointestinal distress, drowsiness, headache, rash, and fever. These effects are usually transient and mild.

Section 7.8 Antiviral Chemotherapy

- **Overview** Viruses are obligate intracellular parasites. They possess relatively few enzymes of their own, relying on the appropriation of the biosynthetic machinery of the host cell for replication. Symptoms of viral infections are not observed until after a major wave of viral proliferation. Consideration of these concepts and of the viral life cycle helps define the targets attacked by pharmacologic agents and explains why effective antiviral therapy is so difficult to achieve.

- **Viral Life Cycle** The life cycle of a virus consists of six separate stages (Fig. 7.1). Although the attachment to a susceptible host cell and the resultant uptake and uncoating of the virus are processes unique to viral infection, these steps often occur before the manifestations of infection. These processes are more appropriate for chemoprophylaxis than for chemotherapy. Most antiviral agents focus on nucleic acid replication. Viral polymerases, especially the reverse transcriptase of retroviruses, are targets for selective toxicity. Modification of host defenses, as elicited by interferons, is another approach to antiviral chemotherapy (Box 7.9).

Box 7.9

ANTIVIRAL AGENTS
Uptake Inhibitors
Amantadine
Rimantadine
Nucleoside Analogs
Ribavirin
Vidarabine
Acyclovir
Ganciclovir
Azidothymidine (AZT)
Dideoxyinosine (ddI)
Endogenous Factor
Interferon-α

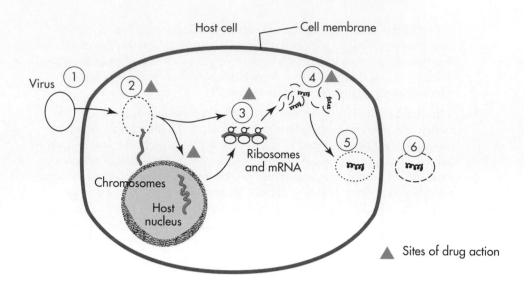

1. Attachment to host cell

2. Uncoating of virus

3. Control of DNA, RNA, or
   protein production

4. Production of viral subunits

5. Assembly of virions

6. Release of virions

Fig. 7.1 Stages of viral life cycle. Sites targeted by antiviral drugs are indicated. *(Adapted from Wingard et al:* Human pharmacology, *St. Louis, 1991, Mosby.)*

■ Inhibitors of Viral Uptake

● Adamantanamines

— ***Amantadine*** A primary symmetric amine, amantadine is an effective antiviral with few serious adverse effects. It is useful only in influenza A infections and rubella. It has high bioavailability after oral administration and is excreted unchanged in the urine. Its half-life is about 12 hours.

Mechanism of action. A virustatic agent, amantadine inhibits viral absorption and uptake. It displays activity in vitro against influenza A, influenza C, Sendai, pseudorabies, and rubella. In patients its activity is limited to influenza A.

Clinical use. Amantadine is approved for the prevention and treatment of influenza A infections. It is used prophylactically for known or expected exposure to influenza A. Therapy should be initiated within 48 hours of onset of influenza A virus symptoms to reduce fever and shorten the course of the disease.

Adverse effects. CNS effects are most common, including insomnia, decreased concentration, nervousness, depression, and drowsiness.

— ***Rimantadine*** Similar to amantadine, rimantadine has a longer half-life. It is eliminated by the liver. It may have a lower incidence of adverse CNS effects than amantadine.

■ Inhibitors of Nucleic Acid Synthesis

● Nucleoside analogues

— ***Ribavirin*** A synthetic nucleoside analog, ribavirin is a competitive inhibitor of DNA and RNA viruses (blocks guanosine-triphosphate

[GTP] formation). It is approved for the treatment of hospitalized infants and young children with severe lower respiratory tract infections caused by respiratory syncytial virus. It is effective when given as an aerosol delivered by head hood or face mask. No serious adverse effects are associated with its use.

Inhibitors of Nucleic Acid Synthesis

Ribavirin
Vidarabine
Acyclovir
Ganciclovir
Azidothymidine
Dideoxyinosine

— *Vidarabine (adenine arabinoside, Ara-A)* A purine nucleoside analog, vidarabine inhibits DNA synthesis by affecting DNA polymerase. It is rapidly deaminated to hypoxanthine arabinoside (ara-Hx) by tissue adenosine deaminase, necessitating constant infusion. Ara-A excretion is primarily renal, with 40% to 53% as Ara-Hx and 1% to 3% as Ara-A. Vidarabine is used for herpes simplex or varicella zoster. It is administered topically or IV. It is the least toxic of the purine analogs. The most frequent adverse effects are nausea and vomiting. Neurologic toxicities may occur.

— *Acyclovir (ACV, acycloguanosine)* A purine nucleoside analog (guanosine), acyclovir is the safest and most widely used antiherpes agent. It is a chain terminator and DNA polymerase inhibitor that must be phosphorylated by viral thymidine kinase, to which it binds 200 times more avidly than to host cell tyrosine kinase. From 50% to 75% of acyclovir is excreted unchanged in urine, mostly by glomerular filtration. Elimination half-life is 2 to 3 hours, except in newborns where it is slightly longer. HSV-1 is more susceptible to acyclovir than HSV-2. It is used topically to limit infectiousness of lesions and to reduce the frequency and severity of the lesions. IV therapy is indicated in all serious HSV infections, including encephalitis and neonatal disease. This route of administration is also indicated as prophylaxis for seropositive transplant patients.

Resistance develops from tyrosine kinase-deficient virus or mutant viral DNA polymerase. Acyclovir is the safest antiherpetic yet marketed. Adverse effects may involve the kidney, skin and soft tissue, and the CNS.

— *Ganciclovir* A deoxyguanosine analog, ganciclovir inhibits DNA polymerase by competitive inhibition. It is activated by thymidine kinase or by deoxyguanosine kinase of cytomegalovirus. The final phosphorylation is by cellular enzymes. IV ganciclovir is mainly eliminated unchanged by renal excretion with a half-life of 3 to 4 hours. It is effective against cytomegalovirus (both retinitis and visceral). Because of its toxicity, it is currently used only for severe or life-threatening cytomegalovirus infections. Ganciclovir-resistant cytomegalovirus strains have been reported. Adverse effects include neutropenia (near 40%), which usually occurs during the second week of treatment and is normally reversible. Other adverse effects include anemia, eosinophilia, headache, behavioral changes, seizure, coma, fever, rash, phlebitis, and nausea.

● Dideoxynucleosides

— *Azidothymidine (AZT, Zidovudine)* A thymidine nucleoside analog, AZT is a competitive inhibitor of reverse transcriptase and a chain terminator of viral DNA synthesis. It is rapidly metabolized and excreted, with 75% of an administered dose eliminated as glucuronide in urine. Its half-life is 1 to 3 hours. It is widely distributed throughout the body, with brain levels approximately 60% of those found in serum.

Azidothymidine has been shown to temporarily reduce the morbidity and mortality associated with HIV infections. Thus early treatment with 500 mg/day of AZT in adults prolongs the time to the first major AIDS-defining event and improves CD4 counts. Adverse effects are common and may be severe. Included are bone marrow depression, headaches, agitation, and insomnia. Its toxicity is enhanced by drugs that compete for glucuronidation, such as acetaminophen and trimethoprin.

— *Dideoxyinosine (ddI)* A purine dideoxynucleoside, ddI is an antiretroviral with a mechanism of action similar to that of AZT. It may be effective against AZT-resistant strains of the virus. Less toxic than AZT, ddI may cause peripheral neuropathy and pancreatitis.

Other dideoxynucleosides are dideoxypyrimidines **dideoxycytidine (ddC)** and **3-deoxythymidin-2-ene (d4T)**. These are used in combination chemotherapy, either as "cocktails" or sequentially.

■ **Endogenous Factor**

● **Interferon-α** An endogenous glycoprotein, interferon-α is produced by leukocytes. It enhances host cell resistance to viral infection, possibly by blocking the release of virions through induction of other cytokines.

Interferon-α has a broad spectrum of activity against RNA and DNA viruses. The human interferons are active against several viral infections and malignancies. Their full potential and role in chemotherapy are not yet defined. Adverse effects include fever, malaise, headaches, anemia, and gastrointestinal distress.

SECTION 7.9 CANCER CHEMOTHERAPY

■ **Overview** Cancer chemotherapy is based on selective toxicity against a target that not only is eukaryotic, but is derived from normal cells of the patient. Although the altered growth, differentiation, and metastatic capacity of tumor cells distinguish them from normal tissue, it is difficult to exploit these differences for selective cytocidal effects.

Tumor cells are initially characterized by a high proliferation rate, and it is this proliferation that is targeted by most anticancer drugs. These drugs either damage DNA, inhibit DNA synthesis, or interfere with the process of mitosis. Although the control of proliferation in tumor cells is altered in some way, the stages of the cell cycle are the same as in normal cells (Fig. 7.2). Drugs that affect DNA synthesis act during the S phase of the cell cycle, whereas those affecting the mitotic apparatus act during the M phase. These are defined as *cell cycle specific* (CCS) drugs. Drugs that damage DNA directly can exert their effects at any point in the cell cycle and thus are defined as *cell cycle nonspecific* (CCNS) drugs. Although CCNS drugs can exert cytocidal effects on any cell, the cells under the metabolic and temporal stress of the S and M phases are more sensitive to this effect than are resting cells. Cycling cells have less time for the detection and repair of DNA damage before replication. Normal cells with a high proliferative rate are also affected by anticancer drugs. Bone marrow, oral and gastrointestinal mucosa, and skin and hair follicles are normal populations with high proliferation rates, and they are also primary sites for dose-limiting adverse effects of anticancer drugs.

The fraction of cells in a normal tissue or a tumor that are either in the S phase or the M phase is called the **growth fraction**. The higher the growth fraction, the more successful (i.e., more cytocidal) the anticancer drugs. Bone mar-

Normal Cells Sensitive to Anticancer Drugs

Bone marrow
Oral mucosa
Gastrointestinal mucosa
Skin follicles
Hair follicles
Gonadal cells

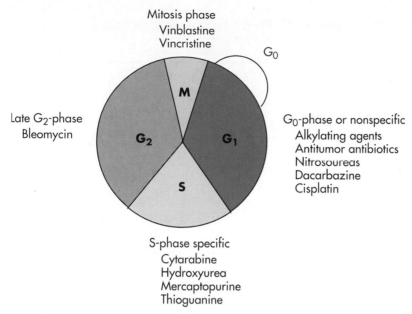

Fig. 7.2 Cell cycle specific and cell cycle nonspecific drug action.

row and oral mucosa have growth fractions of 20% to 30%, whereas tumors have growth fractions ranging from 20% to 70%. The growth fraction for a given tumor is not constant, but instead decreases as tumor mass increases (Fig. 7.3). This decrease in growth rate apparently results from poor vascularization of large tumors. Unfortunately, this also means that large tumors are less susceptible to the effects of anticancer drugs than are smaller, but faster growing, tumors. Poor vascularization also presents a barrier to the delivery of chemotherapeutic drugs.

The tumor cell burden is critical because cure of cancer requires the total eradication of the target cells. Microbial infections are often cured by the elimination of 99.9% of the target cells, but with a typical tumor such a kill rate would leave as many as 10^8 cells. Total eradication of tumor cells requires multiple courses of chemotherapy and the use of multiple drugs (combination chemotherapy).

The principles supporting combination chemotherapy with anticancer drugs are similar to those defined for antimicrobial agents. The use of multiple drugs with different mechanisms of action and different adverse effects can allow lower

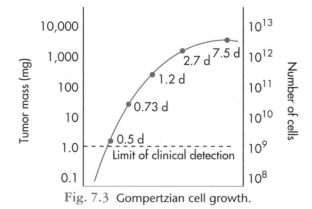

Fig. 7.3 Gompertzian cell growth.

Table 7.3   *Mechanisms of Resistance to Anticancer Drugs*

DRUG	MECHANISM
Alkylating agents	Increased thiols (GSH)
	Increased DNA repair
	Decreased drug uptake
Antimetabolites	
Fluorouracil	Decreased uridine kinase
	Low affinity of thymidylate synthetase for 5FUdR-MP
Methotrexate (MTX)	Increased dihydrofolate reductase (DHFR)
	Low affinity of DHFR for MTX
	Decreased drug uptake
Mercaptopurine	Decreased hypoxanthine-guanine phos-
Thioguanine	phoribosyl transferase
	Increased alkaline phosphohydrolase
	Altered PRPP aminotransferase
Cytarabine	Increased deoxycytidine deaminase
	Decreased deoxycitidine kinase
Vinca alkaloids	Decreased uptake/increased efflux
Antitumor antibiotics	Decreased uptake/increased efflux

doses of individual agents, minimizing dose-dependent toxicities. Synergism in therapeutic responses can occur, particularly when CCS and CCNS agents are combined. Finally, the use of drugs with different mechanisms and targets delays the development of resistant cells.

Resistance is a major problem in cancer chemotherapy. Primary resistance (i.e., resistance without exposure to chemotherapeutic drugs) is seen in colon cancer and in non-small cell lung cancer. Acquired resistance is more widespread, appearing subsequent to initial courses of chemotherapy. Many types of resistance are seen that are specific for particular agents or classes of agents (Table 7.3), but multidrug resistance is also well documented. This usually results from the expression of a plasma membrane phosphoglycoprotein, which actively pumps a broad range of drugs out of the cell. This active process decreases the concentration of drugs in the cell. The calcium channel blocker **verapamil** is a competing substrate for this pump, and trials are under way to determine the clinical utility of this drug in blocking this mechanism of resistance.

■ **Anticancer Drugs**

● **Alkylating agents** The alkylating agents are a large and chemically diverse group that includes **bis(chloroethyl)amines** (nitrogen mustards), **nitrosoureas, aziridines, alkylsulfonates** (busulfan), and the **platinum complexes** (Box 7.10). **Procarbazine** is also classified as an alkylating agent. These drugs have a common mechanism of action and some common adverse effects. They are differentiated by their pharmacokinetics, their clinical applications, and some unique toxic effects.

— *Mechanism of action* Alkylating agents are CCNS drugs (Box 7.11). Their cytotoxic effect is derived from covalent modification of DNA by the agents or their metabolites. Alkylation can lead to abnormal base pairing, blocking of transcription or DNA replication, loss of bases from the DNA strand, or DNA strand breakage, and can cause mutations. Most alkylating agents are bifunctional and can cause cross-linking within or between DNA strands. *Cis*-platin is unique

Box 7.10

PROTOTYPES OF ALKYLATING AGENTS

Bis(chloroethyl)amines
Cyclophosphamide
Mechlorethamine
Chlorambucil
Melphalan

Nitrosoureas
Carmustine (BCNU)
Lomustine (CCNU)

Aziridines
Thiotepa
Triethylenemelamine

Alkylsulfonates
Busulfan

Platinum Complexes
Cis-platin
Carboplatin

Hydrazine
Procarbazine

Box 7.11

ALKYLATING AGENTS—MECHANISMS OF ACTION

Cross-linkage or single-strand binding of DNA, impairing
   its function
Cell cycle nonspecific

---

in that it is a platinating agent; it binds DNA via a bond to the
platinum atom. Platinum complexes are also bifunctional agents, so
crosslinking often occurs. Resistance to the effects of alkylating agents
occurs through increased DNA repair, decreased drug permeability,
or the increased production of trapping agents such as thiols.

— *Pharmacokinetics* Alkylating agents either are inherently reactive or
must be converted to reactive metabolites to allow for their spontaneous reaction with DNA. The former case is illustrated by the direct
cytotoxicity of **mechlorethamine,** an inherently reactive nitrogen
mustard. The reactivity of mechlorethamine raises serious problems
in its use—the half-life is only a few minutes because of its rapid reaction with soluble proteins and other biomolecules, making infusion
directly into arteries supplying a tumor the preferred route of administration. The nitrosoureas, aziridines, alkylsulfonates, and other
nitrogen mustards are activated nonenzymatically but are more stable
than mechlorethamine, with longer half-lives and better distribution. Agents that require conversion to reactive metabolites by host
enzymes, such as the cytochrome P-450-mediated biotransformation
of cyclophosphamide, are more selective. Greater stability and selectivity permit the oral administration of **busulfan, chlorambucil,
melphalan,** and **cyclophosphamide.** Other alkylating agents are administered IV. The high lipophilicity of the nitrosoureas allows them
to cross the blood-brain barrier, which makes them useful for treating brain tumors. Pellets containing nitrosoureas are occasionally im-
planted directly into tumors.

   Most alkylating agents are excreted as inactive metabolites. Urinary excretion is a major route of elimination.

— *Clinical use* The alkylating agents are particularly useful in combination chemotherapy of lymphomas, leukemias, and myelomas. **Cyclophosphamide** and *cis*-**platin** are broad-spectrum alkylating
agents, with important applications in the treatment of many solid
tumors as well, including breast, ovarian, testicular, lung, and bladder
carcinomas.

— *Toxicity* Alkylating agents chemically modify DNA, disrupting its
structure and function. This affects transcription, but may have a
more profound effect on DNA replication. As a result, normal cell
populations with high proliferative rates are often targets for adverse
effects of alkylating agents. General toxic effects of alkylating agents
include bone marrow suppression, loss of gastrointestinal mucosa,
alopecia, and changes in gonadal function. Decreased blood cell counts
are used as an index of effective dosing and as a measure of patient
recovery before resumption of chemotherapy. Nausea and vomiting
also occur, apparently through a direct stimulation of chemoreceptor
zones or the vomiting center in the brain. This effect is minimized

Bioactivation
Cyclophosphamide

Oral
Busulfan
Chlorambucil
Melphalan
Cyclophosphamide
Lomustine

Cis-platin
Nephrotoxicity

Cyclophosphamide
Hemorrhagic cystitis

Box 7.12

PROTOTYPES OF
ANTIMETABOLITES

Methotrexate
Mercaptopurine
Thioguanine
Fluorouracil
Cytarabine

with phenothiazines and with serotonin antagonists such as **ondansetron.**

Specific adverse effects are noted with some alkylating agents. *Cis*-platin, although relatively nontoxic to bone marrow, is associated with a dose-limiting nephrotoxicity. Cyclophosphamide can cause hemorrhagic cystitis. Both are classic dose-related toxicities and result from the high concentrations of the active drugs or the toxic cyclophosphamide metabolite acrolein generated as a consequence of the excretion pathway. Incidence and severity are minimized by aggressive hydration before and during therapy. **Busulfan** can cause adrenal insufficiency, increases in skin pigmentation, and pulmonary fibrosis.

Secondary malignancy is a unique adverse effect of alkylating agents. The ability to covalently modify DNA and thus alter its information content and function is a mechanism not only for these chemotherapeutic agents, but also for many genotoxic carcinogens. Thus alkylating agents may cure the original cancer but cause a new malignancy 10 to 20 years later. The emergence of this new secondary malignancy as a consequence of successful chemotherapy of an original malignancy is of particular importance for young patients. **Procarbazine** is noted to be strongly carcinogenic and leukemogenic.

● **Antimetabolites** Antimetabolites useful in cancer chemotherapy are structurally similar to the endogenous compounds folic acid (**methotrexate**), purines (**mercaptopurine, thioguanine**), and pyrimidines (**fluorouracil, cytarabine**). These agents inhibit DNA synthesis and thus are cell cycle specific agents (Box 7.12).

— *Mechanisms of action* **Methotrexate** and its polyglutamate metabolites inhibit dihydrofolate reductase, thus blocking the synthesis of thymidine, purine nucleotides, and amino acids. The indirect blockade of nucleic acid synthesis is the key chemotherapeutic effect. Tumor resistance arises from decreased drug accumulation, from changes in the affinity of dihydrofolate reductase for methotrexate, or possibly from increased synthesis of dihydrofolate reductase (Box 7.13).

Box 7.13

MECHANISM OF ACTION—ANTIMETABOLITES

Interfere with the synthesis of building blocks for nucleic acids
S-phase specific

Mercaptopurine (6-MP) and **thioguanine** (TG) are converted to nucleotide forms by hypoxanthine-guanine phosphoribosyltransferases (HGPRTase). The activated metabolites inhibit several enzymes involved in purine metabolism. Resistance usually involves decreased HGPRTase activity, but increased levels of alkaline phosphatase inactivate the toxic nucleotides formed from 6-MP or TG.

Fluorouracil (5-FU) is also activated to a nucleotide, specifically 5-F-2′-deoxyuridine-5′-monophosphate (5-FdUMP). This thymidine analogue inhibits thymidylate synthase, leading to thymineless death of cells. Resistance can arise via decreased bioactivation of 5-FU, increased levels of thymidylate synthase, or mutations in thymidylate synthase that lower the affinity of the enzyme for 5-FdUMP.

Cytarabine (cytosine arabinoside, AraC) is phosphorylated by kinases to form the active metabolite AraCTP, an inhibitor of DNA polymerases during the S phase. Resistance results from decreased uptake of AraC by tumor cells or decreased conversion to AraCTP.

— *Pharmacokinetics* **Methotrexate** is well absorbed after oral administration but may also be given intrathecally. Methotrexate is excreted in the urine, primarily as the parent drug. Polyglutamic acid conjugates of methotrexate are retained intracellularly. Purine analogs are effective after oral administration, but the pyrimidine analogs must be given parenterally (usually IV) because of erratic absorption or first-pass effects.

— *Clinical use* Antimetabolites are used in combination regimens, often with CCNS drugs such as alkylating agents. Efficacy has been shown against acute leukemias and against carcinomas of the head, neck, lung, breast, and intestine.

— *Toxicity* Adverse effects for all of these antimetabolites include dose-dependent bone marrow suppression. Nausea and vomiting may occur with the pyrimidine analogs. **Methotrexate** may cause oral and gastric ulceration. Methotrexate toxicity may be treated with folinic acid as part of the leucovorin or citrovorin rescue. This strategy follows high-dose methotrexate with administration of folinic acid to "rescue" normal cells.

● **Plant alkaloids** These natural products include the *Vinca* alkaloids (***vinblastine, vincristine***) podophyllotoxins (***etoposide***), and paclitaxel (***taxol***) (Box 7.14).

Box 7.14

PROTOTYPES OF PLANT ALKALOIDS

Vinca **Alkaloids**
  Vincristine
  Vinblastine

Podophyllotoxins   Etoposide (VP-16)
Paclitaxel (Taxol)

— *Mechanisms of action* **Vinblastine** and **vincristine** bind to tubulin subunits to block the assembly of or to depolymerize the microtubules that make up the mitotic spindle. They are CCS drugs that act in the M phase of the cancer cell cycle, causing metaphase arrest. **Taxol,** in contrast, stabilizes these same mitotic microtubules and thus does not allow cells to pass beyond metaphase. **Etoposide** increases degradation of DNA, primarily via inhibition of topoisomerase II, causing DNA strand breaks. It acts in the late S to early G_2 phases of the cell cycle (Box 7.15). Resistance to the plant alkaloids usually results from removal of these agents by the plasma membrane drug transporter.

Box 7.15

MECHANISMS OF ACTION—PLANT ALKALOIDS

Alter Stability of Mitotic Microtubules (Spindles)
  Vinca alkaloids
  Paclitaxel

Inhibition of Topoisomerase II   Etoposide

— *Pharmacokinetics* All of these agents are given IV. Vincas and paclitaxel are excreted in bile, whereas etoposide is found in the urine. Paclitaxel is extensively metabolized in the liver.

— *Clinical use*

Vincristine is used in acute leukemias, Hodgkin's and non-Hodgkin's lymphomas, and various pediatric and adult solid tumors.

Vinblastine is used in the combination chemotherapy of testicular carcinoma, breast cancer, and lymphomas.

Etoposide is useful against small-cell lung cancers, lymphomas, acute leukemias, and testicular carcinoma.

Paclitaxel is effective against carcinomas of the lung, head, neck, breast, and ovary.

— *Toxicity* The *Vinca* alkaloids and **etoposide** exhibit typical toxicities for anticancer drugs—nausea and vomiting, bone marrow depression, and alopecia. **Vincristine** is less likely to suppress bone marrow than is **vinblastine**. The dose-limiting effect of the vinca alkaloids is neurotoxicity, particularly peripheral neuritis and areflexia. **Paclitaxel** is a bone marrow suppressant and also causes peripheral neuropathy.

● **Antibiotics** This subclass is made up of several structurally dissimilar drugs, including the anthracyclines (*doxorubicin, daunorubicin*), the synthetic anthracycline analog *mitoxantrone, bleomycin, dactinomycin, plicamycin,* and *mitomycin.* With the exception of mitoxantrone, all are natural products (Box 7.16).

Box 7.16

PROTOTYPES OF ANTIBIOTICS
Anthracyclines
Doxorubicin
Daunorubicin
Mitoxantrone
Dactinomycin
Bleomycin
Plicamycin
Mitomycin C

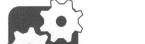

— *Mechanisms of action*

Anthracyclines intercalate between adjacent base pairs in DNA. This noncovalent interaction blocks both DNA and RNA synthesis. Strand breaks also occur, either through free radical mechanisms or the actions of topoisomerase II. Free radical mechanisms involving anthracyclines are also of key importance in the expression of adverse effects.

Mitoxantrone shares the therapeutic mechanism of the naturally occurring anthracyclines.

Bleomycin intercalates between DNA base pairs, but it also chelates iron. This chelated iron, now tethered to DNA, catalytically generates oxygen radicals, which cause strand breaks and DNA fragmentation. Bleomycin is the only CCS antitumor antibiotic.

Dactinomycin tightly intercalates into DNA between adjacent GC base pairs, blocking RNA synthesis. DNA synthesis is only slightly inhibited.

Plicamycin (mithramycin) binds to DNA as a ternary complex with

Mg^{++} and blocks RNA synthesis. More common than its use as an antineoplastic agent is its utilization to reverse hypercalcemia. This apparently results from effects of plicamycin on osteoclasts.

Mitomycin (mitomycin C) is included as an antitumor antibiotic because it is a natural product. Its mechanism of action, however, is derived from initial reductive metabolism, which converts mitomycin to a reactive alkylating agent that cross-links DNA.

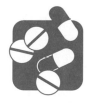

— *Pharmacokinetics* These compounds are administered only parenterally, particularly IV. Mitomycin C may be instilled into the bladder for treatment of bladder papillomas. The anthracyclines and mitomycin undergo extensive metabolism in the liver. Bleomycin is inactivated by bleomycin hydrolase, an enzyme that is found at high levels in the liver and kidneys but that is not present in the skin and lungs. Resistance to anticancer antibiotics often results from active transport out of cells catalyzed by the multidrug resistance membrane phosphoglycoprotein.

— *Clinical use* **Doxorubicin** is a broad-spectrum antitumor agent, often used in combination chemotherapy with alkylating agents for the treatment of many carcinomas, sarcomas, leukemias, and lymphomas. **Daunorubicin** is far narrower in spectrum, used only against acute leukemias. **Mitoxantrone** is useful against acute myelogenous leukemia, non-Hodgkin's lymphoma, and breast cancer. **Bleomycin** is part of a curative combination regimen (with vinblastine and cisplatin) for testicular carcinoma and is also useful against squamous cell carcinomas and lymphomas. **Plicamycin** is used primarily for treatment of malignancy-associated hypercalcemia rather than strictly as an antitumor agent. **Mitomycin C** is used in the treatment of solid tumors of the cervix, stomach, pancreas, lung, bladder, and colon.

— *Toxicity* The antitumor antibiotics cause typical adverse effects such as nausea, bone marrow suppression, and alopecia. Signature toxicities include the potentially fatal cumulative cardiotoxicity of the anthracyclines, the pronounced and long-lived bone marrow suppression of mitomycin C, and the life-threatening irreversible pulmonary fibrosis induced by bleomycin. The latter appears to be a consequence of the absence of bleomycin hydrolase in the lung.

■ **Hormones and Hormone Antagonists** Hormonal control of normal proliferation and differentiation of specific cell and tissue types is common. Tumors derived from such cell populations may retain these control mechanisms. This provides more selective, less toxic mechanisms for the control of proliferative potential than do the general chemotherapeutic targets of DNA and components of the mitotic apparatus. Steroid hormones have been investigated most extensively in this regard. Successful hormonal therapy depends on the presence of functional receptors in the target cells. *Prednisone* suppresses lymphocyte proliferation and thus is used in drug regimens for chronic lymphocytic leukemia, Hodgkin's disease, and other lymphomas. *Sex hormones* (estrogens, progestins, androgens) are used in hormone-dependent cancers to affect changes in proliferation. *Estrogens* can induce remission of prostatic carcinoma, and *progestins* have shown some success in the treatment of metastatic endometrial cancer and more limited success against breast cancer.

Receptor antagonists provide another approach to altering the hormonal stimuli affecting a tumor. *Tamoxifen* is a widely used estrogen receptor antagonist effective against estrogen-dependent breast cancers. ***Flutamide*** is an antiandrogen used in the treatment of prostate cancer. ***Leuprolide*** is a synthetic analog of gonadotropin-releasing hormone that blocks the release of LH and FSH from the pituitary. This leads to a decrease in testicular androgen synthesis and thus removes a growth stimulus for prostatic carcinoma. ***Aminoglutethimide*** is an aromatase inhibitor that decreases the conversion of androstenedione to estrone. This interruption of estrogen synthesis is useful for the treatment of metastatic breast cancer.

MULTIPLE CHOICE
REVIEW QUESTIONS

1. Which antimicrobial drugs may produce hemolysis when given to individuals who have glucose-6-phosphate dehydrogenase deficiency?

    a. Penicillin V
    b. Neomycin
    c. Augmentin (amoxicillin and clavulanic acid)
    d. Cefotaxime
    e. Sulfisoxazole

2. The use of metronidazole and penicillin in treating an abscess caused by beta-lactamase producing bacteroides and anaerobic streptococci is an example of:

    a. synergistic drug treatment.
    b. antagonistic drug effects.
    c. additive drug effects.
    d. none of the above.

3. Which of the following agents is a protein synthesis inhibitor classified as a macrolide antibiotic?

    a. Aztreonam
    b. Erythromyin
    c. Vancomycin
    d. Ceftazidime
    e. Primaxin

4. Which of the following statements is false concerning rifampin?

    a. Rifampin is a macrocyclic antibiotic that inhibits DNA-directed RNA polymerase.
    b. Rifampin is mainly used in the treatment of tuberculosis.
    c. Use of rifampin can permanently discolor contact lenses.
    d. Rifampin has relatively few adverse effects.
    e. Rifampin is often combined with isoniazid for treatment of otitis media.

5. All of the following statements concerning trimethoprim are correct except:

    a. Trimethoprim inhibits bacterial dihydrofolate reductase.
    b. Trimethoprim is active against most grampositive cocci.
    c. Trimethoprim can be combined with sulfamethoxazole and the combination can be used to treat urinary tract infections, otitis media, and gastrointestinal infections caused by *Salmonella*.
    d. High dose trimethoprim-sulfamethoxazole is

    used to treat *Pneumocystis carinii* infection.
    e. Like most sulfonamides, trimethoprim is poorly absorbed from the gastrointestinal tract.

6. A four-year-old child was taken to his pediatrician because of a sore throat. After being placed on ampicillin at the time, the child was taken to the emergency room five days later suffering from a high fever (104° F) and a sore neck. His father indicated that the medication had been taken as prescribed. A diagnosis was made of meningitis probably caused by *H. influenzae*. What antibiotics would be reasonably used in this case at this time?

    a. Continue with ampicillin, but at a higher concentration.
    b. I.V. chloramphenicol
    c. I.V. gentamicin
    d. I.V. streptomycin
    e. All of the above are reasonable approaches.

7. Which of the following drugs is most likely to be effective in treatment of cytomegalovirus (CMV) infection in AIDS patients or other immunosuppressed individuals?

    a. Acyclovir
    b. Amantadine
    c. Vidarabine
    d. Ganciclovir
    e. Zidovudine

8. A 28-year-old white male was found HIV positive during a routine insurance health examination. He did not exhibit physical symptoms of HIV infection; however, his CD_4 cell count was $400/mm^3$. He was started on zidovudine. Three years later he presents to the emergency room complaining of shortness of breath and a low-grade fever. He indicates that he has had the fever for several weeks but only recently has his breathing become labored. His blood gases (pO_2 = 46 mm Hg; pCO_2 = 42 mm Hg) confirm the patient's hypoxic state. Transbronchial biopsy confirmed *Pneumocystis carinii* pneumonia (PCP). The patient was also positive for cytomegalovirus (CMV). What would be appropriate pharmacologic treatment of PCP?

    a. Large doses of penicillin G
    b. I.V. cefotaxime
    c. Trimethoprim/sulfamethoxazole (TMP/SMX)
    d. Pentamidin
    e. Foscarnet

9. Trimethoprim/sulfamethoxazole combination therapy was initiated in the above patient. The patient responded to the treatment and completed a three-week course of therapy. He was prescribed aerosolized pentamidine for prophylaxis of PCP. Eight months later the patient presents to the emergency room having suffered a seizure. Diagnostic testing, including CT examination, supports a diagnosis of toxoplasmosis. Which drug or drug combination is the preferred treatment for toxoplasmosis in this patient?

    a. Trimethoprim/sulfamethoxazole
    b. Penicillin
    c. Pyrimethamine with sulfadiazine
    d. Cefotaxime
    e. None of the above

10. A six-year-old male is brought to the emergency room because of difficulty breathing. The patient is most comfortable sitting and leaning forward in an effort to breathe. His temperature was 103° F with a WBC count of 21000/mm^3. Upon examination, the child's epiglottis is bright red and swollen. What would be the most appropriate therapy?

    a. Corticosteroids
    b. Humidified air
    c. Parenteral antibiotics
    d. None of the above

11. A 72-year-old patient was recovering in the hospital from a partial gastrectomy when, on the fifth post-operative day, he began exhibiting fever and labored breathing. Rales with diminished breath sounds were noted in several lung fields. Blood gases indicated a pO$_2$ of 29 mm Hg which increased to 50 mm Hg with 4L/min of oxygen. A gram stain of lower respiratory tract secretion was positive for gram-negative rods. The diagnosis is hospital acquired pneumonia. Which drugs or drug combinations would be most appropriate for treating this pneumonia?

    a. Gentamicin alone
    b. Ampicillin alone
    c. Gentamicin plus nafcillin
    d. Gentamicin plus nafcillin plus piperacillin
    e. None of these are appropriate

Chapter 8

Hemo/Immunopoietic and Antiinflammatory Drugs

SECTION 8.1 AGENTS TO TREAT ANEMIA

■ **Overview** Anemia is characterized by an abnormally low level of hemoglobin resulting from a decrease in the number of circulating erythrocytes or a decrease in the amount of hemoglobin per red blood cell. The two major types of anemia are microcytic hypochromic anemia, which is caused by iron deficiency, and megaloblastic anemia, which is caused by vitamin B_{12} or folic acid deficiency (Box 8.1). Several diseases and drugs cause anemia by decreasing the synthesis

Box 8.1

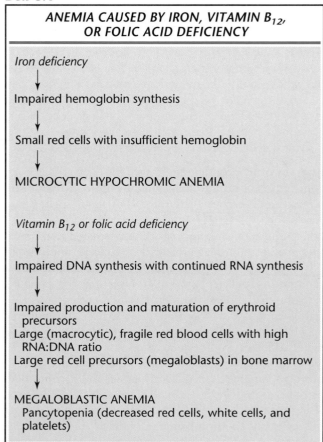

DNA, Deoxyribonucleic acid; *RNA,* ribonucleic acid.

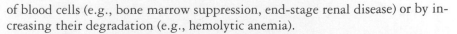

of blood cells (e.g., bone marrow suppression, end-stage renal disease) or by increasing their degradation (e.g., hemolytic anemia).

■ **Iron** Most of the iron in the body is in hemoglobin (70%) and myoglobin (10%), the oxygen-transport proteins in red blood cells and muscle, respectively. Between 10% and 20% of the iron is in storage proteins such as ferritin and hemosiderin, which are found in macrophages in the liver, spleen, and bone marrow. Only 1% of the iron is in cytochromes and the iron-transport protein transferrin.

Approximately 1 mg of iron is required per day, mainly to support hemoglobin synthesis. Iron is obtained from a variety of dietary sources. The average diet contains 10 to 15 mg of elemental iron, of which 5% to 10% is absorbed. In the United States, insufficient dietary iron is rarely the cause of anemia.

Because iron is absorbed in the duodenum and proximal jejunum, surgical removal of the upper small intestine impairs its absorption. Iron absorption is increased by hydrochloric acid, so gastric resection also impairs iron absorption.

Iron present in heme and other organic complexes is absorbed in the ferric (Fe^{3+}) state. Elemental iron, however, must be absorbed in the ferrous (Fe^{2+}) state, which is the form administered therapeutically. Absorption involves active transport of ferrous iron, which is oxidized to ferric iron in the gastric mucosa. Ferric iron is stored as ferritin in the mucosa or is transported by transferrin to other sites. Low iron stores increase iron absorption.

Iron absorption is increased by gastric acid and ascorbic acid and is decreased by food, which increases gastric pH, antacids except for Mylantin, metal chelators, and tetracycline.

Because there is no specific mechanism for excreting iron, iron loss is not regulated. Iron balance is maintained by intestinal absorption. About 1 mg of iron is lost daily by processes such as exfoliation of mucosal cells, which contain ferritin.

Iron deficiency is generally caused by excessive blood loss, frequently from gastrointestinal bleeding or menstruation. The latter can result in the loss of 30 mg of iron, which could take more than a month to replenish. An increase in demand, such as that occurring in pregnancy, can also cause an iron deficiency. Rarely is dietary insufficiency the cause of iron deficiency. Iron deficiency leads to a decrease in hemosiderin and ferritin and an increase in the iron-binding capacity of transferrin, which have diagnostic value (Box 8.2).

● **Treatment of iron deficiency** Iron deficiency is usually corrected by oral administration of iron (ferrous) salts, including **ferrous sulfate, ferrous gluconate,** and **ferrous fumarate.** They should be taken on an empty stomach when gastric pH is at its lowest. Supplementation with vitamin C or other adjuvants is unnecessary. Enteric-coated iron preparations, which are designed to minimize gastric disturbances, should *not* be used because iron is absorbed in the duodenum and proximal jejunum.

During iron deficiency, 50 to 100 mg of iron may be incorporated into hemoglobin daily. Because up to 25% of dietary iron is absorbed during iron deficiency, 200 to 400 mg of dietary iron are required as therapy. Iron therapy is usually continued for 3 to 6 months or longer if the dose of iron is decreased because of intolerance.

Adverse effects associated with oral iron include nausea, epigastric discomfort, abdominal cramps, constipation, and diarrhea. Patients should be informed that iron therapy causes black stools.

Parenteral iron is used to treat iron deficiency after gastric or small bowel resections and in inflammatory bowel disease involving the proximal small intestine. Iron dextran is administered intramuscularly (IM) or in-

Oral Iron Preparations
Ferrous sulfate
Ferrous gluconate
Ferrous fumarate

Box 8.2

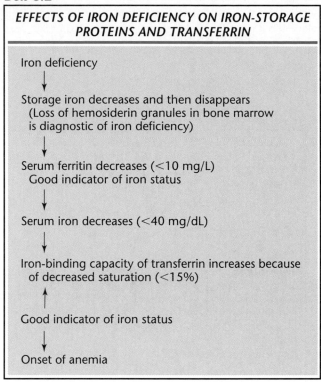

EFFECTS OF IRON DEFICIENCY ON IRON-STORAGE PROTEINS AND TRANSFERRIN

Iron deficiency

Storage iron decreases and then disappears
(Loss of hemosiderin granules in bone marrow
is diagnostic of iron deficiency)

Serum ferritin decreases (<10 mg/L)
Good indicator of iron status

Serum iron decreases (<40 mg/dL)

Iron-binding capacity of transferrin increases because
of decreased saturation (<15%)

Good indicator of iron status

Onset of anemia

travenously (IV) (less painful). Initially, small doses are administered to check for signs of immediate hypersensitivity. The adverse effects of iron dextran include headache, light-headedness, fever, arthralgia, nausea, vomiting, back pain, flushing, urticaria, bronchospasm, and rarely anaphylaxis.

Parenteral Iron Preparations
Iron dextran

- **Acute iron toxicity** Because children are particularly susceptible to the toxic effects of iron, acute toxicity is usually observed in them after accidental ingestion of iron tablets. Iron causes necrotizing gastroenteritis, and as few as 10 tablets can be lethal to children. The symptoms of iron toxicity are vomiting, abdominal pain, and bloody diarrhea (phase 1); shock, lethargy and dyspnea (phase 2); metabolic acidosis, coma, and death (phase 3).

The following steps are taken to treat acute iron toxicity:
  1. Gastric aspiration to remove undissolved iron tablets
  2. Gastric levage with phosphate or carbonate to precipitate iron
  3. **Desferal** instilled in the stomach and administered IM or IV to chelate iron
  4. Supportive therapy (treatment of bleeding, acidosis, shock)

- **Chronic iron toxicity** Iron overload can result in hemochromatosis, which is an inherited disorder characterized by excessive iron absorption, or hemosiderosis, which often results from numerous blood transfusions. The excess deposition of iron in the heart, liver, pancreas, and other organs can lead to organ failure. Iron overload is treated by phlebotomy (1 unit of blood removes 250 mg iron).

■ **Megaloblastic Anemia** Because vitamin B_{12} and folic acid are both required for normal nucleic acid metabolism, a deficiency in either causes megaloblastic

Iron Chelation
Desferal

anemia (see Box 8.1). Inasmuch as a deficiency in vitamin B_{12} also causes neurologic disorders, it is important to determine whether megaloblastic anemia is due to folate or vitamin B_{12} deficiency.

● **Folic acid** Folic acid is converted by dihydrofolate reductase to tetrahydrofolic acid, which is subsequently converted to several cofactors (one-carbon donors) required for purine and pyrimidine synthesis (Box 8.3).

Box 8.3

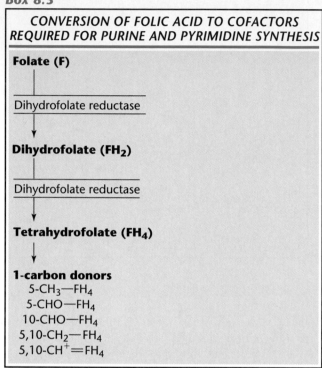

CONVERSION OF FOLIC ACID TO COFACTORS REQUIRED FOR PURINE AND PYRIMIDINE SYNTHESIS

Folate (F)

Dihydrofolate reductase

Dihydrofolate (FH_2)

Dihydrofolate reductase

Tetrahydrofolate (FH_4)

1-carbon donors
$5\text{-}CH_3\text{---}FH_4$
$5\text{-}CHO\text{---}FH_4$
$10\text{-}CHO\text{---}FH_4$
$5,10\text{-}CH_2\text{---}FH_4$
$5,10\text{-}CH^+\text{=}FH_4$

Folic acid is derived from various dietary sources, including yeast, liver, kidney, and green vegetables. Between 50 and 200 µg of folate are absorbed daily, representing 10% to 25% of the dietary intake. Folate is absorbed by active and passive transport in the proximal jejunum.

Dietary folate is mainly in the form of 5-methyl-tetrahydrofolic acid ($5\text{-}CH_3\text{-}FH_4$), one of the many one-carbon donors required for nucleic acid synthesis. It is also the major storage form of folate. Because liver and other tissues store only 5 to 20 mg of folate, serum levels decline within days when intake is diminished. Folates are lost through metabolism and excretion in urine and feces.

Folic acid deficiency usually results from increased demand which occurs during pregnancy, in patients with hemolytic anemia or certain proliferative disorders (e.g., cancers), and in renal dialysis patients. Decreased absorption, which occurs in patients with small bowel resection, sprue, and other malabsorption syndromes, can also cause a deficiency. Dietary insufficiency is common among the elderly and alcoholics. Hepatic disease can lead to folate deficiency because of decreased storage. In addition, drugs that inhibit dihydrofolate reductase, such as **trimethoprim** and **methotrexate,** cause folate deficiency, as does phenytoin and other anticonvulsants, oral contraceptives, and isoniazid, all of which interfere with folate absorption.

Folate Deficiency

Pregnancy
Hemolytic anemia
Cancer
Renal dialysis
Malabsorption syndromes
Hepatic disease

Dihydrofolate Reductase Inhibitors

Trimethoprim
Pyrimethamine
Methotrexate

Folate deficiency leads to megaloblastic anemia in 1 to 6 months. Oral folic acid begins to restore hemoglobin levels during the first week of treatment and fully corrects it in 1 to 2 months. When administered orally, folic acid provokes no adverse effects.

● **Vitamin B$_{12}$** Vitamin B$_{12}$ is composed of a porphyrin-like ring system containing cobalt. Various ligands complex with the cobalt to produce different cobalamins, as follows:

- Active form: R = 5'-deoxyadenoxyl or methyl group
- Drugs: R = Cyano (CN–) or hydroxy (OH–) group
- Food: R = various ligands

Drugs and dietary cobalamins are converted to active forms in the body. Dietary sources of vitamin B$_{12}$ include food of microbial origin, liver, eggs, and dairy products. It is not synthesized in humans.

The absorption of vitamin B$_{12}$, which is also known as *extrinsic factor*, requires *intrinsic factor*, a glycoprotein produced by the parietal cells of the gastric mucosa. Intrinsic factor complexes with vitamin B$_{12}$ in the stomach and duodenum. This complex is absorbed in the distal ileum by a receptor-mediated transport system. Vitamin B$_{12}$ deficiency is invariably due to malabsorption of vitamin B$_{12}$, either from a lack of intrinsic factor or a defective uptake of the vitamin B$_{12}$-intrinsic factor complex in the distal ileum.

In the blood, vitamin B$_{12}$ is transported by transcobalamin II, which binds 50 to 100 μg of the vitamin. When the binding capacity of transcobalamin is exceeded, excess vitamin B$_{12}$ is excreted in the urine.

Vitamin B$_{12}$ is stored in the liver. The amount stored in the liver (up to 5 mg) can meet the daily demand for vitamin B$_{12}$ (2 μg/day) for up to 5 years.

— *Functions of vitamin B$_{12}$* Vitamin B$_{12}$ is a cofactor for methylmalonyl-CoA mutase, which converts methylmalonyl-CoA to succinyl-CoA. Vitamin B$_{12}$ deficiency reduces the activity of this enzyme, resulting in the accumulation of substrate, methylmalonyl-CoA. This leads to the formation of abnormal lipids in the brain, which in turn causes neurologic abnormalities. Another enzyme that requires vitamin B$_{12}$ as a cofactor is 5-methyl-tetrahydrofolate-homocysteine methyltransferase, which converts 5-CH$_3$-FH$_4$ into tetrahydrofolate (Box 8.4).

In vitamin B$_{12}$ deficiency, the levels of 5-CH$_3$-FH$_4$ stored in the liver increase, whereas levels of the other one-carbon factors decrease, leading to an impairment of nucleic acid metabolism. Inasmuch as it blocks the conversion of 5-CH$_3$-FH$_4$ to tetrahydrofolate, vitamin B$_{12}$ deficiency is said to *trap* 5-CH$_3$-FH$_4$ in the liver and other storage sites.

Although tetrahydrofolate cannot be synthesized from 5-CH$_3$-FH$_4$ in the absence of vitamin B$_{12}$, it can be synthesized from folic acid by way of dihydrofolate reductase. Consequently, the defects in nucleotide synthesis caused by vitamin B$_{12}$ deficiency can be corrected with folic acid therapy. For this reason, folic acid corrects the megaloblastic anemia associated with vitamin B$_{12}$ deficiency. However, folic acid treatment cannot correct the neurologic disorders associated with vitamin B$_{12}$ deficiency.

Inhibitors of Folate Absorption

Anticonvulsants
Oral contraceptives
Isoniazid

B$_{12}$ Deficiency

Megaloblastic anemia
Neurologic disorders

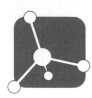

Box 8.4

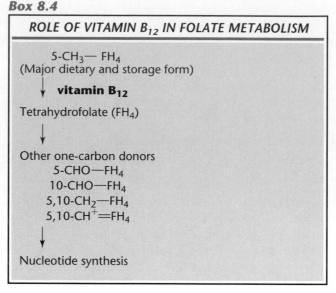

ROLE OF VITAMIN B₁₂ IN FOLATE METABOLISM

5-CH₃— FH₄
(Major dietary and storage form)

↓ **vitamin B₁₂**

Tetrahydrofolate (FH₄)

↓

Other one-carbon donors
    5-CHO—FH₄
    10-CHO—FH₄
    5,10-CH₂—FH₄
    5,10-CH⁺=FH₄

↓

Nucleotide synthesis

Schilling Test
B₁₂ deficiency

● **Vitamin B₁₂ versus folic acid deficiency** It is important to determine the cause of megaloblastic anemia so that corrective therapy can be initiated with either vitamin B₁₂ or folic acid. Diagnosis is based on clinical tests that measure red cell folic acid levels, which are more reliable than serum levels and serum levels of vitamin B₁₂.

The Schilling test, in which radioactive vitamin B₁₂ (with or without pig intrinsic factor) is used, determines whether vitamin B₁₂ deficiency is due to malabsorption. Impaired absorption of free vitamin B₁₂ and vitamin B₁₂ complexed with pig intrinsic factor suggests malabsorption in the distal ileum. This may be due to inflammatory bowel disease or small bowel resection. Impaired absorption of just vitamin B₁₂ indicates malabsorption caused by lack of intrinsic factor which is perhaps due to gastrectomy or pernicious anemia.

■ **(Addisonian) Pernicious Anemia** Pernicious anemia is a megaloblastic anemia resulting from vitamin B₁₂ deficiency caused by decreased production of intrinsic factor by the gastric mucosa. It is accompanied by achlorhydria and is generally observed in older persons of northern European extraction.

Five years or more may elapse between loss of intrinsic factor and the development of megaloblastic anemia because that is the time required to deplete the liver store of vitamin B₁₂.

● **Treatment of vitamin B₁₂ deficiency** Inasmuch as vitamin B₁₂ deficiency invariably results from malabsorption, therapy should involve parenteral administration of the vitamin in the form of hydroxocobalamin or cyanocobalamin. Therapy should be continued for life.

Hydroxocobalamin is highly bound to plasma protein and remains in circulation longer than cyanocobalamin. Because some patients produce antibodies against hydroxocobalamin-transcobalamin II, cyanocobalamin is the drug of choice. There is no risk of cyanide poisoning with this agent.

Hydroxocobalamin and cyanocobalamin are administered IM. The therapeutic objective is to provide the daily requirement and replenish stores of vitamin B₁₂. Doses of 30 to 100 µg are administered daily for 2 to 3 weeks, then every 2 to 4 weeks for life. Daily injections should be continued for up to 6 months if neurologic symptoms occur. Because doses above 100 µg exceed the binding capacity of transcobalamin, 90% of a loading dose of 1000 µg is excreted in urine.

Treatment with parenteral vitamin B_{12} should not be delayed after gastrectomy (or other surgical procedures or diseases that impair B_{12} absorption) and should be continued for life.

The hemopoietic response to vitamin B_{12} therapy is rapid. Bone marrow is normoblastic within 48 hours. Reticulocytosis begins within 2 to 3 days and is maximal within 5 to 10 days, and hemoglobin concentration is normalized in 1 to 2 months. Reticulocytosis should be monitored to confirm the diagnosis and the success of the treatment. Potassium levels should be monitored during the early stages of treatment to ensure that red cell synthesis does not cause hypokalemia.

■ **Erythropoietin** The production of red blood cells in the bone marrow is regulated in part by erythropoietin, a glycoprotein synthesized in the kidney. Erythropoietin produced by recombinant deoxyribonucleic acid (DNA) techniques is useful for treating anemia caused by end-stage renal disease.

Section 8.2 Coagulation Disorders

■ **Overview** Formation of blood clots is an essential part of hemostasis, but their presence within the blood vessels or heart, termed *thrombosis*, is the cause of thromboembolic disease. Failure to form a clot results in bleeding or hemorrhagic disorders. A clot is a hemostatic plug formed from platelets and fibrin. A thrombus is a clot that adheres to a blood vessel wall, and an embolus is an unattached cloth floating in blood.

A thrombus can detach from a vessel wall and become an embolus. Both thrombi and emboli can block blood flow and deprive tissues of oxygen and nutrients (Box 8.5).

There are two types of thrombi: those that form in arteries (white thrombi) and those that form in veins (red thrombi). Arterial thrombi are formed from both platelets and fibrin, whereas venous thrombi are formed mainly from fibrin, with trapped platelets and erythrocytes. Arterial thrombi tend to form in medium-sized arteries in response to vascular damage from atherosclerosis. Their formation can lead to local ischemia, causing myocardial infarction, unstable angina, and stroke. Because blood flow is much slower in veins than in arteries, venous thrombi are characterized by long fibrin tails, which can detach to become emboli that become trapped in the pulmonary arteries, causing an embolism.

Thrombi
White–arteries
Red–vein

■ **Platelet Activation** The recruitment of platelets in the thrombogenic process is regulated by the balance between signals that promote platelet aggregation, such as **collagen, thromboxane,** and **thrombin** (the protease that converts fibrinogen to fibrin), and those that oppose platelet aggregation, such as prostacyclin. When activated, platelets release serotonin and adenosine diphosphate (ADP) stimulating thromboxane synthesis in other platelets, which are then recruited for thrombogenesis.

Damage to the lining of blood vessels promotes platelet aggregation in at least three ways:

1. By decreasing the production of prostacyclin in endothelial cells, which normally inhibits platelet aggregation

Platelet Aggregation
Collagen
Thromboxane
Thrombin

Box 8.5

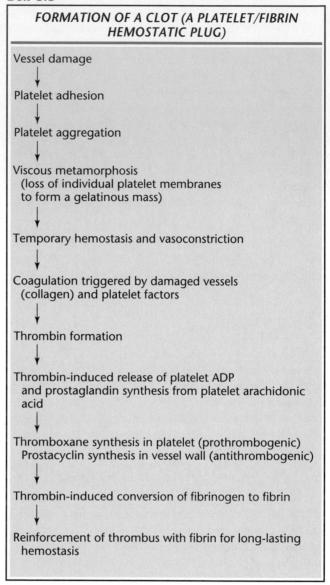

FORMATION OF A CLOT (A PLATELET/FIBRIN
HEMOSTATIC PLUG)

Vessel damage
↓
Platelet adhesion
↓
Platelet aggregation
↓
Viscous metamorphosis
  (loss of individual platelet membranes
  to form a gelatinous mass)
↓
Temporary hemostasis and vasoconstriction
↓
Coagulation triggered by damaged vessels
  (collagen) and platelet factors
↓
Thrombin formation
↓
Thrombin-induced release of platelet ADP
  and prostaglandin synthesis from platelet arachidonic
  acid
↓
Thromboxane synthesis in platelet (prothrombogenic)
  Prostacyclin synthesis in vessel wall (antithrombogenic)
↓
Thrombin-induced conversion of fibrinogen to fibrin
↓
Reinforcement of thrombus with fibrin for long-lasting
  hemostasis

ADP, Adenosine diphosphate.

2. By exposing collagen, which binds platelets and stimulates thromboxane synthesis
3. By activating the coagulation pathway, thrombin, which binds to platelets and stimulates thromboxane synthesis

Measurement

Intrinsic pathway
–partial thromboblastia time
Extrinsic pathway
–one-stage prothrombin time

■ **Coagulation** Fibrin is an important component of blood clots. It is formed from fibrinogen by one of two coagulation pathways known as intrinsic coagulation, for which all the required factors are present in blood, and extrinsic coagulation, which also requires factors derived from tissues, such as thromboplastin and factor III. The **intrinsic pathway** is initiated by collagen, which activates factor XII to factor XIIa (Fig. 8.1). The **extrinsic pathway,** on the other hand, is initiated by tissue thromboplastin, which binds to, and activates factor VII. Both pathways convert factor X to factor Xa, which, in the presence of

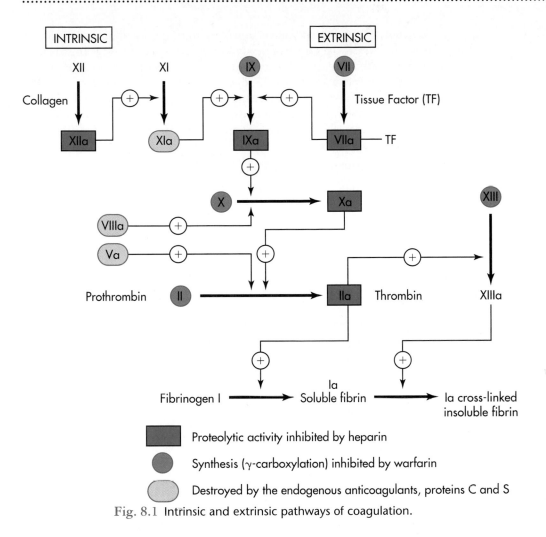

Fig. 8.1 Intrinsic and extrinsic pathways of coagulation.

factor Va, transforms prothrombin (factor II) to thrombin (factor IIa). In addition to converting fibrinogen (factor I) to fibrin (factor Ia), thrombin binds to platelet receptors, which stimulate aggregation. Thrombin is generated at the platelet surface because prothrombin is bound by calcium to cell surface phospholipids.

The intrinsic coagulation pathway is measured as the partial thromboplastin time and is relatively slow. The extrinsic coagulation pathway is measured as the one-stage prothrombin time and is relatively fast.

● **Regulation of coagulation and thrombus formation** Two processes, fibrin inhibition and fibrinolysis, operate to confine blood coagulation and thrombus formation to an area of damage and to prevent disseminated coagulation.

With the exception of fibrin formation, the final step in the process, the coagulation cascade involves sequential activation of clotting factors by proteolytic enzymes. The formation of fibrin at sites remote from an injury is prevented by plasma proteins that inhibit various factors in their activated or proteolytic state. Protease inhibitors include α_1-**antitrypsin**, α_2-**macroglobulin**, α_2-**antiplasmin**, and **antithrombin III**. Failure of fibrin inhibition results in generalized intravascular clotting or disseminated intravascular coagulation.

Protease Inhibitors

α_1-antitrypsin
α_2-macroglobulin
α_2-antiplasmin
antithrombin III

Fibrinolysis involves the conversion of plasminogen to plasmin, a serine protease that limits the spread of newly formed clots and dissolves the fibrin network of established clots during wound healing. With the intrinsic coagulation pathway, activation of plasminogen is catalyzed by factor XII. Thus plasmin forms immediately when coagulation begins. With the extrinsic coagulation pathway, activation of plasminogen is catalyzed by tissue plasminogen activators, ensuring that plasmin forms immediately after tissue damage occurs and the onset of coagulation.

■ **Drugs to Treat Coagulation Disorders**

● **Antiplatelet drugs** Because of the prominent role of platelets in arterial thrombosis, patients with arterial thrombi are treated with antiplatelet drugs, such as aspirin, ticlopidine, sulfinpyrazone, and dipyridamole (Box 8.6).

Box 8.6

DRUGS USED TO TREAT COAGULATION DISORDERS

Antithrombogenic	Prothrombogenic
Platelet inhibitors	Aminocaproic acid
Aspirin	Tranexamic acid
Ticlopidine	Protamine sulfate
Dipyridamole	Vitamin K
Sulfinpyrazone	
Anticoagulants	
Heparin	
Warfarin	
Thrombolytic agents	
Tissue plasminogen activator	
Streptokinase and anistreplase	
Urokinase	

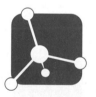

Platelet Inhibitors

Aspirin
Ticlopidine
Sulfinpyrazone
Dipyridamole

Aspirin irreversibly inhibits cyclooxygenase, reducing platelet activity by inhibiting thromboxane synthesis. Aspirin has been approved for prophylaxis of primary myocardial infarction and prevention of arterial thrombosis in patients with a history of such problems. The β-blocker timolol has also been approved as a prophylactic agent for myocardial infarction, but it is not known whether its beneficial effects are due to an effect on platelets.

Ticlopidine inhibits ADP-induced platelet aggregation. It is effective in preventing the recurrence of arterial thrombosis in patients with transient ischemic attacks, strokes, and unstable angina pectoris. It causes gastrointestinal disturbances in 20% of patients, hemorrhage in 5%, and leukopenia and 1%. Regular monitoring of the white blood cell count is required with this agent.

Although generally used as a uricosuric, **sulfinpyrazone** also has antiplatelet properties. Like ticlopidine and aspirin, sulfinpyrazone blocks the chemical mediators of platelet aggregation. Unlike aspirin, however, sulfinpyrazone prolongs platelet survival.

Dipyridamole inhibits cyclic nucleotide phosphodiesterase, potentiating the actions of prostacyclin, which is coupled to a cAMP-generating system in the platelet. In this way, dipyridamole decreases platelet adhesion to thrombogenic surfaces. Although dipyridamole would be expected to potentiate the antiplatelet effects of aspirin, any such effects are marginal. Dipyridamole is effective, when given in conjunction with warfarin, in preventing embolization in patients with prosthetic heart valves.

● **Anticoagulants** Heparin and warfarin are both used to treat established venous thrombosis and pulmonary emboli. Heparin is used for the first 7 to 10 days with an overlap of 3 to 5 days with warfarin, which may be continued for up to 6 months. Heparin, and to a lesser extent warfarin, is the primary treatment for the prevention of venous thrombosis and therefore pulmonary embolism.

Dextran, a branched chain polysaccharide that interferes with platelet function and fibrin polymerization, is used to prevent postoperative venous thrombosis.

Although they have the same therapeutic indications, heparin and warfarin differ in many respects, including their mechanism of action, route of administration, and onset of action (Table 8.1).

— *Heparin* Heparin is a sulfated mucopolysaccharide isolated from pig intestine or cow lung. It is administered IV or subcutaneously (SQ). It cannot be administered orally because it is not absorbed from the gastrointestinal system, and it should not be given IM because of the risk of hematoma at the injection site. Heparin has an immediate onset of action. Its mechanism involves the protease inhibitor, antithrombin III, which forms a 1:1 complex with clotting factor proteases. Although normally slow, this interaction is stimulated 1000-fold by heparin, which binds to antithrombin III.

The therapeutic goal with heparin is to prolong partial thromboplastin time to approximately twice normal.

Heparin is contraindicated in patients with bleeding disorders, conditions that predispose to bleeding such as thrombocytopenia, hemorrhage, and other diseases. Unlike warfarin, heparin does not cross the placental barrier.

Table 8.1   *Comparison between the Anticoagulants Heparin and Warfarin*

FEATURE	HEPARIN	WARFARIN
Mechanism of action	Binds to plasma antithrombin III and accelerates the inhibition of thrombin	Inhibits the hepatic synthesis of the vitamin K–dependent clotting factors
Antidote	Protamine sulfate	Vitamin K or prothrombin (i.e., fresh blood or plasma)
Activity in vitro	Yes	No
Route of administration	Intravenous or subcutaneous	Oral
Onset of action	Immediate	Delayed (until preexisting vitamin K–dependent clotting factors are consumed or degraded)
Duration of action	Hours	Days (reflecting the time needed to synthesize new clotting factors)
Laboratory monitoring	Partial thromboplastin time	Prothrombin time
Major adverse effect	Hemorrhage	Hemorrhage
Clinical use	Prevention and treatment of thromboembolism	Prevention and treatment of thromboembolism

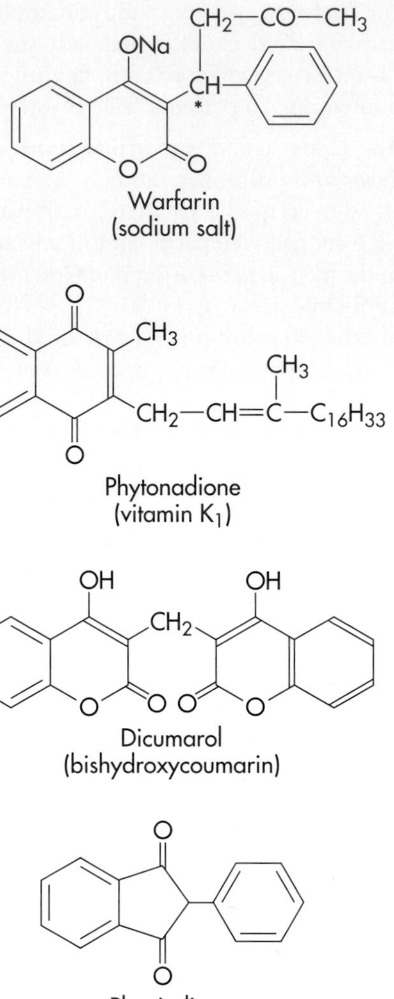

Warfarin
(sodium salt)

Phytonadione
(vitamin K₁)

Dicumarol
(bishydroxycoumarin)

Phenindione

Fig. 8.2 Structures showing the relationship of oral anticoagulants to phytonadione (vitamin K).

Heparin Overdose
Protamine sulfate

Adverse effects of heparin include excessive bleeding, which can be minimized by monitoring the partial thromboplastin time; allergic reactions, which may occur because heparin is an animal product; osteoporosis after long-term therapy; and transient but occasionally severe thrombocytopenia.

Overdose is treated with protamine sulfate, a basic peptide that binds to heparin. Excessive antidote must be avoided because protamine itself is an anticoagulant. One milligram of protamine sulfate is administered IV for each 100 U of heparin remaining in the patient.

— *Warfarin and the coumarin anticoagulants* Warfarin (coumadin) is the most widely used of several oral anticoagulants, most of which are derivatives of coumarin (Fig. 8.2). The oral anticoagulants are structurally related to vitamin K, which accounts for their ability to impair the synthesis of vitamin K-dependent clotting factors, including prothrombin. These drugs differ only in their half-life for producing and maintaining hypoprothrombinemia.

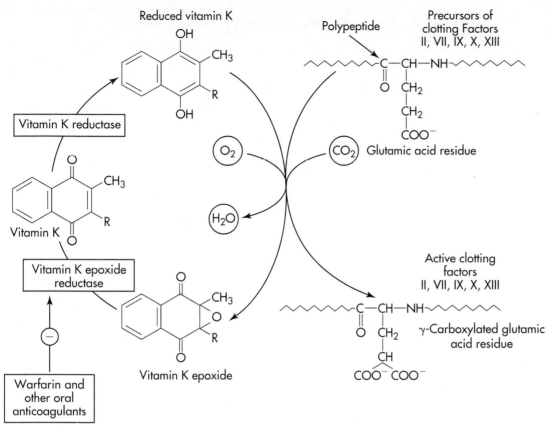

Fig. 8.3 Vitamin K–dependent γ-carboxylation of clotting factors and its inhibition by warfarin and related anticoagulants.

Because of their structural similarity to vitamin K, oral anticoagulants inhibit vitamin K epoxide reductase, which blocks the vitamin K-dependent γ-carboxylation of glutamic acid residues in factors II (prothrombin), VII, IX, X, and XIII, as well as one anticoagulant, protein C (Fig. 8.3).

There is an 8 to 12 hour delay in the onset of the anticoagulant effect, with the maximum effect requiring several days. The delay represents the time necessary to replace normal clotting factors with incompletely γ-carboxylated factors and the time necessary to reach steady-state levels of the drug.

The therapeutic goal with warfarin is to double or treble prothrombin time. This is normally achieved within a week.

In addition to discontinuation of therapy, excessive anticoagulation by warfarin is treated with vitamin K (phytonadione). Restoration of normal coagulation takes about 24 hours, which corresponds to the time required to synthesize new clotting factors. Fresh frozen plasma or factor IX concentrates containing prothrombin complex can be used to normalize coagulation without delay. This may be required to prevent massive warfarin-induced hemorrhage.

Warfarin is contraindicated in patients with bleeding disorders. In contrast to heparin, warfarin crosses the placenta and is therefore contraindicated during pregnancy because of the risk of fetal hemorrhage.

Table 8.2 *Pharmacokinetic Drug Interactions with Warfarin*

DRUGS THAT INHIBIT P-450 AND POTENTIATE THE ANTICOAGULANT EFFECTS OF WARFARIN	DRUGS THAT INDUCE P-450 AND ATTENUATE THE ANTICOAGULANT EFFECTS OF WARFARIN
Amiodarone	Barbiturates
Cimetidine	Glutethimide
Chloramphenicol	Griseofulvin
Cotrimoxazole	Phenytoin
Disulfiram	Rifampin
Metronidazole*	
Miconazole*	
Phenylbutazone*	
Sulfinpyrazone*	
Trimethoprim-sulfamethoxazole*	

*These drugs preferentially inhibit the metabolism of *S*-warfarin.

Because it is extensively bound to plasma protein, warfarin has a low volume of distribution, has a long half-life (36 hours), and may interact with other drugs that bind to albumin.

The elimination of warfarin depends on its metabolism by hepatic cytochrome P-450. Drugs that induce this enzyme increase warfarin metabolism and attenuate its anticoagulant effects. Conversely, drugs that inhibit cytochrome P-450 decrease warfarin metabolism, potentiating its anticoagulant effects (Table 8.2). Inasmuch as warfarin is a racemic mixture, some drugs preferentially inhibit the metabolism of *S*-warfarin, which is four times more efficacious than the *R*-enantiomer as an anticoagulant.

A number of drugs interact with warfarin. Those that potentiate the anticoagulant effects include antiplatelet medications such as aspirin and clofibrate, other anticoagulants, agents that accelerate the turnover of clotting factors such as clofibrate and thyroxine, and drugs that block the synthesis of vitamin K by intestinal bacteria, such as some cephalosporins.

Agents that attenuate the anticoagulant effects of warfarin include vitamin K and diuretics that increase the plasma concentration of clotting factors such as spironolactone and chlorthalidone. Hypothyroidism attenuates the anticoagulant effects of warfarin, as can hereditary resistance to warfarin caused by mutations in vitamin K epoxide reductase. Such mutations do not impede the γ-carboxylation of clotting factors, but rather render the enzyme insensitive to the inhibitory effects of warfarin and the other oral anticoagulants.

Drug interactions that potentiate the anticoagulant effects of warfarin pose the greatest threat because they increase the risk of hemorrhage.

● **Thrombolytic (fibrinolytic) drugs** When coagulation begins, plasminogen is converted to plasmin, a serine protease that limits the spread of new clots and dissolves the fibrin network of established clots during wound healing. This ability to dissolve blood clots is the basis of fibrinolytic therapy, which is directed toward the activation plasmin.

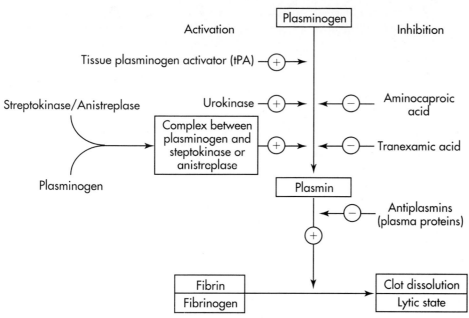

Fig. 8.4 Site of action of drugs acting on the fibrinolytic system.

Plasmin degrades both fibrin and fibrinogen. Degradation of fibrin is beneficial because it confines coagulation to the site of vascular injury and leads to clot dissolution. Degradation of fibrinogen, on the other hand, is detrimental because it leads to a lytic, or hemorrhagic, state. To prevent the degradation of fibrinogen and thereby confine fibrinolysis to newly forming or established clots, the blood contains antiplasmins. Just as the fibrinolytic system controls the coagulation system, so antiplasmins regulate the fibrinolytic system. Circulating antiplasmins preclude the possibility of using plasmin itself for fibrinolytic therapy.

Activators of the fibrinolytic system include **streptokinase, anistreplase, urokinase,** and **tissue plasminogen activator** (Fig. 8.4). They convert plasminogen to plasmin and are used to dissolve hemostatic thrombi and thromboemboli. They are particularly useful for those pulmonary emboli too small to remove surgically. Inhibitors of the fibrinolytic system include **aminocaproic acid** and **tranexamic acid,** which block conversion of plasminogen to plasmin and are used to control fibrinolytic states.

Urokinase, a human kidney protease, and the complex formed between proactivator and **streptokinase,** a streptococcal enzyme, convert plasminogen to plasmin and cause a systemic fibrinolytic state, which can cause bleeding problems. The beneficial effects of urokinase and streptokinase stem largely from activation of plasmin inside the thrombus, where plasmin is protected from the inhibitory effects of circulating antiplasmins.

Acylating the plasminogen streptokinase-activated complex produces **anistreplase,** which preferentially converts plasminogen to plasmin in thrombi, rather than converting free plasminogen to plasmin. Anistreplase has a longer half-life than streptokinase, urokinase, or tissue plasminogen activator.

Preferential conversion of fibrin-bound plasminogen to plasmin is also achieved with **tissue plasminogen activator,** which is more efficacious than streptokinase or anistreplase for thrombolytic therapy in myocardial

Fibrinolytic Activators

Streptokinase
Anistreplase
Urokinase
Tissue plasminogen activator

Fibrinolytic Inhibitors

Aminocaproic acid
Tranexamic acid
Antiplasmins

infarction. However, it is associated with a higher incidence of hemorrhagic stroke than the others. Currently, tissue plasminogen activator is approved only for the treatment of myocardial infarction. Other indications are being considered.

The fibrinolytic agents are administered by intracoronary or, more commonly, IV infusion. Ideally, therapy is initiated within 6 hours of clot formation because clots become more resistant to lysis over time. Fibrinolytic agents were once used only for deep-vein thrombosis and serious pulmonary embolism, but they are now used increasingly for the treatment of acute peripheral arterial thrombosis and emboli and for unclogging catheters and shunts. To prevent reformation of a blood clot, some fibrinolytic agents are administered simultaneously with heparin.

After an IV loading dose, streptokinase is administered for 24 to 72 hours with the aim of at least doubling thromboplastin time. After an initial loading dose, urokinase is administered for 12 hours, whereas tissue plasminogen activator is administered for 2 hours. The longer-lasting anistreplase is administered as a single IV injection lasting 3 to 5 minutes. Fibrinolytic therapy is expensive. It is followed by anticoagulant therapy with heparin and then warfarin.

Fibrinolytic agents do not distinguish between desirable and undesirable blood clots. In addition, by converting both free and fibrin-bound plasminogen to plasmin, streptokinase and urokinase cause a systemic fibrinolytic state. For these reasons, hemorrhage is the major adverse effect of this therapy. Lesions, such as ulcers, may hemorrhage during fibrinolytic therapy. Because of the risk of hemorrhage, fibrinolytic therapy is contraindicated during pregnancy, after a recent cerebrovascular accident, and in patients with a healing wound. Severe hemorrhage is countered by administering aminocaproic acid or tranexamic acid, which block the conversion of plasminogen to plasmin.

In patients with antistreptococcal antibodies (approximately 3%), the bacterial protein streptokinase is neutralized or causes an allergic reaction, such as fever, rash, and rarely anaphylaxis.

■ **Coagulation (Hemorrhagic) Disorders** Bleeding problems can be genetically determined or acquired. Hemophilias are caused by heritable deficiencies in the synthesis of a clotting factor. Most commonly these are factor VIII or IX, which result in hemophilia A and B, respectively. Hemophilias are treated by administering the defective factor, often derived from human blood, with a risk of viral infection. **Desmopressin acetate** and **danazol** increase factor VIII activity and are useful in cases of mild hemophilia. Inhibitors of the fibrinolytic system, aminocaproic acid and its analog tranexamic acid, are used as adjunctive therapy in hemophilia.

Acquired coagulation disorders can result from the following:

1. A deficiency of vitamin K, which is required to synthesize prothrombin and several other clotting factors that require γ-carboxylation
2. Liver failure, which impairs the synthesis of several clotting factors
3. Procedures that cause excessive bleeding, such as gastrointestinal surgery and prostatectomy
4. Overdose of anticoagulants of fibrinolytic drugs

Vitamin K is a fat-soluble vitamin found in green vegetables and produced by intestinal bacteria. Its absorption from the gastrointestinal tract requires bile acids. Vitamin K is given to all newborns to safeguard against nutritional deficiency and before gall bladder surgery. Because of a lack of bile acids, such patients are often vitamin K deficient and prone to excessive bleeding during surgery. Vitamin K is an antidote for oral anticoagulant overdose, although 24 hours are required to synthesize new clotting factors. Heparin overdose is treated with protamine sulfate, whereas overdose of fibrinolytic agents is treated with aminocaproic acid or tranexamic acid.

SECTION 8.3 ANTIINFLAMMATORY DRUGS

■ **Overview** Inflammation is a normal response to tissue damage and infection and may be associated with pain and fever. In some cases, such as allergies to pollen, and with certain autoimmune disorders, such as rheumatoid arthritis, the inflammatory response is detrimental. Inflammation is triggered by chemicals released from damaged tissues and circulating blood cells (Box 8.7).

Box 8.7

CHEMICALS INVOLVED IN THE INFLAMMATORY RESPONSE
Lipids
Prostaglandins
Leukotrienes
Thromboxane
Platelet-activating factor
Amines
Histamine
Serotonin (5-hydroxytryptamine)
Small peptides
Bradykinin
Large peptides
Interleukin-1

Agents that modify the inflammatory response are classified as nonsteroidal antiinflammatory drugs (NSAIDs), nonopioid analgesics, slow-acting antiinflammatory drugs to treat arthritis, and drugs to treat gout (Box 8.8).

■ **Nonsteroidal Antiinflammatory Drugs** To understand the mechanism of action of NSAIDs, it is necessary to appreciate the role of eicosanoids in the inflammatory response. Eicosanoids are not stored in the body but rather are synthesized on demand from arachidonic acid, released by the action of phospholipase A_2 on phospholipids in cell membranes (Fig. 8.5). This initial step in eicosanoid synthesis is inhibited by corticosteroids, which are antiinflammatory, and stimulated by bradykinin and angiotensin, which are proinflammatory. Arachidonic acid is converted to eicosanoids by the lipoxygenase pathway, which converts arachidonic acid to leukotrienes, and the cyclooxygenase pathway, which converts arachidonic acid to thromboxane, prostacyclin, and a variety of prostaglandins. The NSAIDs inhibit cyclooxygenase, blocking the formation of eicosanoids derived from this pathway. With few exceptions, however, NSAIDs do not block the lipoxygenase pathways.

By inhibiting cyclooxygenase, NSAIDs have antiinflammatory, analgesic, and antipyretic actions. The NSAIDs are analgesic because pain receptors are sensitized by prostaglandins, bradykinin, and histamine. The NSAIDs have antipyretic effects because bacterial pyrogens, by increasing interleukin-1 and other

Box 8.8

ANTIINFLAMMATORY DRUGS

Nonsteroidal Antiinflammatory Drugs
Aspirin (acetylsalicylic acid)
Ibuprofen, fenoprofen, ketoprofen, sulindac
Piroxicam, nabumetone, oxaprozin, naproxen
Indomethacin, phenylbutazone

Nonopioid Analgesics
Acetaminophen
Phenacetin

Drugs to Treat Arthritis (Slow-Acting)
Gold salts
Chloroquine
D-Penicillamine
Methotrexate

Drugs to Treat Gout
Colchicine
Allopurinol
Probenecid
Sulfinpyrazone

cytokines, induce the synthesis of PGE_2 in the hypothalamus, increasing body temperature. By blocking the synthesis of thromboxane in the platelet more than the synthesis of prostacyclin in the endothelial lining of blood vessels, NSAIDs prolong bleeding time.

The NSAIDs differ in their antiinflammatory, analgesic, and antipyretic effects. For example, acetaminophen exerts analgesic and antipyretic effects comparable to aspirin but displays negligible antiinflammatory activity. These variations may reflect differences in the extent to which NSAIDs block the cyclooxygenase and lipoxygenase pathways.

There are two isozymes of cyclooxygenase: COX I, which is present in a variety of tissues, and COX II, which is present only in cells involved in the inflammatory response. The NSAIDs are known to differ in their ability to inhibit these isozymes, which could account for some of the differences in their therapeutic effects. Low doses of NSAIDs exert analgesic and antipyretic effects, with much higher doses being required to reduce inflammation.

Not all NSAIDs have the same adverse effects, even when inhibition of cyclooxygenase appears to the mechanism of toxicity. For example, there is a high incidence of gastric irritation with aspirin, but little or no interstitial nephritis. The opposite is generally true of all other NSAIDs.

● **Aspirin (acetylsalicylic acid)** Aspirin is the prototypical NSAID. It is inexpensive and effective, although poorly tolerated by about 15% of patients because of gastric irritation. Like all NSAIDs, aspirin inhibits cyclooxygenase and blocks the synthesis of prostaglandins, thromboxane, and prostacyclin. However, aspirin differs from all other NSAIDs by binding irreversibly to cyclooxygenase. Thus restoration of eicosanoid synthesis after administration of aspirin requires the synthesis of new enzyme. Because it is the acetyl group on aspirin that binds to and irreversibly inhibits cyclooxygenase, salicylic acid, a metabolite of aspirin, does not cause prolonged inhibition of eicosanoid synthesis.

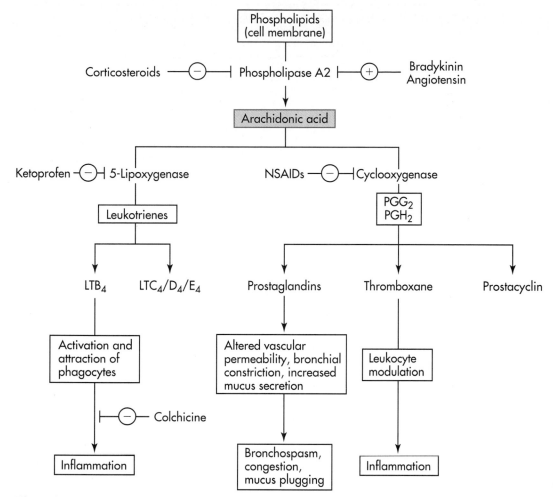

Fig. 8.5 Synthesis of eicosanoids from arachidonic acid. *NSAIDs,* Nonsteroidal antiinflammatory drugs.

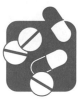

— **Pharmacokinetics** Aspirin is absorbed from the stomach and small intestine. It has a pK_a of 3.5, whereas salicylic acid has a pK_a of 3.0; therefore, absorption of both is favored by low pH. Bufferin contains aspirin in a formulation intended to raise gastric pH in an effort to protect the gastric mucosa from irritation. Alkalinization of urine increases the renal excretion of salicylate.

Acetylsalicylic acid is hydrolyzed (deacetylated) by esterases to salicylic acid, which is extensively conjugated with glucuronic acid and glycine. Small amounts (1%) are hydroxylated to gentisic acid. When the conjugation pathways become saturated, small increases in dose can produce large increases in the plasma levels of salicylate. Salicylates bind to albumin, but the proportion of free drug increases with dose. The pharmacokinetics of salicylic acid are dose dependent (Table 8.3).

— **Pharmacotherapeutics**

Antiinflammatory effects. At high doses (about 4 g/day) aspirin has antiinflammatory effects and is the initial drug of choice in the treatment

Table 8.3	Dose-Dependent Pharmacokinetics of Salicylate	
DOSE	**THERAPEUTIC ACTION**	**PHARMACOKINETICS**
Low (600 mg)	Analgesic, antipyretic	First order, half-life 3-5 hr
High (4 g)	Antiinflammatory	Zero order, half-life greater than 12 hr

of rheumatoid arthritis, rheumatic fever, and other inflammatory joint diseases.

Analgesic effects. Aspirin is a useful analgesic for pain associated with skeletal muscles, vasculature, toothache, arthritis, and bursitis. However, it is not effective for visceral pain, such as renal, colic, pericarditis, and myocardial infarction.

Antipyretic. Aspirin lowers fever but has a negligible effect on normal body temperature. During fever, aspirin adjusts body temperature, promoting heat loss through vasodilation of superficial blood vessels. This can cause profuse sweating.

Antiplatelet effects. By preferentially blocking the synthesis of thromboxane over the synthesis of prostacyclin, low doses of aspirin inhibit platelet aggregation, prolonging bleeding time. Because aspirin causes an irreversible inhibition of cyclooxygenase, its antiplatelet effects persist for 1 week after discontinuation of treatment. To prevent bleeding complication, aspirin should be withheld for 1 week before surgery.

Other therapeutic effects. Aspirin is used to reduce the formation of cataracts, to decrease the incidence of transient ischemic attacks and unstable angina, and to reduce the incidence of recurrent myocardial infarction. Because aspirin appears to prevent myocardial infarction, it is used prophylactically by people over 50 years old, especially those with signs of coronary disease.

— *Adverse effects* Aspirin is a relatively safe agent. At therapeutic doses the main adverse effect is disturbance of the upper gastrointestinal tract.

Gastrointestinal tract. The gastric irritation experienced by about 15% of patients taking aspirin is thought to result from inhibition of cyclooxygenase in the stomach. This decreases the synthesis of prostaglandin, which inhibits acid secretion, and prostaglandin PGE_2 and $PGF_{2\alpha}$, which stimulate the synthesis of the protective mucosa in the stomach and small intestine. The gastrointestinal irritation is reduced somewhat by taking aspirin after meals, with antacids, or with the PGE_1 analog misoprostol. Buffers added to some formulations of aspirin have little effect on gastric pH and therefore do little to reduce the incidence of aspirin-induced gastrointestinal irritation. Other NSAIDs are less likely than aspirin to irritate the gastrointestinal tract.

Kidney. Cyclooxygenase inhibitors block the synthesis of prostaglandin PGE_2 and prostacyclin in the kidney. These substances help maintain blood flow to the kidney, particularly in the presence of vasoconstrictors. In some patients decreased prostaglandin synthesis results in edema and hyperkalemia because of increased water and sodium retention. As a result, aspirin decreases the response to spironolactone. With the exception of aspirin, all NSAIDs cause interstitial nephritis.

Hypersensitivity. Approximately 15% of patients develop a hypersensitivity to aspirin which may appear as urticaria or bronchoconstriction. There is little risk of fatal anaphylactic shock. Patients allergic to aspirin are generally allergic to other NSAIDs.

Toxicity. Mild aspirin toxicity (salicylism) usually requires plasma concentrations that exceed those required for antiinflammatory effects. Symptoms include decreased hearing, tinnitus, nausea, vomiting, hyperventilation, dizziness, and mental confusion. At higher doses there is fever, dehydration, delirium, hallucinations, metabolic and respiratory acidosis, convulsions, and coma. Death from aspirin overdose is caused by respiratory and renal failure. Children are more prone than adults to the toxic effects of aspirin.

Treatment of overdose. Treatment of aspirin poisoning should be guided by measurements of plasma salicylate levels and pH. In mild cases, salicylate levels can be reduced by maintaining high urine volume and alkalinizing the urine with sodium bicarbonate. In severe cases it may be necessary to remove salicylate by hemodialysis or peritoneal dialysis to normalize acid-base disturbances and to ventilate the patient.

— **Drug interaction** The antiplatelet effects of aspirin can complicate therapy with anticoagulants and other inhibitors of platelet aggregation. Severe hemorrhage can result from such interactions. Aspirin decreases the response to spironolactone, and alcohol increases the gastric bleeding caused by salicylates. Pharmacokinetic interactions include the following:

Absorption. Antacids reduce the rate of aspirin absorption.

Excretion. Acidifying agents such as acetazolamide and ammonium chloride reduce the renal excretion of aspirin and enhance its toxicity.

Renal secretion. Aspirin competes with penicillin and uric acid for renal tubular secretion and blocks the uricosuric effects of sulfinpyrazone and probenecid.

Protein binding. Aspirin is highly protein bound and displaces several drugs from albumin, such as tolbutamide, chlorpropamide, methotrexate, phenytoin, and probenecid.

— **Contraindications** Aspirin crosses the placental and blood-brain barriers and is therefore not recommended for pregnant women or children with viral infections because of an increased risk of Reye's syndrome. As a weak acid, aspirin competes with uric acid for renal secretion. Because low doses increase plasma uric acid levels, aspirin is not recommended for use in patients with gout, even though high, antiinflammatory doses are uricosuric.

● **Other nonsteroidal antiinflammatory drugs** There are a large number of structurally diverse NSAIDs that exert varying degrees of antiinflammatory, analgesic, antipyretic, and antiplatelet effects. Like aspirin, all other NSAIDs block the synthesis of certain eicosanoids by inhibiting cyclooxygenase, but, in contrast to aspirin, they do so reversibly. Other NSAIDs generally have the same therapeutic uses as aspirin. As with aspirin, analgesia can be achieved with low doses of NSAIDs, whereas much higher doses are required for antiinflammatory effects.

— *Advantages of other NSAIDs over aspirin* Other NSAIDs cause fewer disturbances of the upper gastrointestinal system, although all cause some gastric irritation and bleeding. The antiplatelet effects of other NSAIDs are terminated rapidly after drug administration.

— *Advantages of aspirin over other NSAIDs* Aspirin is less expensive and is unlikely to cause interstitial nephritis or other serious adverse effects.

— *Ibuprofen and other propionic acid derivatives* Ibuprofen is an over-the-counter NSAID. Like other propionic acid derivatives (fenoprofen, ketoprofen), ibuprofen has a short half-life (about 2 hours) and therefore must be given four times a day to treat rheumatoid arthritis. A longer-acting NSAID in this class, naproxen, with a half-life of about 13 hours, need be given only twice a day. In general, the propionic acid NSAIDs are better tolerated than aspirin. They are contraindicated in individuals with hypersensitivity to aspirin.

Ketoprofen is an unusual NSAID in that it inhibits both cyclooxygenase and lipoxygenase.

Long-Acting NSAIDs

Piroxicam
Nabumetone
Oxaprozin

— *Long-acting nonsteroidal antiinflammatory drugs* Three NSAIDs, **piroxicam, nabumetone,** and **oxaprozin,** have such long half-lives that they need be given only once a day to treat rheumatoid arthritis. Although this regimen improves compliance, it does not reduce the adverse effects associated with NSAID use. For example, piroxicam causes gastrointestinal disturbances in about 20% of patients.

When the dose of piroxicam, nabumetone, and oxaprozin is altered, several days are required to reach a new steady-state level. This is also true of antiinflammatory doses of aspirin, because at high doses the half-life of salicylate is greater than 12 hours (See Table 8.3).

— *Indomethacin and phenylbutazone* Indomethacin is more toxic than aspirin and many of the other NSAIDs but is often superior in the treatment of special inflammatory conditions, such as acute gouty arthritis, ankylosing spondylitis, and osteoarthritis of the hip. Indomethacin is also used to treat patent ductus arteriosus. Indomethacin usually is not given to children or to pregnant women because of its toxicity. Adverse effects with indomethacin are numerous, common, and frequently severe. Included are pancreatitis, hepatitis, neutropenia, thrombocytopenia, and aplastic anemia. Patients with hypersensitivity to aspirin are allergic to indomethacin.

Phenylbutazone is a relatively weak analgesic and antipyretic, but it is a potent antiinflammatory agent. It is used to treat acute gout and acute rheumatoid arthritis if aspirin and other NSAIDs fail. In addition to numerous other adverse effects, phenylbutazone can cause agranulocytosis and aplastic anemia. For this reason treatment is limited to 1 week or less.

■ **Nonopioid Analgesics** Acetaminophen and phenacetin exert analgesic and antipyretic effects equivalent to aspirin but display no significant antiinflammatory effects. Both inhibit cyclooxygenase in the brain, which accounts for their analgesic and antipyretic properties. Because they cause less inhibition of prostaglandin synthesis in peripheral tissues than aspirin, they have weak antiinflammatory and antiplatelet effects. As analgesics, both have an advantage over opioids in that neither causes physical dependence or tolerance. Phenacetin can be con-

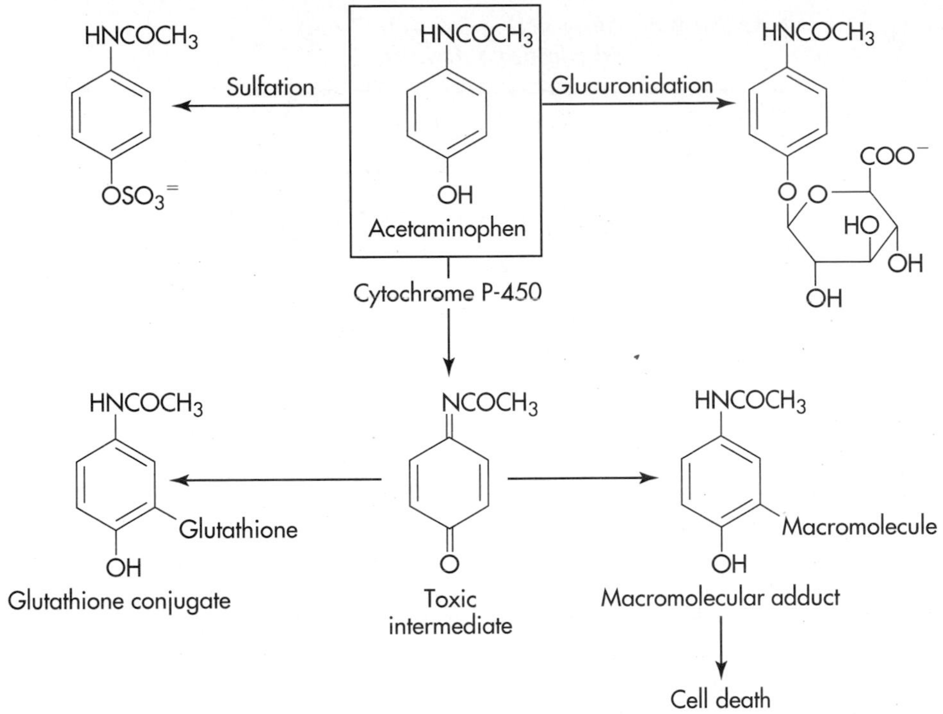

Fig. 8.6 Metabolism of acetaminophen, including the formation of a toxic intermediate.

sidered a prodrug because it is rapidly converted to acetaminophen by cytochrome P-450. Despite this rapid conversion, phenacetin causes a severe nephrotoxicity that is rarely seen with acetaminophen. For this reason, only acetaminophen is available in the United States.

● **Acetaminophen** Acetaminophen is used as an analgesic and antipyretic
for the same indications as aspirin and the other NSAIDs. Acetaminophen
can be used in situations where aspirin is contraindicated, such as in patients with upper gastrointestinal disturbances and in children with viral
infections who are at risk of developing Reye's syndrome if they take
aspirin. It can also substitute for aspirin in patients who must avoid a prolongation of bleeding time, such as those scheduled for surgery, in patients
taking anticoagulants, and in patients with gout.

Acetaminophen is extensively conjugated (sulfated and glucuronidated)
in the liver, where it is also oxidized by cytochrome P-450 to N-acetyl-*p*-
benzoquinoneimine (Fig. 8.6). This reactive metabolite binds to cellular
macromolecules and causes centrilobular hepatic necrosis unless detoxified
by glutathione. Factors such as alcohol that increase the P-450-depen-
dent activation of acetaminophen or decrease glutathione levels are predis-
posing to the hepatotoxic effects of acetaminophen. **N-Acetylcysteine**,
which mimics glutathione, is used to treat acetaminophen poisoning if
therapy can be initiated within 20 hours of overdose.

● **Drugs to treat rheumatoid arthritis** When given at high, antiinflammatory doses, aspirin or another NSAID is the initial drug of choice to treat
rheumatoid arthritis. When these cyclooxygenase inhibitors provide inadequate control of rheumatic inflammation and articular degeneration, one
of the slow-acting remittive (remission-inducing) drugs is used (Table 8.4).

Table 8.4   *Slow-Acting Drugs to Treat Rheumatoid Arthritis*

Gold salts
   Aurothiomalate, aurothioglucose, auranofin
Antimalarials
   Chloroquine, hydroxychloroquine
Penicillamine
Immunosuppressants
   Methotrexate
Corticosteroids
   Prednisone
Immunostimulants
   Levamisole

Although these drugs do not repair existing damage, they can prevent further degenerative changes.

— *Gold salts*   Gold salts reduce the symptoms and slow the progression of rheumatoid arthritis, although therapeutic effects are usually modest. Gold salts may also retard the progression of bone and articular destruction. The mechanism of action appears to involve uptake by macrophages and suppression of phagocytic and lysosomal activity. There are three major formulations of gold salts, two of which must be administered IM (Table 8.5).

Gold therapy should follow treatment with aspirin or NSAIDs and ideally should be used early in the treatment of rapidly progressive rheumatoid diseases with signs of active synovitis or erosive changes.

Gold salts are highly bound (95%) to plasma proteins and concentrate in synovial membranes, liver, kidney, spleen, bone marrow, lymph nodes, and adrenals. Long-term therapy is possible despite the accumulation of gold in various organs, but therapy is contraindicated during pregnancy and in individuals with disorders of the liver, kidney, or blood-forming organs, where gold accumulates.

The adverse effects of gold salts include dermatitis and diarrhea. Accumulation of gold in the kidney can lead to proteinuria and possibly nephrosis. Gold salts may also cause eosinophilia and other hematologic disturbances, including aplastic anemia.

Therapy with gold salts should not be resumed in individuals who have exhibited signs of toxicity. Gold salts should not be administered with penicillamine, another slow-acting antiinflammatory drug, because penicillamine is a metal chelator used to treat overdose with gold and other metals.

Table 8.5   *Formulation of Gold Salts*

Aurothiomalate	50% elemental gold	Intramuscular
Aurothioglucose	50% elemental gold	Intramuscular
Auranofin	29% elemental gold	Oral

— *Antimalarial drugs: chloroquine, hydroxychloroquine* Chloroquine and hydrochloroquine are used to treat rheumatoid arthritis if NSAIDs are ineffective or in conjunction with NSAIDs. The precise mechanism of the antiinflammatory action of antimalarials is unknown. The antiinflammatory effects are apparent only after a 1 to 3 month latency period.

Because only low doses of chloroquine and hydrochloroquine are used to treat rheumatoid arthritis, adverse effects are typically not observed. Their use is contraindicated in patients with porphyria and in those with psoriatic arthritis because of the possibility of exfoliative dermatitis.

— *Penicillamine* Penicillamine is an analog of cysteine and a metabolite of penicillin (Fig. 8.7). Only the D-isomer of penicillamine is used clinically to avoid incorporation into proteins, which are synthesized from L-amino acids. Although penicillamine retards the progression of bone and articular destruction associated with rheumatoid arthritis, it has serious adverse effects. Accordingly, its use is usually reserved for active and progressive erosive rheumatoid disease that cannot be controlled by more conservative treatments, including gold therapy.

The mechanism of actions of penicillamine is unknown. Antiinflammatory effects occur only after a 3 to 4 month latency period.

Adverse effects include leukopenia/thrombocytopenia, which may progress to aplastic anemia. Thus blood counts and urinalysis must be performed every 2 weeks during the first 6 months, then every month. Most patients relapse within 6 months after terminating penicillamine therapy.

Penicillamine is contraindicated during pregnancy and renal insufficiency. It impedes absorption of many drugs and should not be given to patients receiving gold unless used to treat gold intoxication. It should not be used with cytotoxic drugs or phenylbutazone.

— *Immunosuppressive drugs* The immunosuppressant **methotrexate** has been approved for the treatment of severe rheumatoid arthritis in patients who have failed to respond to conventional therapy. Lower doses of methotrexate are used to treat rheumatoid arthritis than are used for cancer chemotherapy. Although this minimizes adverse effects, cytopenia, cirrhosis, and a pneumonia-like condition can occur in arthritic patients.

— *Corticosteroids* Corticosteroids (e.g., **prednisone**) provide prompt and dramatic relief from the inflammatory symptoms of rheumatoid arthritis. However, they do not alter the progressive destruction of bone and cartilage, and symptoms return immediately after the drug is withdrawn, precluding alternate-day therapy. For long-term treatment the dose of prednisone should not exceed 10 mg per day and should be reduced over time. In severe cases of rheumatoid arthritis,

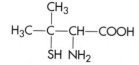

Fig. 8.7 Structure of penicillamine.

intraarticular administration is preferable to increasing the dose of corticosteroid.

— *Immunostimulatory drugs*   Paradoxically, the immunostimulant **levamisole** is effective in the treatment of rheumatoid arthritis, although this use has not been approved by the Food and Drug Administration (FDA). Like other slow-acting agents, levamisole exerts its beneficial effects after a latency of 3 to 4 months.

— *Diet*   Polyunsaturated fatty acids, such as eicosapentaenoic acid, show promise in the relief of various symptoms of rheumatoid arthritis. The mechanism is thought to involve inhibition of arachidonic acid metabolism.

● **Drugs to treat gout**   Gout is caused by high blood levels of uric acid, a product of purine metabolism. Hyperuricemia can result in the crystallization of sodium urate in the kidneys, producing renal calculi, and in the joints and cartilage, which initiates an inflammatory response leading to arthritis (Box 8.9).

Box 8.9

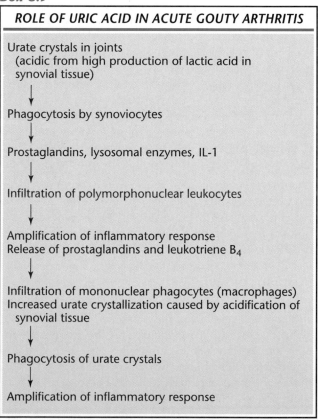

ROLE OF URIC ACID IN ACUTE GOUTY ARTHRITIS

Urate crystals in joints
(acidic from high production of lactic acid in synovial tissue)

↓

Phagocytosis by synoviocytes

↓

Prostaglandins, lysosomal enzymes, IL-1

↓

Infiltration of polymorphonuclear leukocytes

↓

Amplification of inflammatory response
Release of prostaglandins and leukotriene B_4

↓

Infiltration of mononuclear phagocytes (macrophages)
Increased urate crystallization caused by acidification of synovial tissue

↓

Phagocytosis of urate crystals

↓

Amplification of inflammatory response

The treatment of acute gouty arthritis is aimed at decreasing circulating levels of uric acid and suppressing the inflammatory response. Drugs used include colchicine, which blocks granulocyte infiltration and phagocytosis; NSAIDs (except aspirin), which inhibit cyclooxygenase and the production of proinflammatory eicosanoids; allopurinol, which blocks the synthesis of uric acid from purines; and uricosuric agents such as probenecid and sulfinpyrazone, which promote the renal excretion of uric acid.

— *Colchicine in acute gouty arthritis* Colchicine provides prompt and dramatic relief of the pain and inflammation associated with acute gouty arthritis. It would be the drug of choice to treat and prevent acute gouty arthritis were it not for undesirable adverse effects, such as diarrhea, nausea, vomiting, abdominal pain, and, with chronic administration, alopecia, myopathy, agranulocytosis, and aplastic anemia.

Colchicine binds to tubulin, depolymerizing microtubules, which in turn prevents granulocyte migration and phagocytosis. Colchicine also inhibits the lipoxygenase pathway from arachidonic acid, inhibiting leukotriene B_4 formation. Although colchicine is effective in treating acute gouty arthritis, it is relatively ineffective in other types of arthritis, which do not depend on phagocytosis of urate crystals by granulocytes.

Although it is effective orally, colchicine is usually administered IV to minimize gastrointestinal disturbances. To minimize adverse effects, low doses (0.5 mg) of colchicine are given IV every 2 hours. A total dose of 8 mg in a 24 hour period can be fatal.

— *Nonsteroidal antiinflammatory drugs* **Indomethacin,** which has potent antiinflammatory effects, is the drug most widely used to treat acute gouty arthritis. **Phenylbutazone** is also effective in treating acute gouty arthritis. Both drugs inhibit urate crystal phagocytosis by blocking the synthesis of prostaglandins. Treatment with indomethacin or phenylbutazone is limited to 3 days to minimize serious adverse effects.

With the exception of aspirin, all NSAIDs can be used to treat acute gouty arthritis, provided they are administered at high, antiinflammatory doses. Aspirin is not used because at low doses it blocks the tubular secretion of uric acid, increasing uric acid levels in the blood. At high doses, aspirin lowers uric acid blood levels by blocking resorption of uric acid at the proximal tubules. High doses of aspirin, such as those used to treat inflammation, could be used for acute gouty arthritis. However, the risk of increasing uric acid levels and the availability of other effect agents preclude the use of aspirin.

— *Uricosuric agents: probenecid and sulfinpyrazone* Probenecid and sulfinpyrazone are organic acids that promote the renal excretion of uric acid by blocking its resorption at the proximal tubule. Like aspirin, probenecid and sulfinpyrazone block both the resorption and secretion of uric acid by anion transporters in the kidney. At high doses the net effect is to decrease resorption, lowering uric acid levels in blood. At low doses, however, aspirin, probenecid, and sulfinpyrazone increase blood levels of uric acid by blocking its renal secretion.

During therapy with uricosuric agents, the risk of renal calculi formation increases because of the higher levels of uric acid in the kidney. This is minimized by maintaining a large urine volume and by treating patients with sodium bicarbonate to maintain the urine pH above 6. Uricosuric agents should not be used in patients excreting large amounts of uric acid. Uricosuric agents are typically given 2 or 3 weeks after an acute attack of gouty arthritis to prevent the formation of renal calculi.

Probenecid and sulfinpyrazone have few adverse effects and can be used almost indefinitely. Some patients take a uricosuric agent for years. Because both drugs can cause gastrointestinal disturbances, they are given in divided doses with meals. Both can also cause allergic dermatitis.

— *Allopurinol* As a substrate of xanthine oxidase, allopurinol competitively inhibits the formation of uric acid from purines (Fig. 8.8). Allopurinol is converted to alloxanthine, which also inhibits xanthine oxidase. Because uric acid is less water soluble than its precursors, the precursors are less likely to precipitate in the kidney and joints.

Allopurinol is used to treat the primary hyperuricemia of gout. It is effective even in patients on a purine-free diet. In the case of chronic tophaceous gout, allopurinol causes a quicker reabsorption of tophi than do uricosuric agents. Allopurinol is particularly useful in the treatment of patients with gout and a high urinary excretion of uric acid. Probenecid and sulfinpyrazone are avoided in such cases because, as discussed, uricosuric agents should not be used in patients excreting large amounts of uric acid given the risk or renal calculi.

Allopurinol is often taken for life. The drug is generally well tolerated, although hypersensitivity can develop at any time in a small

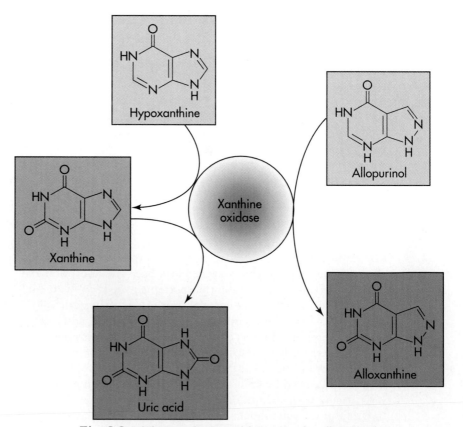

Fig. 8.8 Inhibition of uric acid formation by allopurinol.

number (3%) of patients. When first administered, allopurinol can precipitate an attack of acute gouty arthritis caused by resorption of uric acid from tissues. This is prevented by giving colchicine during the first weeks of allopurinol therapy, unless allopurinol is being used with probenecid or sulfinpyrazone.

Allopurinol inhibits the metabolism of mercaptopurines (anticancer agents) by xanthine oxidase. It also inhibits the metabolism of probenecid and oral anticoagulants.

SECTION 8.4 IMMUNOPHARMACOLOGY

■ **Overview** Immunopharmacology deals with drugs that affect the immune system. This system is involved in almost every aspect of human health and disease, with numerous interactions existing between the immune system and the rest of the body (Fig. 8.9). Because of this, it is difficult to modify the immune system in a selective manner to avoid adverse effects.

■ **Organs of the Immune System**

● **Primary** The bone marrow is the site of pluripotent stem cells. These cells differentiate along any of the hematopoietic lineages. After initiation of dif-

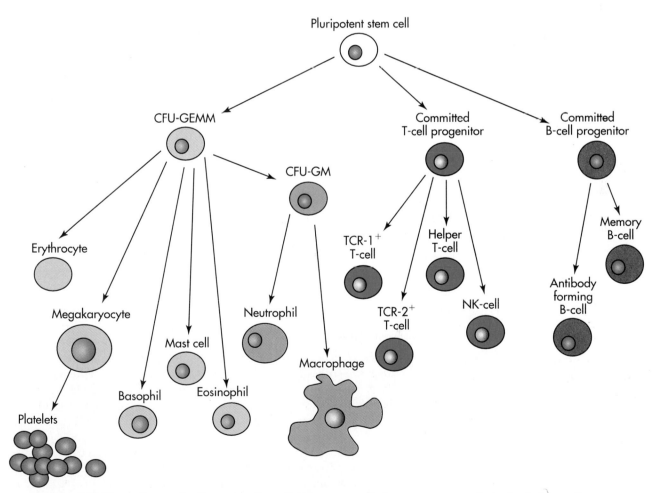

Fig. 8.9 The pathways for the generation of all immune cells from a common pluripotent stem cell.

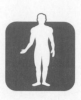

ferentiation a cell is committed to a selected pathway. Most blood cells, including B-cells, develop in bone marrow. The B-cells that generate self-antibodies are eliminated by apoptosis before leaving the bone marrow.

The thymus is the site of T-cell maturation of CD1$^+$ thymocytes. It contains long-lived T-cells that recognize and bind antigen. Self-reacting T-cells are eliminated by apoptosis before leaving the thymus.

- **Secondary** The spleen, lymph nodes, and lymphatic vessels are sites where B-cells and T-cells react with foreign antigens.

    The gastrointestinal tract, lung, and skin are barriers for penetration of foreign antigens and are sites where macrophages and specific B-cells guard against intruders.

    The liver is a fetal immune organ. In the unborn, islets of pluripotent stem cells give rise to lymphocytes and red blood cells. The adult liver retains some immune function by providing accessory proteins (acute phase proteins), such as complement.

■ **The Immune Response** Foreign particles, such as viruses, bacteria, fungi, protozoa, and proteins, are phagocytized by macrophages, monocytes, or other virgin antigen presenting cells (APCs). After phagocytosis the particles are destroyed and specific protein determinants appear on the cell surface as processed antigen with a major histocompatibility complex (MHC) molecule. The antigen/MHC form the recognition surface for receptors on B-cells and T-cells, which dock to the APC. The cell-cell interaction, in combination with the action of lymphokines secreted by the APC, activates the docked cells. The B-cells are stimulated to proliferate and differentiate into plasma cells, producing antibodies. Activated B-cells also trigger the complement cascade, which ultimately destroys the target cell. The T-cells are stimulated to proliferate and differentiate into cytotoxic T-cells, which kill foreign cells by releasing perforin, or by inducing apoptosis. Some T-cells may also proliferate and differentiate into T-helper or T-suppressor cells, depending on the nature of the MHC molecule present on the APC. These cells modulate B-cell and T-cell function. Some B-cells and T-cells are retained as memory cells. Because these cells are specific for the activating antigen, they are rapidly activated and need only to proliferate to destroy foreign cells. This mechanism is used in vaccination.

■ **Sites of Pharmacologic Intervention** Most drugs inhibit cell proliferation or differentiation to suppress an immune response (Fig. 8.10).

■ **Immunosuppression versus Cancer Chemotherapy** Drugs used in immunosuppression and cancer therapy suppress growth or differentiation. However, different principles govern their use (Table 8.6).

■ **Immunosuppressive Drugs (Box 8.10)**

- **Corticosteroids**

    — *Mechanism of action* Corticosteroids reduce prostaglandin and leukotriene synthesis by inhibiting the formation of arachidonic acid. They are lympholytic in that they decrease the size and cell content of the lymph nodes, spleen, and thymus. They suppress both cellular and humoral immunity and are cytotoxic to certain T-cell subpopulations, both helper and suppressor.

        Because precursor lymphoid cells are more sensitive than plasma cells to corticosteroids, they are more effective against the primary response than against an established immune response.

        Corticosteroids are nontoxic to proliferating myeloid or erythroid

Box 8.10

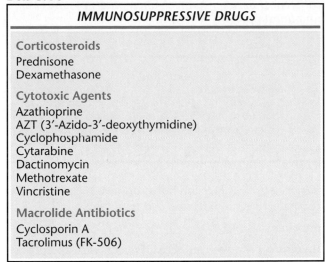

IMMUNOSUPPRESSIVE DRUGS

Corticosteroids
Prednisone
Dexamethasone

Cytotoxic Agents
Azathioprine
AZT (3'-Azido-3'-deoxythymidine)
Cyclophosphamide
Cytarabine
Dactinomycin
Methotrexate
Vincristine

Macrolide Antibiotics
Cyclosporin A
Tacrolimus (FK-506)

stem cells in bone marrow. Thus high doses are used during organ transplant rejection without bone marrow toxicity.

— *Clinical use* Corticosteroids are used to treat a variety of conditions involving the immune system. Included are organ transplantation, autoimmune diseases (autoimmune hemolytic anemia, idiopathic thrombocytopenia purpura, inflammatory bowel disease, lupus erythematosus, rheumatoid arthritis, Hashimoto's thyroiditis) and allergies (bronchial asthma).

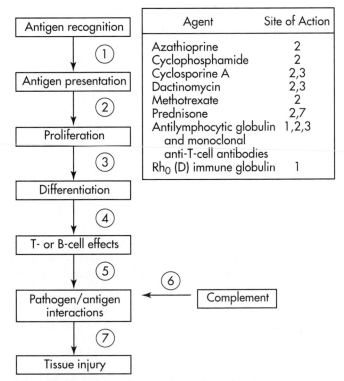

Agent	Site of Action
Azathioprine	2
Cyclophosphamide	2
Cyclosporine A	2,3
Dactinomycin	2,3
Methotrexate	2
Prednisone	2,7
Antilymphocytic globulin and monoclonal anti-T-cell antibodies	1,2,3
Rh$_0$ (D) immune globulin	1

Fig. 8.10 The sites of action for selected immunosuppressive agents.

Table 8.6	*Differences Between Cancer Chemotherapy and Immunosuppressive Therapy*	
	CANCER	IMMUNOSUPPRESSION
Onset	Spontaneous, unstimulated	Antigen stimulated
Growth characteristics	Nonsynchronous	Stimulated synchronous burst of mitosis
Drug delivery	High dose every 3-6 wk to allow recovery of the immune system	Daily low doses to maintain immunosuppression

— *Adverse effects* Corticosteroids suppress the adrenal glands and predispose patients to infection and lymphoma.

● Azathioprine

— *Mechanism of action* A derivative of 6-mercaptopurine, azathioprine is an antimetabolite that interferes with nucleic acid metabolism and synthesis, inhibiting cell proliferation. It is toxic to proliferating lymphocytes after antigen exposure.

— *Basic pharmacology* Azathioprine is well absorbed from the gastrointestinal tract. It is converted to 6-mercaptopurine by glutathione S-transferases and then to 6-thiouric acid by xanthine oxidase. The 6-mercaptopurine, as well as some of the azathioprine, are excreted in urine.

 The toxicity of azathioprine is augmented by kidney disease and inhibitors of xanthine oxidase, such as allopurinol. Thus the dose is reduced in anemic/anuric patients and in patients receiving allopurinol to treat hyperuricemia.

— *Clinical use* Azathioprine is used in kidney transplantation and a host of autoimmune diseases, such as acute glomerulonephritis and hemolytic anemia.

— *Adverse effects* The use of azathioprine is associated with bone marrow suppression, skin rashes, fever, nausea, vomiting, diarrhea, and occasionally liver dysfunction and jaundice.

● Cyclophosphamide

— *Mechanism of action* Cyclophosphamide is an alkylating agent after activation by cytochrome P-450. It is the most potent immunosuppressive drug available. It destroys proliferating lymphoid cells and some quiescent cells.

— *Clinical use* Cyclophosphamide is used in bone marrow transplantation and to treat a variety of autoimmune disorders, including antifactor VIII coagulation disorder, antibody-induced red cell aplasia, and Wegener's granulomatosis.

— *Adverse effects* Cyclophosphamide causes bone marrow suppression, and high doses may induce tolerance to new antigens if administered during or shortly after antigen exposure.

● Methotrexate

— *Mechanism of action* Methotrexate is an inhibitor of dihydrofolate reductase, which is required for folate synthesis. It blocks folate-requiring reactions in the biosynthesis of nucleotides, interfering with nucleic acid metabolism, and blocks growth of proliferating cells. It is cytotoxic to proliferating lymphoid cells after antigen exposure.

— *Clinical use* Methotrexate is used prophylactically for treating graft versus host syndrome for bone marrow transplantation. It also has antileukemic effects and is used to treat rheumatoid arthritis and psoriasis.

● Cyclosporin

— *Mechanism of action* Cyclosporin is a lipophilic, cyclic peptide of fungal origin (*Tolypocladium inflatum*). It binds to cyclophillins (peptidyl proline *cis-trans* isomerase) and blocks the differentiation and activation of T-cells by inhibiting production of modulating factors such as IL-2 by helper T-cells that stimulate T-cell growth.

— *Basic pharmacology* Cyclosporin is incompletely absorbed from the gastrointestinal tract (20% to 50%) and extensively metabolized (hydroxylation) by cytochrome P-450 in the intestines and liver. The metabolism is blocked by erythromycin or ketoconazole, which is often given to reduce the dose of cyclosporin. Its metabolism is enhanced by rifampin and anticonvulsants.

— *Clinical use* Cyclosporin is used primarily to suppress organ rejection after transplantation. It is also used for selected autoimmune disorders, including type I diabetes (antiislet cell autoimmune disease). Cyclosporin alone or in combination with prednisolone may be as effective, and less toxic, when administered with cyclophosphamide, azathioprine, prednisone, or antilymphocytic antibodies.

— *Adverse effects* Cyclosporin predisposes the patient to viral infections and lymphoma. It is nephrotoxic, but this can be prevented with mannitol diuresis.

● Tacrolimus (FK-506)

— *Mechanism of action* Tacrolimus is a macrolide antibiotic of fungal origin. It is chemically distinct from cyclosporin but is similar in its use.

— *Clinical use* Tacrolimus is used in situations where cyclosporin is ineffective or toxic.

— *Adverse effects* Administration of tacrolimus is associated with nausea and vomiting.

● AZT (3′-azido-3′-deoxythymidine)

— *Mechanism of action* The main action of AZT is to block retroviral reverse transcriptase.

— *Clinical use* AZT is used primarily to treat HIV infection.

— *Adverse effects* Adverse effects associated with AZT include anemia, neutropenia, nausea, and vomiting.

  Resistance develops to AZT by changes in reverse transcriptase activity or by alterations in its metabolism.

■ **Antibodies as Immunosuppressive Agents (Table 8.7)**

● Anti-T-cell antibody OKT3

— *Mechanism of action* The mouse monoclonal antibody OKT3 inhibits the interaction between antigen-presenting cells and T-cells, sup-

Table 8.7   *Key Features of Monoclonal and Polyclonal Antibodies*

	MONOCLONAL ANTIBODY	POLYCLONAL ANTIBODY
Specificity	One kind of antibody directed against a single epitope	A diverse collection of antibodies with various affinities directed against numerous antigenic determinants (epitopes) on an antigen (immunogen)
Source	Produced in cell culture by fusing an antibody-secreting plasma B-cell (from an immunized animal) and an immortal myeloma cell to generate an immortal, antibody-secreting hybridoma cell	Derived from antiserum isolated from immunized animals by purification (IgG preparation and immunoaffinity purification)
Production	Unlimited, provided the hybridoma cell is stable	Limited by the amount of antigen available to generate antiserum in animals
Variability	Theoretically no variation	Potentially large batch-to-batch variation in specificity or affinity in antisera derived from different animals immunized with the same immunogen
Dosage	Theoretically constant	Varies from batch to batch depending on specificity and affinity
Examples	Anti–T-cell antibodies	Antithymocyte globulin Antilymphocyte globulin $Rh_0(D)$ immune globulin

pressing T-cell activation and proliferation. The antibody is directed against the CD3 T-cell receptor.

— *Clinical use* The anti-T-cell antibody is used in kidney transplantation.

● Antithymocyte globulin

— *Clinical use* Antithymocyte globulin is used in the treatment of idiopathic aplastic anemia and autoimmune disorder resulting from hematopoietic suppression caused by overproduction of the γ-interferon by activated $CD8^+$ suppressor cells.

● Antilymphocyte globulin

— *Mechanism of action* Antilymphocyte globulin targets T-cells involved in antigen recognition. Acutely it targets long-lived, circulating peripheral lymphocytes. When given chronically, it affects thymus-dependent lymphocytes. The binding of the antibody to cell surface antigens activates the complement-mediated destruction of lymphocytes. This results in decreased cellular immunity (delayed hypersensitivity). There is little effect on humoral immunity.

— *Clinical use* Antilymphocyte globulin is used in organ transplantation and graft-versus-host syndrome.

— *Adverse effects* Adverse effects include pain, erythema and possibly lymphoma at the site of injection, anaphylactic shock, and serum sickness.

● $Rh_0(D)$ immune globulin

— *Mechanism of action* When an Rh-negative mother gives birth to an Rh-positive child, fetal red blood cells enter the maternal circulation (parturition) and induce a primary immune response. The mother develops antibodies against the $Rh_0(D)$ antigen that, during a second pregnancy, enter the fetal circulation during the third trimester, and cause lysis of fetal red blood cells (erythroblastosis fetalis). The $Rh_0(D)$ immune globulin is administered to the mother, not the infant, within 72 hours or parturition to suppress the immune response against the foreign $Rh_0(D)$-positive cells.

— *Clinical use* $Rh_0(D)$ immune globulin is used in the prophylactic treatment of Rh hemolytic disease (erythroblastosis fetalis).

— *Adverse effects* The use of $Rh_0(D)$ immune globulin is associated with relatively few adverse effects. Care must be taken to ensure that the mother is Rh(D)-negative and D^u-negative and not already immune to the Rh(D) factor.

■ **Immunomodulating Agents** This area of pharmacology aims at modulating, rather than suppressing, the immune response. This approach is of potential importance in the treatment of immunodeficiency disorders, chronic infectious diseases, and cancer.

● **Thymosin** Thymosin is a 10 kDa protein produced in the thymus. It induces and stimulates the maturation of T-cells. Peptide fractions with lower molecular weight than thymosin have been found to possess thymic hormone-like activity.

Thymosin stimulates the differentiation of uncommitted lymphoid stem cells into T-cells or the maturation of pre-T-cells into mature T-cells.

Thymosin levels decrease with age and are reduced in DiGeorge's syndrome, a condition characterized by a lack of thymic hormone, underdeveloped thymus, and low T-cell numbers. Thymosin is used in the treatment of DiGeorge's syndrome and other disorders of T-cell deficiency.

● **Adjuvants** Bacille Calmette-Guérin (BCG) is a viable strain of *Myobacterium bovis* used to immunize against tuberculosis. It is employed as an immunostimulant in cancer therapy. It appears to activate macrophages, making them more efficient killer cells in concert with lymphoid cells.

● **Drugs**

— *Levamisole* Developed for the treatment of parasitic infections, levamisole also enhances cellular, T-cell mediated immunity. Potential uses of levamisole include treatment of Hodgkin's disease and rheumatoid arthritis.

— *Inosiplex* Inosiplex enhances T-cell and monocyte activities and natural killer cytotoxicity. It may be useful in the treatment of AIDS.

● **Cytokines**

— *Colony-stimulating factors (CSF)* These agents are synthesized using cloned human genes. Members include GM-CSF, M-CSF, and G-CSF, which regulate the proliferation and differentiation of bone marrow progenitor cells along specific lineages. They may be useful in treating burn patients and patients suffering from leukopenia secondary to cancer chemotherapy.

— *Interleukins* These cytokines have many stimulatory and some suppressive effects on T-cell and B-cell proliferation and differentiation.

— *Interferons (α, β, γ)* The interferons display antiviral properties. Interferon-α has been approved for the treatment of hematologic neoplasms and hepatitis.

■ **Vaccines**

● Active immunization—bacterial vaccines

— *Pertussis (whooping cough)* This vaccine is composed of an inactivated phase of *Bordatella pertussis* adsorbed onto aluminum hydroxide or precipitated with aluminum. It is injected IM during the first year of life to protect against whooping cough. Adverse effects include febrile reaction.

— *Cholera* A suspension of killed cholera vibriae is injected SQ or IM to stimulate partial resistance to cholera. Booster injections are required every 6 months. Adverse effects include local pain, swelling, and a febrile reaction.

— *Typhoid* This vaccine consists of a suspension of acetone-killed *Salmonella typhii*. It is administered by repeated SQ injections to stimulate partial resistance to typhoid infection. Adverse effects include local pain, swelling, and a febrile reaction.

— *Tuberculosis* Vaccination for tuberculosis entails multiple intradermal injections, or dermal puncture for partial resistance, of live, avirulent, *Bacillus tuberculosis* strain BCG. Such vaccination usually results in conversion of a tuberculin skin test from negative to positive. This may last from 3 to 7 years. The BCG vaccination is recommended only for tuberculin-negative persons with a high risk of exposure to the pathogen.

Adverse effects include local pain, swelling, and a febrile reaction. Concern exists about the increased incidence of infection with drug-resistant strains in industrialized countries. This may be due in part to the indiscriminate use of antibiotics.

— *Plague* The vaccine for plague is a suspension of inactivated *Pasteurella pestis.* It is administered by repeated IM injections to induce partial resistance. Adverse effects include local pain, swelling, and a febrile reaction.

● Active immunization—rickettsial vaccines

— *Epidemic typhus* This vaccine is a suspension of inactivated *Rickettsia prowazeki* grown in the yolk sacs of chicken egg embryos. It is administered by repeated IM injection to induce protection against louseborne typhus. Frequent booster injections are required. Adverse effects include hypersensitivity, especially in persons allergic to egg proteins.

— *Rocky Mountain Spotted Fever* This vaccine is a suspension of inactivated purified *Rickettsia rickettsii* grown in the yolk sacs of chicken egg embryos. It is administered by repeated IM injections to induce protection against infection in persons likely to be exposed to tick bites. Adverse effects include hypersensitivity, especially in persons allergic to egg proteins.

● Active immunization—viral vaccines

— *Influenza* A suspension of inactivated egg-grown *Influenza* virus, this vaccine is administered IM to induce partial protection against the flu. Because of frequent changes in the viral antigenic determinants, full protection cannot be achieved and frequent booster injections are needed with polyvalent vaccine.

Treatment is recommended for high-risk patients, such as elderly persons with chronic respiratory diseases, patients with serious mitral valve disease, and children with cystic fibrosis. These individuals should be injected every year with polyvalent vaccine.

Adverse effects include hypersensitivity, especially in persons allergic to egg proteins.

— *Poliomyelitis* This vaccine is a suspension of attenuated live strains of *Poliomyelitis* virus types 1, 2, and 3 grown in cell culture. It is administered orally to immunize against polio. Adverse effects include hypersensitivity and febrile reaction.

— *Smallpox* Active *Vaccinia* virus is suspended in the form of glycerolated calf lymph or grown on chick embryos to prepare smallpox vaccine. It is administered to dry skin by the multiple pressure method. Adverse effects include hypersensitivity. It is contraindicated in patients with eczema or other widespread skin diseases and in patients with immunodeficiencies.

— *Measles* Measles vaccine is a suspension of attenuated live *Rubeola* virus grown in cell culture. It is administered IM to immunize against Rubeola measles. Adverse effects include hypersensitivity. The vaccine is not well tolerated in adults and is contraindicated in pregnant women because the virus may infect the fetus.

— *Mumps* Mumps vaccine is a suspension of attenuated live strains of the mumps virus grown in cell culture. It is administered SQ or IM. Adverse effects include hypersensitivity.

— *Yellow fever* To prevent yellow fever, subjects are injected SQ with a suspension of attenuated live strains of yellow fever virus grown in chicken embryos.

— *Rabies* A suspension of tissue from rabies-infected animals is inactivated with phenol and administered SQ for 14 to 21 days to patients bitten by animals suspected of having rabies. Adverse effects include allergic encephalomyelitis and paralysis of one or more extremities.

There are numerous vaccines available and recommended. Although active immunization is generally better than passive, it carries greater risks for complications. Many of these risks are unavoidable, but, on balance, patients are safer accepting the risk of vaccination.

● **Passive immunization** Passive immunization is the administration of antibodies, or antiserum, to a patient incapable of producing antibodies at all or at the time needed. To this end, human or animal immunoglobulins (antibodies) of varying degrees of purity are used. The preparations may contain high titers of one specific antibody or antibodies found in most of the population, as with pooled immunoglobulins. Animal antisera injected into humans have much shorter half-lives than human antisera.

— *Clinical use* Passive immunization is used in individuals who are unable to produce their own antibodies, such as those suffering from congenital agammaglobulinemia or AIDS. It is also used for the prevention of disease when time does not permit active immunization, such as after exposure. Passive immunization is used for the treatment of diseases after an outbreak that would normally be prevented by immunization, such as tetanus, or for conditions for which active immunization is impractical, such as for snake bite.

— *Adverse effects* There are frequent hypersensitivity reactions (anaphylaxis or serum sickness) to animal sera.

- **Toxoids** Toxoids are prepared from the exotoxins of bacteria by treatment with formaldehyde followed by purification. This results in denatured material that has lost its toxic properties but maintains the antigenic specificity of the active toxin.

  — *Diphtheria toxoid* This toxoid is prepared from *Corynebacterium diphtheriae* treated with formaldehyde. It is administered by SQ injection to immunize against diphtheria. Adverse effects include hypersensitivity reactions.

  — *Tetanus toxoid* Tetanus toxoid is prepared from *Clostridium tetani* treated with formaldehyde and administered by SQ injection. Adverse effects include hypersensitivity reactions.

- ■ **Drug Allergies** Some drug reactions, such as those to penicillin, iodides, phenytoin, and sulfonamides, have an immunologic basis and are therefore classified as drug allergies. Four types of allergic reactions can be distinguished (Table 8.8).

- **Type I drug allergy** Examples of Type I allergic responses are IgE-mediated acute reactions to pollens, stings, and drugs. This results in vasodilation, edema, inflammatory response, urticaria, rhinitis, and anaphylaxis.

  — *Mechanism of action* Drug bound to plasma protein, such as albumin, serves as the antigenic determinant on macrophages and is recognized by reaginic (IgE) B-cell precursors that, in the presence of IL-4 from T-helper cells, are converted to IgE-secreting cells. The IgE reaginic antibodies are fixed on mast cells and basophilic leukocytes by binding to the Fc receptor (FcϵR). Thus, the drug antigen triggers IgE-mediated release of histamine, leukotrienes, prostaglandins, and other mediators of the allergic response from cytoplasmic granules in mast cells.

  — *Treatment* The T-helper effect is blocked by interferon-γ and the proliferation and differentiation of B-cells can be blocked by prednisone. The effect of histamine on smooth muscle cells is inhibited by antihistamines, and isoproterenol, epinephrine, and theophylline are used to inhibit the release of mediators from mast cells and basophils. **Cromolyn sodium** is used to treat allergic asthma because cromolyn appears to inhibit liberation of mediators of anaphylaxis.

Table 8.8	*Classification of Immunologic Reactions to Drugs*
Type	**Mechanism**
Type I	IgE-mediated acute allergic reactions to stings, pollens, and drugs. Reactions include inflammatory response, anaphylaxis, urticaria, and angioedema.
Type II	Autoimmune or cytolytic. Complement-dependent allergic reactions involving IgG or IgM. Reactions include complement-dependent T-cell lysis.
Type III	Arthus. Serum sickness involving IgG or IgM and complement. Reactions include complement-dependent vasculitis.
Type IV	Delayed hypersensitivity. Cell-mediated allergic reaction involving allergic contact dermatitis.

- **Type II drug allergy (autoimmune or cytotoxic)** Type II is characterized by complement-fixing IgG or IgM (Box 8.11).

Box 8.11

COMPLEMENT-DEPENDENT LYSIS OF CELLS IN THE CIRCULATION	
Systemic lupus erythematosus	Hydralazine, procainamide
Lupoid hepatitis	Cathartic sensitivity
Hemolytic anemia	Penicillin
Autoimmune hemolytic anemia	Methyldopa
Thrombocytopenia purpura	Quinidine
Agranulocytosis	Carbamazepine, clozapine

- — *Treatment* Drug withdrawal and, in severe cases, immunosuppression with corticosteroids are the primary treatments.

- **Type III drug allergies (arthus)** Type III drug allergies are complement-dependent allergic reactions involving IgG or IgM. Symptoms include urticaria, arthralgia, arthritis, lymphadenopathy, and fever.

  - — *Mechanism of action* Antibody-antigen complexes are deposited in the vascular epithelium and trigger destructive inflammatory response such as vasculitis or serum sickness. Drugs most frequently associated with precipitating a type III response include sulfonamides, penicillin, thiouracil, anticonvulsants, and iodides. Sulfonamides can cause Stevens-Johnson syndrome, a severe form of vasculitis.

  - — *Treatment* Drug withdrawal and, in severe cases, immunosuppression with corticosteroids are the primary treatments.

- **Type IV drug allergies (delayed hypersensitivity)** This is a cell mediated allergic response to topically applied antigens. An example is contact dermatitis caused by poison ivy. Likewise, topical exposure to drugs (e.g., penicillins) or chemicals (e.g., chromium) can often cause contact dermatitis.

MULTIPLE CHOICE
REVIEW QUESTIONS

1. A middle-aged man is taking high, antiinflammatory doses of aspirin to control his rheumatoid arthritis. To alleviate occasional stomach pain, he takes Zantac (rantidine) or Rolaids. The aspirin is helping to control the pain from an impacted wisdom tooth, but eventually he elects to have his wisdom tooth pulled. The surgery is accompanied by excessive bleeding, which surprises the patient because he had no previous bleeding disorders. The likely cause of the patient's excessive bleeding is:

   a. activation of the fibrinolytic system by ranitidine.
   b. late onset (adult form) hemophilia.
   c. inhibition of thromboxane synthesis by aspirin.
   d. ranitidine-induced thrombocytopenia.
   e. antacid-induced deficiency of vitamin K.

2. A patient is being treated for small pulmonary emboli with warfarin (after treatment with fibrinolytic agents and heparin). The patient begins taking aspirin for a recurrent headache and neck pain. The aspirin causes gastric irritation, which the patient treats himself with his wife's Tagamet (cimetidine), which she takes for her peptic ulcer. The patient cuts himself shaving and cannot stop the bleeding. Which of the following drug interactions best explains the excessive bleeding?

   a. Inhibition of warfarin metabolism by cimetidine combined with the antiplatelet effects of aspirin
   b. Displacement of aspirin and warfarin from serum protein binding sites by cimetidine
   c. Enhanced absorption of warfarin due to acid suppression by cimetidine
   d. Activation of the fibrinolytic system by cimetidine combined with the antiplatelet effects of aspirin
   e. Synergy of the antiplatelet effects of cimetidine and aspirin

3. The drug of choice for relief of symptoms of rheumatoid arthritis is:
   a. levamisole.
   b. aspirin.

   c. penicillamine.
   d. gold thiomalate.
   e. acetaminophen.

4. An effective drug in rheumatic disease that does not respond to treatment with cyclooxygenase inhibitors is:

   a. ibuprofen (Motrin).
   b. phenylbutazone (Butazolidin).
   c. colchicine.
   d. gold (e.g., auranofin).
   e. allopurinol (Zyloprim).

5. Which of these drug allergies is primarily dependent on IgE?

   a. Type I (immediate)
   b. Type II (cytolytic)
   c. Type III (serum sickness)
   d. Type IV (delayed)
   e. All of the above

6. Which drug is used for immunosuppressive therapy but not for cancer chemotherapy?

   a. Vincristine
   b. Cyclophosphamide
   c. Methotrexate
   d. Cyclosporine
   e. None of the above

7. A patient with rheumatoid arthritis was treated for 3 months with aspirin, but signs of active inflammation and erosive bone changes were still evident and apparently worsening. The situation remained unchanged after an additional month of more aggressive therapy with aspirin. Blood analysis confirmed compliance and adequate dosing with aspirin. Which of the following treatments should be initiated to treat the patient's persistent and active synovitis?

   a. Phenylbutazone
   b. Indomethacin
   c. Chloroquine
   d. Gold salts (e.g., auranofin)
   e. *N*-acetylcysteine

8. Which of the following pairs of agents does not describe a drug-antidote relationship?

   a. Heparin-protamine sulfate
   b. Iron-desferal (desferoxaine)
   c. Warfarin-vitamin K
   d. Vitamin B_{12}-intrinsic factor
   e. Bishydroxycoumarin-vitamin K

9. A 43-year-old woman has been treated with aspirin for rheumatoid arthritis. Her menstrual bleeding has increased, possibly as a result of the therapy. To relieve her stomach pains, which began shortly after taking aspirin, she takes bicarbonate of soda (sodium bicarbonate) 3 to 4 times a day and drinks plenty of milk. She takes laxatives because her stools have become dark and uncomfortably hard. After several months she complains of fatigue and shortness of breath. She looks pale and tired. The patient's fatigue and shortness of breath are likely due to:

a. metabolic acidosis.
b. iron deficiency anemia.
c. interstitial nephritis.
d. lactose intolerance.
e. disseminated intravascular coagulation.

Chapter 9

Toxicology

SECTION 9.1 OVERVIEW

Toxicology is the study of adverse effects of chemicals. Toxicologists are divided into different areas:

- *Descriptive toxicologists* determine what adverse effects are produced by chemicals and the dose required to produce such effects.
- *Mechanistic toxicologists* attempt to determine how a chemical produces the toxic effects.
- *Regulatory toxicologists* judge the amount of chemical people should be exposed to.
- *Forensic toxicologists* establish the probable cause of human death for someone exposed to toxic substances to determine whether criminal actions have occurred.
- *Clinical toxicologists* treat patients who are poisoned by drugs and other chemicals and develop new techniques for the diagnosis and treatment of such conditions.

The Food and Drug Administration (FDA) is responsible for regulating and approving for sale food, drugs, and cosmetics.

The Environmental Protection Agency (EPA) is responsible for monitoring and regulating the amount of pesticides, toxic chemicals, hazardous wastes, and pollutants in water and air.

The Occupational Safety and Health Administration (OSHA) is responsible for regulating chemicals in the workplace. The maximum allowable concentration (MAC) and threshold limit value (TLV) are examples of limits set on the concentration of airborne substances. These limits are based on animal experiments and human exposures.

■ **Dose Response** Paracelsus (1493–1541) noted that "all substances are poisons; there is none which is not a poison. The right dose differentiates a poison and a remedy."

Just as there is a dose response to the therapeutic effect of drugs, toxic effects are also dose related (Fig. 9.1). The LD_{50} is the dose that is lethal to 50% of the subjects. The therapeutic index (TI) is the LD_{50} divided by the dose that produces a therapeutic effect in 50% of the subjects (ED_{50}).

■ **Definitions**

- *Lethal concentration time,* or LCT_{50}, is the average airborne concentration of a substance causing death in 50% of the animals over a given period of time.
- *Idiosyncrasy* is a genetically determined abnormal reaction to a chemical.
- *Toxicity* is the capacity of a substance to produce injury under defined conditions.

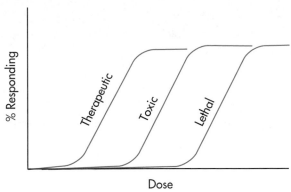

Fig. 9.1 Dose response to the therapeutic, toxic, and lethal effects of a drug.

- *Risk* is the probability that injury will result from exposure to a substance under specified conditions of dose and route of administration.
- *Acute toxicity* is an adverse effect resulting from a single, usually large, exposure to a toxin.
- *Chronic toxicity* is the harmful effect resulting from repeated exposures to a toxin for 3 months or more.
- *Iatrogenic disease,* or toxicity, is an adverse effect associated with the inappropriate use of a drug.
- *Local toxicity* occurs at the site of contact with a poison, such as acid burn.
- *Systemic toxicity* occurs after absorption and distribution of a toxic substance to different parts of the body.
- *Delayed toxicity* is an adverse effect that occurs weeks, months, or years after exposure to a toxin. Chemical-induced neurotoxic effects are often not immediately apparent. Likewise, cancer often requires 20 years to develop after exposure to a carcinogen.

■ **Spectrum of Undesired Effects** Side effects of drugs are nondeleterious, such as the xerostomi associated with tricyclic antidepressant therapy (Fig. 9.2). Toxic ef-

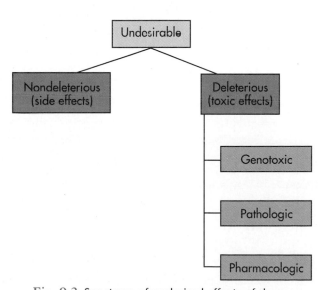

Fig. 9.2 Spectrum of undesired effects of drugs.

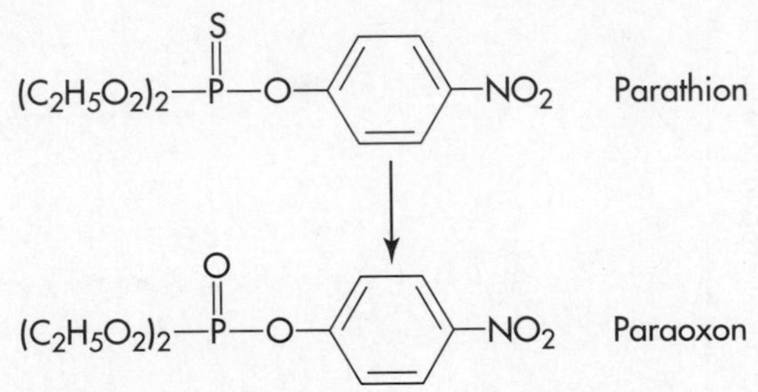

$$(C_2H_5O_2)_2 - \overset{\overset{S}{\parallel}}{P} - O - \langle\!\!\bigcirc\!\!\rangle - NO_2 \quad \text{Parathion}$$

$$(C_2H_5O_2)_2 - \overset{\overset{O}{\parallel}}{P} - O - \langle\!\!\bigcirc\!\!\rangle - NO_2 \quad \text{Paraoxon}$$

Fig. 9.3 The bioactivation of parathion to paraoxon.

fects may be an extension of the pharmacologic action, such as the coma associated with barbiturate overdose. Other deleterious effects of drugs include pathologic responses such as the liver injury that results from acetaminophen overdose. A chemical may produce genotoxic effects, resulting in mutations, cancer, or birth defects.

■ **Chemical Forms of Drug-Producing Toxicity** The parent, or administered, drug is usually responsible for the desired effect, but it can also be toxic. Some chemicals are biotransformed to toxic metabolites. For example, the nontoxic insecticide parathion is biotransformed to paraoxon, a toxic substance (Fig. 9.3). Acetaminophen is biotransformed to a reactive-toxic metabolite (Fig. 9.4). In this case the toxic metabolite is an electrophile that binds to and depletes glutathione, after which it attaches to macromolecules in cells to produce liver injury. Some chemicals, such as the herbicide paraquat, are biotransformed to reactive oxygen species that mediate toxicity (Fig. 9.5).

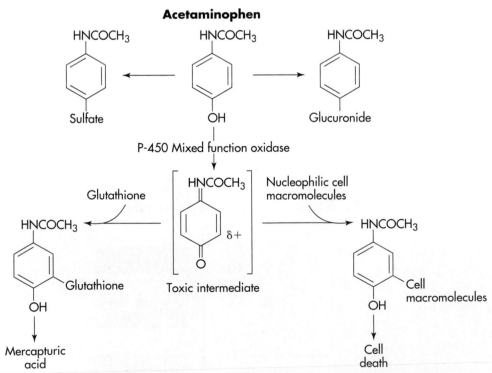

Fig. 9.4 Toxicity can be mediated by a toxic intermediate formed during biotransformation.

Paraquat

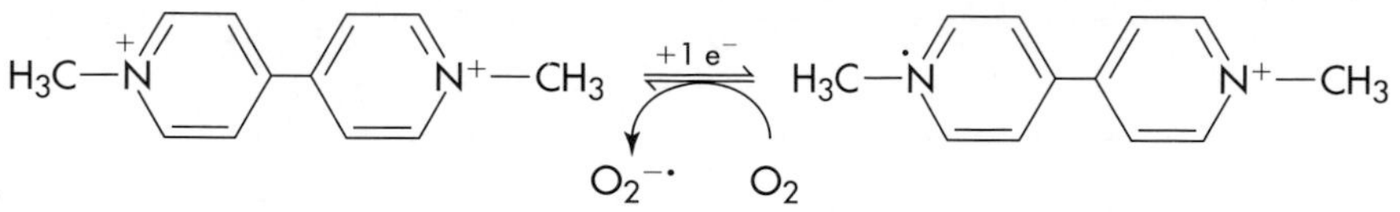

$$H_3C-\overset{+}{N}\text{◯}\text{◯}\overset{+}{N}-CH_3 \underset{}{\overset{+1\,e^-}{\rightleftharpoons}} H_3C-\overset{\cdot}{N}\text{◯}\text{◯}\overset{+}{N}-CH_3$$

$$O_2^{-\cdot} \quad O_2$$

Fig. 9.5 Toxicity can be mediated by reactive oxygen species formed during the biotransformation of some chemicals.

Section 9.2 Treatment of Poisoning

■ **Incidence of Acute Poisoning** The actual incidence of poisoning in the United States is unknown. Approximately 2 million cases of poisoning are voluntarily reported yearly to the American Association of Poison Control Centers, with some 700 deaths each year attributed to poisonings.

Chemicals most frequently involved in human poisoning are cleaning substances, followed by analgesics, cosmetics, and cough and cold preparations (Table 9.1).

The highest incidence of poisoning (59%) is in children between 1 and 2 years of age. Fortunately, most substances available to them are not too toxic because only 16% of the deaths belong to this age category.

Drugs are not the most frequent cause of acute poisoning, but they are in the top four categories of chemicals that produce death (Table 9.2). Most people who die from poisoning are adults, with the deaths often resulting from intentional rather than accidental exposure.

■ **Major Sources of Toxicology Information** Because of the large number of poisons, it is important to have available reference materials for diagnosing and treating poisons. Useful texts include the following:

Table 9.1 *Substances Most Frequently Involved in Human Exposure*

SUBSTANCE	NUMBER	PERCENT*
Cleaning substances	196,022	10.5
Analgesics	178,284	9.76
Cosmetics	153,721	8.2
Cough and cold preparations	107,980	5.8
Plants	106,939	5.7
Bites/envenomations	74,906	4.0
Pesticides (includes rodenticides)	70,687	3.8
Topicals	70,458	3.8
Hydrocarbons	64,041	3.4
Foreign bodies	63,297	3.4
Antimicrobials	63,025	3.4
Sedative/hypnotics/antipsychotics	58,582	3.1
Chemicals	52,499	2.8
Food poisoning	50,511	2.7
Alcohols	50,276	2.7
Vitamins	43,187	2.3

*Percentages are based on total number of known ingested substances rather than the total number of human exposure cases. (From Litovitz et al, 1992. Courtesy of the *American Journal of Emergency Medicine.*)

Table 9.2 *Categories with Largest Numbers of Deaths*

CATEGORY	NUMBER	PERCENT OF ALL EXPOSURE IN CATEGORY
Antidepressants	194	0.497
Analgesics	186	0.104
Stimulants and street drugs	81	0.364
Cardiovascular drugs	80	0.301
Alcohols/glycols	59	0.117
Gases and fumes	42	0.144
Asthma therapies	35	0.198
Chemicals	24	0.046
Pesticides	20	0.028
Cleaning substances	19	0.010
Anticonvulsants	18	0.150

(From Litovitz et al, 1992. Courtesy of the *American Journal of Emergency Medicine.*)

- Amdur M, Doull J, Klaassen CD: *Casarett and Doull's toxicology: the basic science of poisons,* 4 ed, New York, 1991, McGraw-Hill.
- Allenhorn MJ, Barceloux DG: *Medical toxicology,* New York, 1988, Elsevier-North Holland.
- Goldfrank LR et al: *Goldfrank's toxicologic emergencies,* 4 ed, Norwalk, Conn, 1990, Appleton & Lange.
- Gosselin RE, Smith RP, Hodge HC: *Clinical toxicology of commercial products,* 5 ed, Baltimore, 1984, Williams & Wilkins.
- Haddad LM, Winchester JF, editors: *Clinical management of poisoning and drug overdose,* 2 ed, Philadelphia, 1990, Saunders.
- A computerized system for information on acute exposure to chemicals is **POISINDEX** (Micromedex, Inc., Denver, Colorado).
- In addition, there are about 120 poison control centers in the United States. Information can be obtained from these centers by telephone.

■ **Treatment of Poisoning** The adage "treat the patient, not the poison" is the most important principle in clinical toxicology. Support of respiration and cardiovascular function are essential.

An accurate history and physical examination can help considerably in determining the offending agent. For example, odor, pill fragments, needle tracks, and evidence of trauma are all clues. Routine laboratory tests are useful, but the most definitive diagnosis is made with analytic toxicology testing. Because such tests can be time consuming, initiation of treatment must sometimes precede a definitive diagnosis. For example, if the patient is in coma, the stage of coma must be determined to ensure that it does not deepen (Table 9.3).

The first goal in the treatment of poisoning is to maintain vital function. The second is to prevent further absorption of the toxin or to enhance its excretion. A third objective, when possible, is to decrease the pharmacologic and toxicologic effects of the substance, such as with chemical antagonists.

● **Prevention of further absorption** Ipecac is most commonly used to prevent absorption of toxicants from the gastrointestinal tract by inducing vomiting. Fluids should be administered with the ipecac to facilitate vom-

Treatment Goals

Maintain vital functions
Prevent further absorption
Enhance excretion
Chemical antagonists

Table 9.3	**Stages of Coma**	
0	Asleep	Arousable, can talk
I	Comatose	Withdraws from pain, reflexes intact
II	Comatose	Unresponsive to pain, reflexes intact
III	Comatose	Reflexes absent, respiration and circulation not depressed
IV	Comatose	Reflexes absent, respiratory or circulatory depression with apnea, cyanosis, shock

iting. Chronic use of ipecac for weight loss can result in cardiomyopathy, ventricular fibrillation, and death. Other chemicals, such as apomorphine, are used to induce vomiting. Apomorphine stimulates dopamine chemoreceptors in the brain that cause vomiting. If apomorphine-induced vomiting is excessive, naloxone, an opioid antagonist, can be used to stop it. Gastric lavage is a popular procedure for removing toxins from the gastrointestinal system. Large tubes should be used because large pills may need to be removed. There are four contraindications to the use of vomiting or gastric lavage:

— *Caustics* If a corrosive substance, such as a strong acid or base (e.g., drain cleaners) is ingested, vomiting may cause further damage to the esophagus and a gavage tube may perforate the esophagus. Acid and base burns should be diluted with water.

— *Convulsions* If the patient has been exposed to a convulsant, such as strychnine, the stress associated with vomiting or lavage may precipitate convulsions.

— *Coma* If the patient is comatose, there is the possibility of aspiration into the lungs with vomiting.

— *Solvents or petroleum* In this case vomiting should be avoided because the solvent may be aspirated into the lungs, causing chemical pneumonitis. This is especially a problem with volatile hydrocarbons, such as mineral oil found in liquid furniture polishes.

Chemical absorption is another means for decreasing the absorption of chemicals. Activated charcoal adsorbs many chemicals, preventing their absorption and toxicity. Recent studies have shown that activated charcoal is as effective as ipecac or lavage plus charcoal in reducing the absorption of an ingested substance.

Purgation is used to enhance the passage of the chemical through the gastrointestinal tract. Few if any clinical studies have been performed to determine the effectiveness of this procedure, but it is not likely to do harm. Cathartics most often used are sodium sulfate, magnesium sulfate, and sorbitol.

● **Enhanced elimination of the poison** Biotransformation usually reduces the lipid solubility and increases the excretion of drugs. Although, in general, there is no way to rapidly increase the activity of drug-metabolizing enzymes, thiosulfate does enhance the detoxification of cyanide to thiocyanate.

The urinary excretion of some drugs can be enhanced. Nonionized chemicals filtered at the glomerulus are reabsorbed into the renal tubules.

With some weak organic anionic drugs, such as phenobarbital and salicylates, alkalinizing the urine maintains a large percentage of the drug in the ionized form. This retains the drug in the lumen, enhancing its excretion in urine. Renal excretion of basic drugs such as amphetamine can theoretically be increased by acidification of the urine. This phenomenon is referred to as ion trapping. The urine can be acidified with ascorbic acid or ammonium chloride. Sodium bicarbonate is used for alkalinization.

Dialysis, although not used routinely, can be life saving in certain situations. Both peritoneal dialysis and hemodialysis are dependent on having a significant fraction of free drug in blood. That is, they work best with substances that have a low volume of distribution and that are not bound avidly to plasma proteins. Hemoperfusion entails the passage of blood through a column of charcoal or resin. This technique can also remove chemicals that are bound to plasma proteins.

● **Antagonists** Antidotes are seldom used to treat poisonings. The impression that there is an ideal antidote for every chemical is false. In fact, there are few antidotes (Table 9.4).

There are four classes of antagonists: functional, chemical, dispositional, and receptor (Fig. 9.6). *Functional,* or *physiologic, antagonism* occurs when two different chemicals produce opposite effects on the same system. For example, dopamine infusion is used to combat severe hypotension.

Chemical antagonism is when two substances chemically neutralize each other. An example is the use of chelators to treat metal toxicity.

Dispositional antagonism is when one substance alters the absorption, biotransformation, or excretion of another. The inhibition of toxin absorption by charcoal is one example, and the use of sodium bicarbonate to increase the urinary excretion of salicylate is another.

Receptor antagonism is when one chemical blocks the biologic site through which the toxin works. The use of naloxone to treat a heroin overdose is an example of this approach.

Table 9.4   *Common Antidotes*

Toxin	Antidote
Anticholinergic agents	Physostigmine
β-Blockers	Glucagon
Benzodiazepines	Flumazenil
Calcium channel blockers	Calcium
Carbon monoxide	Oxygen
Cyanide	Nitrite and thiosulfate
Digitalis	Digoxin-specific antibody fragments
Ethylene glycol	Ethanol
Isoniazid	Pyridoxine
Lead	Ethylenediaminetetraacetic acid
Methanol	Ethanol
Opioids	Naloxone
Organophosphate or carbamate insecticides	Atropine
Tricyclic antidepressants	Bicarbonate

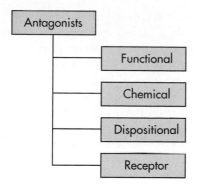

Fig. 9.6 Classification of antagonists.

Section 9.3 Heavy Metals
and Heavy Metal Antagonists

■ **Lead** Lead is the most common metal poison in the United States. The primary sources of lead are the environment, as a result of tetraethyl lead added to gasoline; lead-based paint in older homes; water, because of lead pipes and solder; improperly glazed earthenware; and the workplace, such as smelters and battery factories.

● **Toxicokinetics** Lead absorption from the gastrointestinal tract varies with age. About 10% of an ingested dose is absorbed in adults and up to 40% is absorbed in children. Up to 90% of inhaled lead is absorbed.

Once in the blood, about 99% of lead is in the red blood cells bound to hemoglobin. It distributes to soft tissues, such as the kidneys and liver. Eventually it redistributes to bone, where, because of its chemical similarity to calcium, about 95% is eventually deposited. The deposition of lead in bones can be detected by x-ray examination.

Lead is excreted into the urine and bile. It has a half-life of 1 to 2 months in soft tissue and 20 to 30 years in bone.

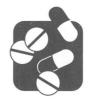

● **Acute lead poisoning** Acute lead poisoning is rare.

● **Chronic lead poisoning** Lead poisoning from chronic exposure, sometimes referred to as plumbism, is relatively common. The most common cause in children is exposure to lead paint or lead in water. For adults, occupational exposure is the primary culprit. Chronic lead exposure has effects on numerous organ systems.

— *Gastrointestinal effects* Lead affects intestinal smooth muscle, resulting in vague symptoms such as anorexia, malaise, and constipation. With more severe poisoning, intestinal pain, sometimes referred to as lead colic, is observed. The colic is important diagnostically because it is the symptom for which the patient may seek relief. The pain can be relieved by administration of **calcium gluconate.**

— *Neuromuscular effects* Skeletal muscle weakness during extended activity is a consequence of chronic lead toxicity. Wristdrop, and sometimes footdrop, is seen. This is often referred to as lead palsy.

— *Central nervous system* The most serious toxic effect in children is on the central nervous system (CNS), referred to as **lead encephalopathy.** Early symptoms include irritability, headache, insomnia, restlessness, and ataxia, followed by convulsions, lethargy, and coma. Capillary damage, along with signs and symptoms of increased intracranial pressure, are evident. Many survivors have permanent neurologic sequalea, such as mental retardation or seizures.

Children with blood lead levels too low to produce lead encephalopathy may have mild neurologic dysfunction, such as learning disabilities, decreased IQ, and behavioral abnormalities. As a result, the Center for Disease Control and Prevention suggests screening of children beginning at 6 months of age. Those with blood levels greater than 10 μg/dl are considered to have excessive exposure to lead. When blood levels exceed 25 μg/dl, chelation therapy should be considered.

— *Hematologic effects*   One sign of lead intoxication is the appearance of basophilic stippled red blood cells. These juvenile forms of erythrocytes are not diagnostic for lead poisoning because they are evident in a variety of blood dyscrasias.

Low concentrations of lead interfere with the synthesis of hemes, which are necessary for incorporation into hemoglobin, myoglobin, cytochromes, and catalase (Fig. 9.7). This results in enzyme inhibition and the accumulation of protoporphyrin IX in red blood cells, the ac-

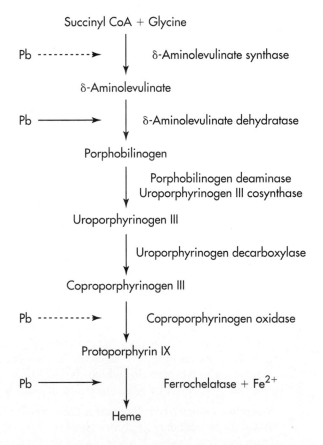

Steps that are definitely inhibited by lead are indicated by →; steps at which lead is thought to act but evidence is inconclusive are indicated by --►.

Fig. 9.7   Effects of lead on heme synthesis.

cumulation of δ-aminolevulinic acid (ALA) in plasma, and an increased urinary excretion of ALA and coproporphyrin III (oxidation product of coproporphyrinogen III).

Because lead inhibits ferrochelatase, an enzyme that normally incorporates iron into hemoglobin, lead exposure causes a hypochromic microcytic anemia. This is more common in children than in adults.

— *Renal effects* Lead has significant effects on the kidneys, although they are less severe than on other organs. Proteinuria, hematuria, and cysts are often found in the urine with chronic lead exposure. Hyperuricemia and gout are often seen in lead-induced chronic renal injury.

— *Other effects* A black or blue-black line along the gingival margin sometimes occurs. Because of better dental hygiene, this sign is less common today. The line is not specific for lead in that it is also encountered with bismuth, mercury, tin, and arsenic. Lead also changes skin coloration, resulting in an ash-gray color of the face and pallor of the lips. This is sometimes referred to as the lead hue or lead pallor.

● **Diagnosis of lead poisoning** Patient history of lead exposure coupled with signs of the toxic effects are significant clues that lead toxicity has occurred, although the diagnosis needs to be confirmed (Fig. 9.8). Because lead decreases heme synthesis at several steps, an accumulation of diagnostically important substrates, such as ALA and coproporphyrin in urine and zinc protoporphyrin in red blood cells, supports the diagnosis. The most sensitive and specific test is blood lead measurement.

The average blood lead concentration is about 5 μg/dl. Children with levels above 10 μg/dl are at risk for developmental disabilities. Adults with blood lead concentrations below 30 μg/dl exhibit no apparent injury or symptoms, although their heme synthesis would be altered.

Lead Chelation
CaNa$_2$ EDTA
BAL
D-penicillamine
Succimer

● **Treatment of lead poisoning** Although prevention of further exposure is most important, the mainstay of treatment for lead poisoning is the use of chelators to enhance lead excretion. Four chelators are commonly used: edetate calcium disodium (CaNa$_2$EDTA), dimercaprol (British anti-Lewisite, BAL), D-penicillamine, and succimer. Because the combination of CaNa$_2$EDTA and dimercaprol is more effective than either alone, it is often used to treat lead encephalopathy.

■ **Mercury** Mercury was once an important therapeutic agent. It was used as a diuretic, antiseptic, antibacterial, and cathartic. It has now been replaced by more specific agents. However, because mercury still has a number of industrial uses, environmental pollution is a problem (Table 9.5).

With regard to toxicity, three categories of mercury compounds are distinguished: mercury vapor (elemental mercury), mercury salts, and organic mercurials.

Elemental mercury exposure is usually occupational. For the general population, most exposure comes from dental amalgams (Table 9.6). The amount of mercury released from dental amalgams is not believed to have any biologic significance.

Inorganic mercury exists as monovalent mercurous salts or as divalent mercuric salts. **Mercurous chloride (calomel)** is used in acne skin creams and was used as a diuretic and cathartic. Because it is more irritating, **mercuric chloride** has been used as an antiseptic. Mercuric salts are widely used in industry. Because of industrial discharge into rivers, environmental pollution is a problem.

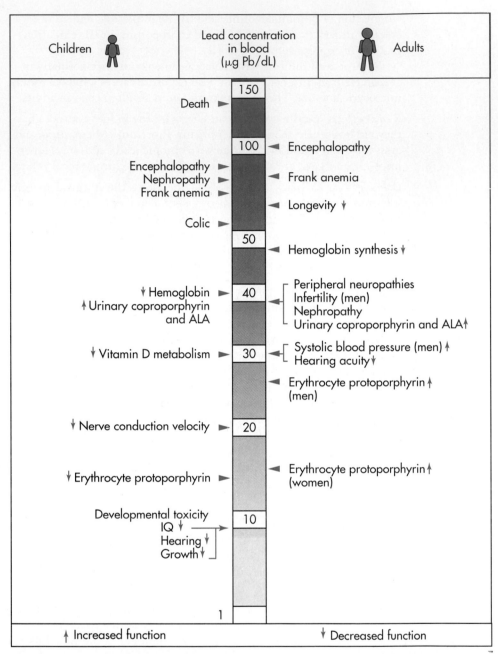

Fig. 9.8 The relationship between the lead concentration in blood and toxicologic symptoms in children and adults. *ALA*, δ-aminolevulinic acid.

All the organomercurial compounds in use today have one covalent bond to a carbon atom. Of these, alkylmercury salts are the most dangerous, and **methylmercury** is the most common. Organomercurials have been used as fungicides on seed grain and inadvertently consumed, resulting in major incidents of human poisoning. In addition, microorganisms convert inorganic mercury into methylmercury, which is accumulated by algae and concentrated in fish through the food chain. Thus discharge of inorganic mercury into rivers and lakes results in fish containing high concentrations of methylmercury.

Table 9.5 *Industrial Uses of Mercury*	
INDUSTRIAL USES OF MERCURY	PERCENT OF TOTAL CONSUMPTION
Chlor-alkali	25
Electrical equipment	20
Paints	15
Thermometers	10
Dental	3
Laboratory	2

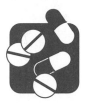

- **Mechanism of action** Mercury has a high affinity for the sulfur atom in thiol groups in enzymes and proteins, resulting in their inactivation. This interaction of mercury with sulfur is responsible for the toxicity of all mercury compounds. The organic moiety of the organomercurials and the dissociable anion in the mercury salts alter the volatility and solubility of mercury. The affinity of mercury for thiols provides the rationale for using chelators to treat mercury poisoning.

- **Toxicokinetics**

  - *Elemental mercury* Elemental mercury is relatively nontoxic when ingested because it does not dissociate but remains as droplets. However, it is readily absorbed by inhalation and enters the brain before being oxidized.

  - *Inorganic mercury salts* Inorganic mercury salts are absorbed by the gastrointestinal tract. It distributes equally between blood cells and plasma, with high concentrations found in the kidneys. Little is found in the brain because it does not readily cross the blood-brain barrier. It has a half-life of 2 months in humans.

  - *Organic mercurials* Organic mercurials, such as methylmercury, are readily absorbed (about 90%) from the gastrointestinal tract (Fig. 9.9). Methylmercury distributes much more evenly throughout the body than the mercury salts and readily enters the brain. Methylmer-

Table 9.6	*Estimated Average Daily Retention of Total Mercury and Mercury Compounds in the General Population Not Occupationally Exposed to Mercury*		
	ESTIMATED MEAN DAILY RETENTION OF MERCURY COMPOUNDS (MG MERCURY/DAY)		
EXPOSURE	MERCURY VAPOR	INORGANIC MERCURY	METHYLMERCURY
Air	0.024	0.001	0.0064
Food			
Fish	0.0	0.04	2.3
Other	0.0	0.25	0.0
Drinking water	0.0	0.0035	0.0
Dental amalgams	3-17	0.0	0.0
Total	3-17	0.3	2.31

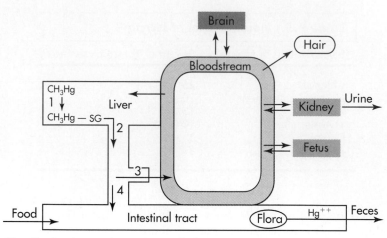

Fig. 9.9 The distribution pathway for methylmercury (CH_3Hg) in the body. *1*, Glutathione metabolite of methylmercury. *2*, Biliary secretion. *3*, Enterohepatic circulation. *4*, Excretion.

cury is believed to enter the brain by the methionine amino acid carrier after it complexes with methylmercury (Fig. 9.10). Methylmercury also readily crosses the placenta (Fig. 9.9). It is excreted into the bile as a complex with glutathione and undergoes an enterohepatic circulation. The half-life of methylmercury in humans is about 2 months.

● **Toxicity**

— *Elemental mercury* Mercury vapor produces neuropsychologic effects (Fig. 9.11). Tremors are common, as well as psychologic changes such as depression, insomnia, excessive shyness, irritability, reduced self-confidence, and uncontrolled blushing (erethism).

— *Inorganic salts of mercury* Because inorganic mercury precipitates proteins, oral exposure produces an ashen-gray appearance in the mouth, intestinal pain, and vomiting. After absorption, the target organs of toxicity are the kidneys.

A hypersensitive reaction to mercury may be noted after chronic exposure. This condition, known as acrodynia or pink disease, consists

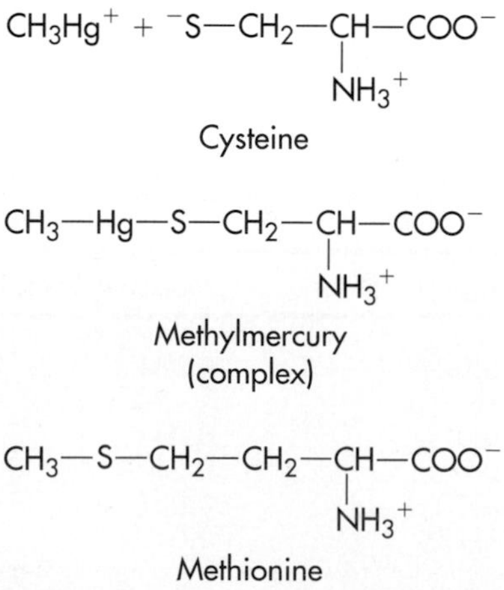

$$CH_3Hg^+ + {}^-S-CH_2-\underset{\underset{NH_3^+}{|}}{CH}-COO^-$$

Cysteine

$$CH_3-Hg-S-CH_2-\underset{\underset{NH_3^+}{|}}{CH}-COO^-$$

Methylmercury
(complex)

$$CH_3-S-CH_2-CH_2-\underset{\underset{NH_3^+}{|}}{CH}-COO^-$$

Methionine

Fig. 9.10 Methylmercury readily binds to sulfhydryl molecules in the body.

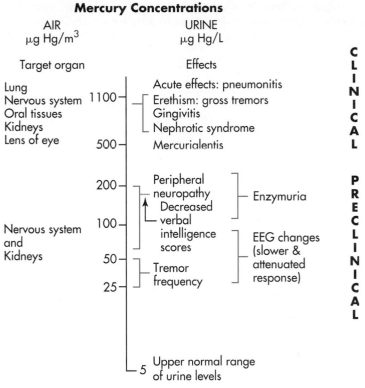

Fig. 9.11 The correlation of mercury concentrations in air and urine with toxicologic symptoms.

of erythema of the extremities, face, and chest, as well as photophobia and tachycardia. It was a significant problem in the 1980s when phenylmercuric fungicide was used in a commercial diaper service.

— *Organic mercurials* Methylmercury is a neurotoxicant and at low concentrations produces paresthesias, visual defects, and ataxia (Table 9.7). The visual cortex is especially sensitive to methylmercury, resulting in visual field constriction. Likewise, the brain of the develop-

Table 9.7 *Frequency of Symptoms of Methylmercury Poisoning in Relation to Concentration of Mercury in Blood[*]*

Concentration of Mercury in Blood µg/ml (µM)	Cases with Symptoms (%)					
	Paresthesias	Ataxia	Visual Defects	Dysarthria	Hearing Defects	Death
0.1-0.5 (0.5-2.5)	5	0	0	5	0	0
0.5-1.0 (2.5-5.0)	42	11	11	5	5	0
1-2 (5-10)	60	47	53	24	5	0
2-3 (10-15)	79	60	56	25	13	0
3-4 (15-20)	82	100	58	75	36	17
4-5 (20-25)	100	100	83	85	66	28

[*]Based on data in Bakir et al: Clinical and epidemiological aspects of methylmercury poisoning, *Postgrad Med J* 56:1–10, 1980.

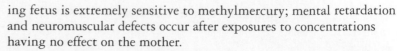

ing fetus is extremely sensitive to methylmercury; mental retardation and neuromuscular defects occur after exposures to concentrations having no effect on the mother.

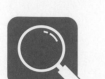

- **Diagnosis of mercury poisoning** A history of exposure to mercury, either industrial or environmental, is most helpful in making this diagnosis. Analytic chemistry is used to confirm the diagnosis because mercury may be quantified in blood, plasma, urine, and hair. Methylmercury concentrates in erythrocytes and inorganic mercury does not. Therefore the distribution of mercury between red blood cells and plasma indicates whether exposure was due to inorganic or organic mercury. The concentration in urine is a good index of the body burden of inorganic mercury, but not organic mercury because it is excreted mainly in the bile. Because hair is rich in sulfhydryl groups, the concentration of mercury is about 300-fold higher in hair than in blood.

- **Treatment of mercury poisoning**

  — *Elemental mercury vapor and inorganic mercury* Immediate termination of exposure is essential. Removal from the mercury vapor and gastric lavage of inorganic mercury should be instituted. Chelators, such as dimercaprol, are given to symptomatic patients, whereas penicillamine is used for low-level exposure. Inasmuch as penicillamine-mercury chelate is excreted into urine, it should be used with caution when renal function is impaired. The new orally effective chelator, succimer, also appears to be effective for mercury chelation.

  — *Organic mercury* Dimercaprol is contraindicated for organic mercury poisoning because it increases the concentration of mercury in the brain. Although penicillamine facilitates the excretion of organic mercury, its effects are not impressive. Because methylmercury undergoes an enterohepatic recirculation, the use of a nonabsorbable polythiol resin that interrupts this process enhances the fecal excretion of methylmercury.

- ▪ **Arsenic** Arsenic was historically used as a chemotherapeutic agent but is now of concern solely because of industrial and environmental exposure. Arsenic is an active ingredient in many pesticides. In addition, arsanilic acid is fed to poultry and livestock to enhance growth rates. Arsenic from natural sources is found in water in Argentina, Chile, Taiwan, and the western United States.

  Arsenic exists in a number of chemical forms, which determine its toxicity. In general, the toxicity increases in the sequence of: organic arsenicals $< As^{5+} < As^{3+} <$ arsine (AsH_3). Organic arsenicals can contain arsenic in the trivalent or pentavalent state. The pentavalent arsenates are more toxic than organic arsenicals but less toxic than the trivalent arsenicals. Arsine (AsH_3) is a highly toxic gas that produces different effects (hemolysis) than other arsenic compounds.

- **Mechanism of action** The pentavalent form of arsenic (arsenate) substitutes for inorganic phosphate in the formation of adenosine triphosphate, which is not stable and is rapidly hydrolyzed. The more toxic trivalent form of arsenic (arsenite) has a high affinity for thiol groups and therefore inhibits many sulfhydryl-containing enzymes. It has particular affinity for closely aligned sulfhydryl groups, such as in lipoic acid (Fig. 9.12), forming a stable six-membered ring. Because lipoic acid is an essential cofactor for pyruvate dehydrogenase, arsenic causes a blockade of energy metabolism and accumulation of pyruvic acid in plasma.

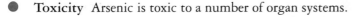

Fig. 9.12 The binding of arsenite to lipoic acid.

- **Toxicokinetics** Arsenic is relatively well absorbed from the gastrointestinal tract and is initially distributed to the liver and kidney. However, because of high affinity for sulfhydryl groups, it eventually collects in skin, hair, and nails. It readily crosses the placenta.

    Arsenate (pentavalent) is biotransformed to arsenite (trivalent) and then methylated to methylarsenite and dimethlyarsenite (Fig. 9.13), which is readily eliminated in the urine. Dimethylarsenite has a half-life of 3 to 5 days.

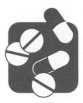

- **Toxicity** Arsenic is toxic to a number of organ systems.

    — *Cardiovascular system* Arsenic induces vasodilation and increases capillary permeability. Long-term exposure results in gangrene in the extremities, especially in the feet, and is referred to as Blackfoot disease.

    — *Gastrointestinal tract* Arsenic causes capillary damage in the intestines, especially in the splanchnic area. The loss of plasma proteins produces blisters under the gastrointestinal mucosa. Eventually these rupture, and due to the cathartic action of arsenic and an increase in peristalsis, the so-called ricewater stools result.

    — *Kidneys* Arsenic injures the glomeruli first and then the renal tubules.

    — *Skin* Arsenic causes vasodilation and increases capillary permeability, leading to what is referred to as the "milk and roses complexion". Longer use results in hyperkeratosis, especially on the palms and soles, as well as hyperpigmentation. Skin cancer may also occur.

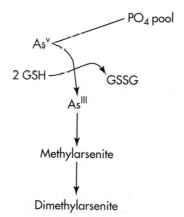

Fig. 9.13 The biotransformation pathway for arsenic. *GSH*, glutathione.

— *Nervous system* Although arsenic can cause encephalopathy, peripheral neuropathy is more common.

— *Carcinogenesis* Occupational exposure to arsenic in sheep-dip or vineyard sprays may result in intraepidemal squamous-cell and superficial basal-cell carcinomas. It also produces lung cancer.

● **Acute arsenic poisoning** Arsenic trioxide (As_2O_3, arsenous acid) used to be a common cause of poisoning because it was readily available, is nearly tasteless, has the appearance of sugar, and is quickly absorbed from the gastrointestinal tract. Gastrointestinal symptoms are the first observed after acute arsenic poisoning, including stomach pains, vomiting, and diarrhea. Depressed urine flow and hypovolemic shock may develop. Death usually occurs within 24 hours. Survivors often have peripheral neuropathies, with severe crippling.

Acute inhalation of arsine gas results in hemolysis, with subsequent anemia, reduced red blood cell count, and hemoglobin in urine. The released hemoglobin results in jaundice and kidney injury.

● **Chronic arsenic poisoning** If the patient survives the severe hemolysis, fewer gastrointestinal effects are observed after chronic than acute exposure to arsenic. Skin abnormalities are often observed, including increased pigmentation, hyperkeratosis, and edema. Mees' lines (white transverse lines of deposited arsenic) are found in the fingernails. Garlic odor on the breath may arouse suspicion. Liver and kidney injury often follow, along with the development of peripheral neurites and encephalopathy. The bone marrow is injured and all hematologic elements may be altered (aplastic anemia). Lung and skin carcinomas may result from long-term exposure.

● **Treatment of arsenic poisoning** Prevention of further exposure and treatment of severe effects, such as hypotension, are vital. Chelators, such as dimercaprol, penicillamine, and succimer, are effective in treating arsenic toxicity.

■ **Cadmium** Because it is resistant to corrosion, cadmium is used in alloys. It is also used as a yellow pigment in inks, in nickel-cadmium rechargeable batteries, plastics, and other items. As a result, it has become an environmental pollutant. Cadmium concentrates in plants such as tobacco and rice. As a result, smokers have higher body burdens of cadmium. Rice grown on contaminated soil in Japan resulted in *Itai-Itai* (ouch-ouch) disease.

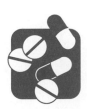

● **Toxicokinetics** Although less than 5% of ingested cadmium is absorbed from the gastrointestinal tract, 10% to 40% is absorbed after inhalation. It is distributed mainly to the liver and kidney, where it is bound to a low-molecular-weight protein, metallothionein. The half-life of cadmium in the body is very long, from 10 to 30 years. As a result, it is a cumulative poison.

● **Acute cadmium poisoning** Acute exposure to cadmium by inhalation can produce respiratory problems. Acute oral exposure causes only local irritation and vomiting.

● **Chronic cadmium poisoning**

— *Kidney* The main target organ of chronic cadmium exposure is the kidney. Cadmium is initially accumulated by the liver, where it is conjugated with glutathione (GSH) and excreted into bile or bound to metallothionein (Fig. 9.14). Metallothionein acts as a scavenger for cadmium in the liver, protecting hepatocytes. However, some of the

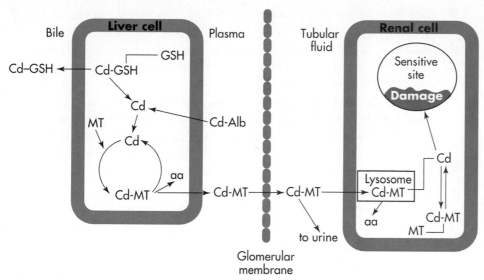

Fig. 9.14 Cadmium-metallothionein complexes leak from the liver and are taken up by the kidney, where they cause renal damage.

cadmium metallothionein complex leaks out of the liver and, in this form, is avidly taken up by the kidney. The cadmium metallothionein complex is degraded in the kidney lysosomes, releasing cadmium and damaging the kidney.

— *Lung* When inhaled, cadmium causes emphysema and pulmonary fibrosis.

— *Cardiovascular system* Epidemiologic data show a correlation between hypertension and the concentration of cadmium in the kidney. It is uncertain whether this indicates a cause-and-effect relationship.

— *Bone* One of the hallmarks of *Itai-Itai* disease was osteomalacia. Although the mechanism is unknown, osteomalacia was most common in multiparous, postmenopausal women, suggesting an interaction among cadmium, nutrition, and bone disease.

— *Cancer* Laboratory and clinical studies indicate that cadmium is a carcinogen. These investigations have identified tumors of the lungs, prostate, and to a lesser extent the kidney and stomach.

● **Treatment of cadmium poisoning** There are no chelators available for treating cadmium toxicity. In fact, some studies indicate that chelators can enhance the distribution of cadmium to the kidney, enhancing nephrotoxocity.

■ **Other Metals: Nonessential**

● **Aluminum** Aluminum has many industrial uses, and it is used as an antacid. By inhalation it produces lung fibrosis, referred to as Shaver's disease. Because aluminum salts are used in dialysis patients, it is believed by some that dialysis encephalopathy is due to this metal. This remains an issue of dispute.

● **Antimony** Antimony toxicity is similar to that encountered with arsenic.

● **Barium** Although soluble salts of barium (e.g., chloride) produce cardiovascular and CNS effects, insoluble barium salts (e.g., sulfate) are poorly absorbed and display minimal toxicity.

- **Beryllium** Beryllium produces skin lesions, dermatitis, and granulomas. It is a carcinogen in laboratory animals.

- **Fluoride** Fluoride is often added to drinking water to decrease dental caries. Higher concentrations cause discoloration of teeth, and at extremely high concentrations it causes brittle bones.

- **Nickel** Nickel jewelry may cause dermatitis (nickel itch). Nickel carbonyl $[Ni(CO)_4]$ is the most toxic form of the metal and can cause pneumonia, hyperthermia, and delirium. Nickel subsulfate is a human carcinogen (nose). The chelator most effective for nickel is dithiocarbamate.

- **Silver** Silver can cause a discoloration of the skin known as argyria.

- **Thallium** Thallium is used as a rodenticide. Its distribution in the body is similar to potassium. Acute exposure produces gastrointestinal and cardiovascular effects.

Other Metals: Essential

- **Chromium** Chromium exists in several valences. Whereas Cr^{3+} is essential as a glucose tolerance factor, Cr^{6+} is a carcinogen of the respiratory tract.

- **Cobalt** Although cobalt is an essential part of vitamin B_{12}, in excess it causes polycythemia, and in combination with alcohol it causes cardiomyopathy.

- **Iron** Iron is a common poison because of the availability of iron pills. It produces severe damage to the gastrointestinal tract, as well as acidosis. Iron pills in the gastrointestinal tract can often be localized by x-ray examination. The specific chelator for iron is **deferoxamine**.

- **Manganese** Chronic exposure to manganese produces a Parkinson-like syndrome. The condition is treated similarly to Parkinson's disease.

Heavy Metal Antagonists
The primary treatment for heavy metal toxicity is the use of chelators. The toxicity is due to binding the metals with endogenous ligands, thereby inhibiting some biochemical processes. The chelator competes with the endogenous ligands. The complex of the chelator and the metal is water soluble and is excreted in the urine.

- **Edetate calcium disodium** Edetate calcium disodium is the calcium chelate of the disodium salt of ethylenediaminetetraacetic acid (EDTA) (Fig. 9.15).

  — *Chemistry and mechanism of action* EDTA binds many cations. Sodium and potassium are held weakly, but calcium, lead, and copper have higher stability constants. If the disodium salt of EDTA (Na_2EDTA) is given, it chelates calcium and causes hypocalcemic tetany. Therefore $CaNa_2EDTA$ is used for treatment of poisoning by

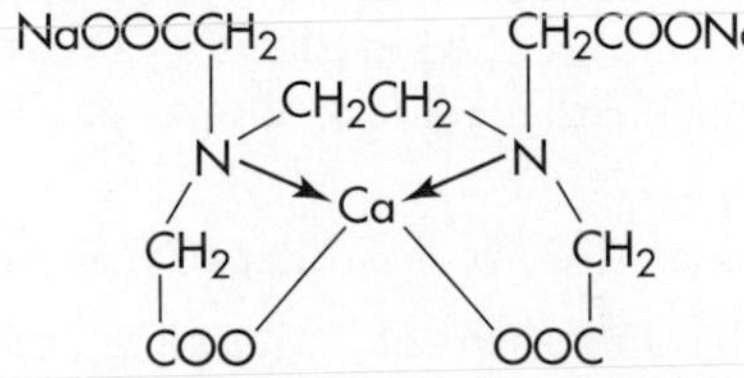

Treatment of Iron Poisoning
Deferoxamine

Fig. 9.15 Structure of edetate calcium disodium.

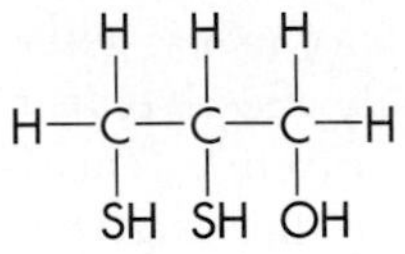

H H H

H—C—C—C—H

SH SH OH

Fig. 9.16 Structure of dimercaprol.

metals that have higher affinity for the chelating agent than does calcium. **Lead** is the main metal for which $CaNa_2EDTA$ is used. It is not effective for mercury, arsenic toxicity, or most other metals.

— *Pharmacokinetics* Because less than 5% of $CaNa_2EDTA$ is absorbed from the gastrointestinal tract, it is usually administered intravenously (IV) or occasionally intramuscularly (IM). It is water soluble, and does not readily enter into cells. It has a half-life of 20 to 60 minutes. Most of it is excreted unchanged in urine.

— *Toxicity* The principal toxic effect of $CaNa_2EDTA$ is on the kidney. Proximal tubular injury is observed and is usually reversible after cessation of treatment. The most common complaint is pain at the site of injection.

● **Dimercaprol** Dimercaprol, 2,3-dimercaptopropanol, is also known as British antilewisite (BAL) because is was originally synthesized as an antidote for lewisite, a vesicant arsenical war gas (Fig. 9.16).

— *Mechanism of action* Dimercaprol forms stable complexes with mercury, arsenic, and gold, promoting the excretion of these metals. Dimercaprol reactivates sulfhydryl enzymes inhibited by metals, but it is more effective in preventing this inhibition. It is routinely used for the chelation of mercury, arsenic, and gold and in combination of $CaNa_2EDTA$ for lead poisoning, especially when there is evidence of lead encephalopathy.

— *Pharmacokinetics* Dimercaprol is administered in oil by deep IM injection. Peak blood concentrations are attained within 1 hour, with excretion almost complete within 4 hours. Dimercaprol more readily enters tissues than does $CaNa_2EDTA$.

— *Toxicity* Although therapeutic doses of dimercaprol are usually quite safe, it can produce nausea, vomiting, headache, and a burning sensation of the lips. The most pronounced and consistent effects are increased blood pressure and tachycardia.

Because metal chelators dissociate in an acid medium, production of an alkaline urine protects against kidney injury.

● **Succimer** Chemically similar to dimercaprol, succimer also contains two carboxylic acids that greatly alter its distribution and spectrum of chelation (Fig. 9.17).

CaNa₂ EDTA
Lead

BAL
Mercury
Arsenic
Gold
Lead

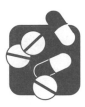

Succimer
Lead

COOH
|
CHSH
|
CHSH
|
COOH

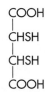

Fig. 9.17 Structure of succimer.

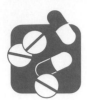

— *Pharmacokinetics* Succimer is a new lead chelator. One of its advantages is that it is orally effective. It is biotransformed in humans to a mixed disulfide with cysteine. The succimer-lead chelate is eliminated in urine and bile, with that excreted in bile undergoing enterohepatic circulation.

— *Mechanism of action* Succimer is used to treat children with lead blood levels greater than 45 µg/dl. Because it is orally effective and it does not mobilize essential metals such as zinc, copper, and iron, it is a particularly useful chelator. In laboratory animals it has been shown effective in chelating arsenic, cadmium, and mercury.

— *Toxicity* The adverse effects of succimer are considerably less than dimercaprol. This might be due to its lower lipid solubility, which limits its penetration into cells. The most common adverse effects are gastrointestinal, including nausea, vomiting, diarrhea, and loss of appetite. Transient elevation of hepatic enzymes and rashes have also been reported.

● **Penicillamine** Penicillamine is a D-β,β-dimethylcysteine (Fig. 9.18).

— *Mechanism of action* Penicillamine effectively chelates copper, mercury, zinc, and lead. It promotes the excretion of these metals in the urine.

Penicillamine
Mercury
Lead
Arsenic

— *Pharmacokinetics* Penicillamine is well absorbed from the gastrointestinal tract.

— *Clinical use* Penicillamine is used for the treatment of Wilson's disease, which is characterized by hepatolenticular degeneration caused by an excess of copper. It is also used as an adjunct in lead, mercury, and arsenic poisoning. It is particularly appropriate for the treatment of cystinuria because it reacts with the poorly soluble cysteine and forms a water-soluble cysteine-penicillamine mixed disulfide. It is also used in rheumatoid arthritis.

— *Toxicity* Penicillamine induces a number of cutaneous reactions manifested by maculopapular or erythematous rash with generalized edema, pruritus, and fever.
Cross-sensitivity to penicillin may exist.

● **Deferoxamine** Deferoxamine is a natural iron chelator isolated from *Streptomyces pilosis* (Fig. 9.19).

— *Pharmacokinetics* Deferoxamine is poorly absorbed after oral administration.

— *Toxicity* Deferoxamine causes a number of allergic reactions, including pruritus, wheals, rash, and anaphylaxis.

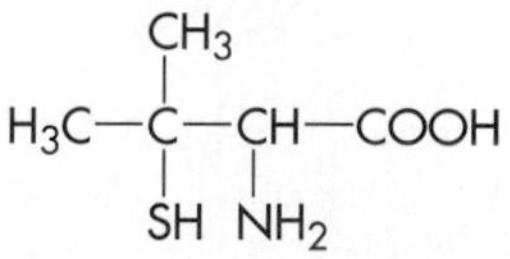

Deferoxamine
Iron

$$H_3C-\underset{\underset{SH}{|}}{\overset{\overset{CH_3}{|}}{C}}-\underset{\underset{NH_2}{|}}{CH}-COOH$$

Fig. 9.18 Structure of penicillamine.

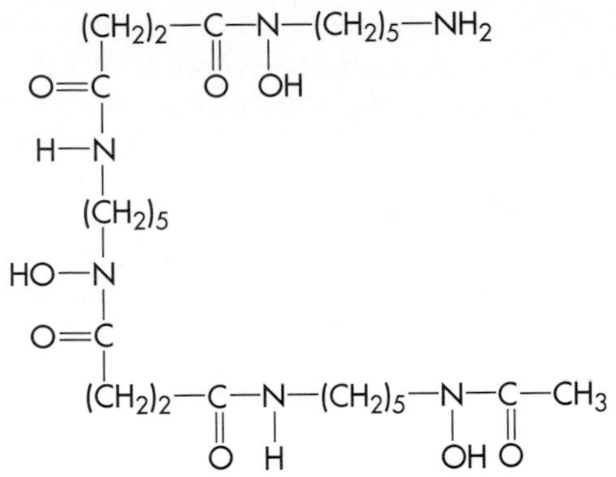

$$(CH_2)_2—C—N—(CH_2)_5—NH_2$$

Fig. 9.19 Structure of deferoxamine.

SECTION 9.4
AIR POLLUTION, SOLVENTS,
AND VAPORS

■ Nonmetallic Environment and Toxicants

● **Air pollution** Air pollution is the result of human activity. Although pollutants contaminate not only the air, but also the water and soil, they enter the body mainly through the lungs. Particles less than 1 μm in diameter remain suspended in air and reach the alveoli, where they are readily absorbed because the surface area is large, blood flow is high, and blood is in close contact with the air. Larger particles (>5 μm) are deposited in the upper respiratory tract, and smaller particles (1 to 5 μm) accumulate in the tracheobronchial tree and are cleared by the upward movement of mucus by the cilia.

● **Air pollutants** Five pollutants make up 98% of air pollution: **carbon monoxide** (52%), **sulfur dioxide** (18%), **hydrocarbons** (12%), **particulate matter** (10%), and **nitrogen oxides** (6%). Five sources account for 90% of pollutants: transportation (60%), industry (18%), electric-power generation (13%), space heating (6%), and refuse disposal (3%).

  There are two kinds of pollution. The **reducing type** is caused by sulfur dioxide and smoke resulting from incomplete combustion of coal, especially in the presence of fog and cool temperatures. Reducing-type pollution can be dangerous, especially for individuals with cardiac or respiratory diseases and for the elderly: 30 people died in Belgium in 1930, 20 in Pennsylvania in 1948, and 4000 in London in 1952 as a result of reducing-type pollution.

  Oxidizing, or photochemical, pollution contains hydrocarbons, oxides of nitrogen, and photochemical oxidants produced by automobiles. Oxidizing air pollutants are not known to produce death, but they can cause irritation and correlate with allergic disorders, upper respiratory tract infections, influenza, and bronchitis.

● **Sulfur dioxide** Sulfur dioxide (SO_2) is a gas generated by the combustion of fossil fuels containing sulfur. It forms sulfurous acid on contact with moist membranes, giving rise to irritation. Sulfur dioxide causes bronchial constriction, with asthmatics being more sensitive to this effect.

- **Ozone** There is little margin between the concentrations of ozone in urban air and that known to decrease respiratory function in humans. Ozone causes shallow, rapid breathing, a decrease in pulmonary compliance, and symptoms such as cough, tightness in the chest, and dryness of the throat. The pulmonary injury resulting from ozone exposure is due to free-radical intermediates.

- **Carbon monoxide** The most common cause of accidental and suicidal poisoning is carbon monoxide (CO). It has been estimated that over 4000 people die in the United States each year as a result of CO poisoning. In addition, CO exposure can cause permanent disability, such as subtle neurologic problems.

  - *Sources* CO is a colorless, odorless, tasteless, and nonirritating gas. It has recently been implicated as a gaseous neurotransmitter in the brain, similar to nitric oxide. However, more work is necessary to conclusively determine whether CO has a normal physiologic function. It is produced in the body during the catabolism of heme. The normal carboxyhemoglobin (COHb) levels in blood seldom exceed 0.4% to 0.7%, but in hemolytic anemia they may be as high as 8%. Heavy smokers (two packs a day) may have COHb levels of 6%.

    Automobile exhaust is the largest source of CO. However, the use of catalytic converters and modified fuels has decreased the amount of CO released. Running the automobile engine in a closed garage is a common cause of poisoning.

    Another major source of CO is inadequate ventilation of heating equipment. This is true for all stoves, whether they are fueled by gas, coal, wood, or oil. Heating equipment must be well ventilated to allow adequate oxygen and to eliminate the CO.

  - *Mechanism of action* The toxicity of CO is largely due to a decrease in delivery of oxygen to tissues. The CO combines with hemoglobin, which, in this form, cannot carry oxygen. CO has an affinity 220 times greater for hemoglobin than does oxygen. In addition, COHb has an inhibitory influence on the dissociation of oxyhemoglobin.

    The two most critical determinants in CO toxicity are its concentration in air and duration of exposure. Other factors, such as hemoglobin concentration and oxygen demand of the tissues, are also important.

  - *Signs and symptoms* Inasmuch as the brain and heart are the organs with the greatest oxygen demand, they are the sites for most of the toxic effects of CO.

    The signs and symptoms of CO poisoning are characteristic of hypoxia (Fig. 9.20). The severe headache after exposure to CO is believed to be caused by excessive transudation across hypoxic capillaries, resulting in cerebral edema and increased intracranial pressure. The fetus is more susceptible to CO and often displays neurologic sequelae.

  - *Treatment* In treating CO poisoning it is essential to prevent further absorption of the gas. Therefore the patient should be transferred immediately to fresh air.

    CO is eliminated from the body by the lungs, with a half-life of 320 minutes. Because oxygen competes with CO for hemoglobin, in-

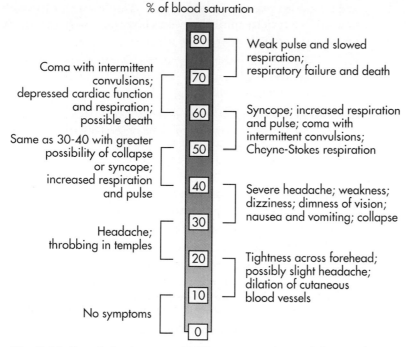

Fig. 9.20 Correlation between COHb concentration and signs and symptoms of carbon monoxide poisoning.

creasing the concentration of oxygen from 21% to 100% reduces the half-life to 80 minutes, and hyperbaric oxygen decreases the half-life to 25 minutes. Although administration of 100% oxygen is extremely beneficial, hyperbaric oxygen is the preferred treatment, but often it is not readily available. Other supportive therapy, such as respiration, hydration, and maintenance of acid-base balance, are sometimes required.

■ **Particulate Matter** Pneumoconiosis is a disorder caused by the inhalation of dusts. **Silicosis** is the most common example of pneumoconiosis. Silica dusts of 2 to 3 μm are phagocytized by alveolar macrophages, resulting in fibrotic nodules throughout the lungs. This often requires 10 to 25 years to develop, at which time the patient experiences shortness of breath. Silicosis enhances the susceptibility to tuberculosis.

Asbestosis results from long-term inhalation of asbestos dust. Asbestosis, a form of pulmonary fibrosis, develops first in areas adjacent to the bronchioles, where the longer fibers deposit. Bronchial cancer is associated with asbestos, with the incidence being much higher in cigarette smokers. In addition, mesothelioma, a rapidly fatal malignancy, is also caused by asbestos fibers.

Other pulmonary diseases caused by dust are coal workers' pneumoconiosis, or black lung disease, aluminosis, or bauxite lung, and byssinosis, which is caused by cotton.

■ **Solvents and Vapors** Organic solvents and their vapors are present in gasoline, lighter fluids, spot removers, aerosol sprays, and glues. Solvents are widely used in industry. Because of improper disposal, some contaminate our drinking water.

● Aliphatic hydrocarbons

— C_1-C_2 Methane and ethane are present in natural gas, and propane and butane are present in bottled gas. As asphyxiants these carbons do not produce toxicity until their concentration is so high that they decrease the amount of available oxygen.

— C_5-C_8 These higher-molecular-weight hydrocarbons depress the CNS. In addition, *n*-hexane is a neurotoxin. This was discovered in workers making sandals using a glue containing *n*-hexane.

● **Gasoline and kerosene** Gasoline and kerosene are CNS depressants, producing signs and symptoms similar to those observed with ethyl alcohol. CNS depression is seen after exposure by either inhalation or ingestion. Ingestion is more hazardous because the low surface tension of gasoline makes it easily aspirated into lungs. Death from hemorrhagic pulmonary edema can occur within 24 hours of aspiration. Because of the danger of aspiration, emesis or gastric lavage is usually contraindicated.

Chronic exposure to gasoline is of concern, because it contains benzene, a carcinogen in humans.

■ **Halogenated Hydrocarbons** Because halogenated hydrocarbons have low flammability, they are widely used in industry. Some halogenated hydrocarbons, such as chloroform, bromodichloromethane, dibromochloromethane, and bromoform, are produced during the chlorination of water. Correlations between water chlorination and the incidence of colon, rectal, and bladder cancers have been noted.

CCl$_4$ Toxicity

CNS depression
Sensitize heart to
  catecholamines
Kidney injury
Lliver injury
Liver cancer

● **Carbon tetrachloride** Carbon tetrachloride (CCLU) has been used for many purposes, including medicinally and as a cleaning agent. Because of its toxicity it is rarely used today except as a fumigant.

There are five major toxic effects of carbon tetrachloride: it produces CNS depression, as do all the solvents; it can sensitize the heart to catecholamines and produce arrhythmias; it causes kidney injury; in laboratory animals it produces liver cancer; and it causes liver injury.

The mechanism of CCl$_4$ hepatotoxicity has been extensively examined. It is metabolized by cytochrome P-450 to the trichloromethyl free radical ($\bullet$CCl$_3$). This radical attacks membrane lipids, resulting in lipid peroxidation and a decrease in membrane function. This causes an increase in intracellular Ca^{++} and cell death.

Because hepatotoxicity depends on biotransformation to the free radical, increases in P-450, such as those produce by phenobarbital and ethanol, potentiate CCl$_4$ hepatotoxicity.

● **Other halogentaed hydrocarbons** All halogenated hydrocarbons produce CNS depression at high doses (Table 9.8). However, there is a difference in the ability of these agents to sensitize the heart to catecholamines, to produce liver and kidney injury, and to cause cancer.

Although chloroform has a toxicity profile similar to carbon tetrachloride, it produces more kidney injury. In contrast, methylene chloride, a common paint stripper, is relatively safe. It is biotransformed to CO, which can be measured in blood when used with poor ventilation. 1,1,1-Trichloroethane is also a relatively safe chemical and is widely used as an industrial solvent.

Vinyl chloride is especially hazardous because it is a known carcinogen in humans. Although other chlorinated hydrocarbons produce liver tumors in mice, epidemiologic data does not indicate that they are human carcinogens.

Trichloroethylene and tetrachloroethylene are also relatively safe. Tri-

Table 9.8   *Other Halogenated Hydrocarbons*

	CENTRAL NERVOUS SYSTEM DEPRESSION	SENSITIVE HEART	LIVER INJURY	KIDNEY INJURY	CANCER
Methanes					
Carbon tetrachloride	+	+	++++	++	+
Chloroform	+	+	+++	+++	+
Dichloromethane (methylene chloride)	+	−	+−	−	+
Ethanes					
1,1,1-Trichloroethane	+	+	+−	−	+
1,1,2-Trichloroethane	+		++	+	+
Ethylenes					
Chloroethylene (vinyl chloride)	+		++	−	+++
1,1-Dichloroethylene (vinylidine chloride)	+		+++	−	+
Trichloroethylene	+	+	+−	−	+
Tetrachloroethylene (perchloro-ethylene)	+	−	+−	+−	+

chloroethylene is used extensively as an industrial solvent, and tetrachloroethylene is used for dry cleaning.

Chlorinated hydrocarbons, like the chlorofluorocarbons, have a detrimental effect on the ozone layer, which shields the earth from solar radiation. As a result, their use is decreasing to comply with the Montreal Protocol, an international agreement to phase out the use of ozone-depleting chemicals.

■ Aliphatic Alcohols

● **Ethanol** This agent is discussed in Chapter 6.

● **Methanol** Methanol is a common industrial solvent and is found in canned fuels, some paints, paint removers, and some antifreeze fluids.

The distribution and biotransformation of methanol is similar to ethanol in that it distributes in total body water and is biotransformed by alcohol and aldehyde dehydrogenases.

— *Toxicity* Methanol is a CNS depressant similar to ethanol. However, it is less inebriating than ethanol.

The most severe toxic effects of methanol poisoning are acidosis and blindness. Although methanol is biotransformed by the same enzymes as ethanol, the products are different. With methanol, formaldehyde and formic acid are formed (Fig. 9.21). Both the acidosis and blindness are thought to be due to the accumulation of formic acid. Formic acid is eliminated slowly because of the low amounts of tetrahydrofolate in humans.

— *Treatment* Correction of acidosis is the primary approach to the treatment of methanol poisoning. In addition, inhibitors of alcohol dehydrogenase decrease the formation of formic acid. The most common inhibitor used to treat methanol poisoning is ethanol because it has a 100-fold greater affinity than methanol for dehydrogenase. In

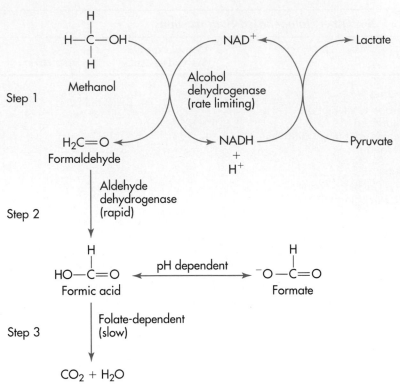

Fig. 9.21 Methanol metabolism to toxic intermediates.

addition, 4-methylpyrazole, a specific inhibitor of alcohol dehydrogenase, is used. In severe cases of methanol poisoning, dialysis may be necessary.

● **Isopropanol** Isopropanol is used in rubbing alcohol, hand lotions, and de-icing preparations. It produces CNS depression and severe gastritis.

■ **Glycols**

● **Ethylene glycol** Ethylene glycol is widely used as an antifreeze solution for automobile radiators. It is a CNS depressant.

The target organ of ethylene glycol toxicity is the kidney. The renal toxicity is due to oxalic acid, a metabolite. As with ethanol and methanol, ethylene glycol is biotransformed by alcohol and aldehyde dehydrogenase. Therefore treatment of ethylene glycol poisoning is similar to methanol poisoning, namely inhibiting the formation of the toxic metabolite by the administration of ethanol.

● **Diethylene glycol** Diethylene glycol was used as a solvent for a sulfonamide preparation in the 1930s, when it caused the death of over 100 children from renal injury. The mechanism of the renal toxicity for diethylene glycol is the same as for ethylene glycol.

● **Propylene glycol** Because propylene glycol does not produce renal injury, it is commonly used for many purposes, including as a solvent for drugs.

■ **Glycol Ethers** Glycol ethers are used in films, insulation of high voltage wires, paints, fingernail polish, semiconductors, fuel deicers, inks, and other products. Both ethylene glycol monomethyl ether and ethylene glycol monoethyl ether are teratogenic and produce testicular atrophy. These effects appear to be due to metabolites rather than the parent compound. Propylene glycol monomethyl ether is neither a reproductive toxin nor a teratogen.

■ Aromatic Hydrocarbons

● **Benzene** Because gasoline contains 1% to 2% benzene, there is exposure to this aromatic hydrocarbon when pumping gas into an automobile. As a result of leaking gasoline storage tanks, gasoline, and thus benzene, has contaminated drinking water.

    Acute exposure to benzene produces CNS depression. Of greater concern with benzene is its chronic toxicity, which is characterized by aplastic anemia and leukemia. Benzene is classified as a human carcinogen by the EPA and the International Agency for Research on Cancer. It is metabolized to a number of phenolic and ring-opened products. The aplastic anemia and leukemia are probably not due to any one metabolite but rather to the combined action of a number of metabolites.

Benzene
Aplastic anemia
Leukemia

● **Toluene** Toluene does not produce aplastic anemia or leukemia. Because it is a CNS depressant, glue sniffers inhale it for its effect on the sensorium.

SECTION 9.5 PESTICIDES

The term *pesticide* is a general classification that includes insecticides, fumigants, rodenticides, herbicides, and fungicides. Over one billion pounds of pesticides are sold in the United States, and over 4.5 billion pounds are sold around the world each year. Pesticides are used to destroy some form of life. The aim is to have pesticides that are selective for the target organism. (Fig. 9.22).

■ Insecticides All of the insecticides are neurotoxins.

● **Organochlorine insecticides**

— *DDT* Chlorophenothane, or DDT, is the best-known organochlorine insecticide (Fig. 9.23).

    DDT is one of the most effective and one of the safest insecticides. In fact, there is not one documented human fatality associated with DDT. It has a wide margin of safety for humans and has been used on humans to control lice. However, DDT is a cytochrome P-450 microsomal enzyme inducer. At very high doses in laboratory animals it produces seizures that are treated with diazepam. The mechanism

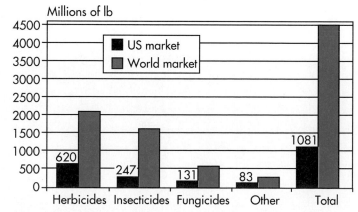

Fig. 9.22 Millions of pounds of pesticides sold per year in the United States and world markets.

Fig. 9.23 Structure of chlorophenothane (DDT).

of action of the CNS stimulation appears to be a delay in the closing of Na^+ channels and prevention of the opening of the K^+ gate. This results in prolongation of the falling phase of the action potential and repetitive neuronal discharge.

Because of its lipid solubility and persistence, DDT has created environmental problems. Biomagnification, an increase in the concentration of DDT in animals as they rise on the food chain, resulted in eggshell thinning and a decrease in the population of fish-eating birds. This, together with the observation that DDT produces hepatomas

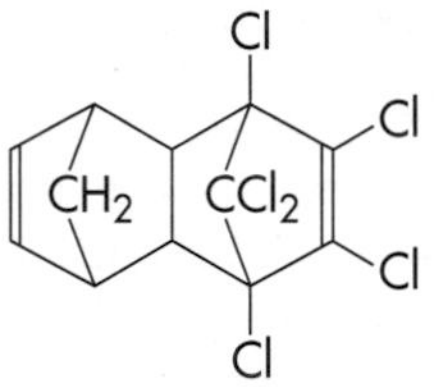

Aldrin

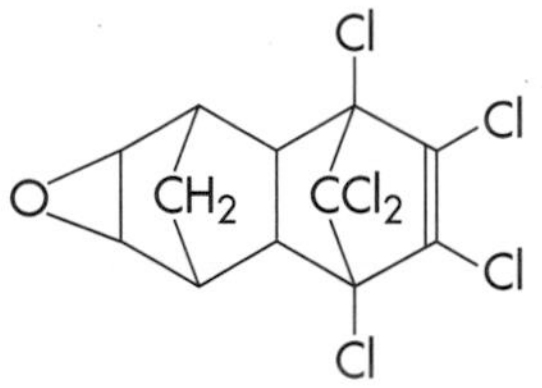

Dieldrin*

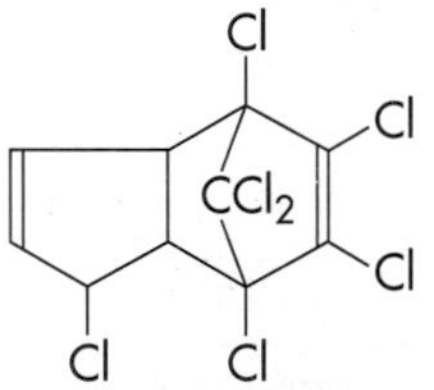

Heptachlor

Chlordane

*Endrin is a stereoisomer of dieldrin

Fig. 9.24 Chemical structures of some chlorinated cyclodienes.

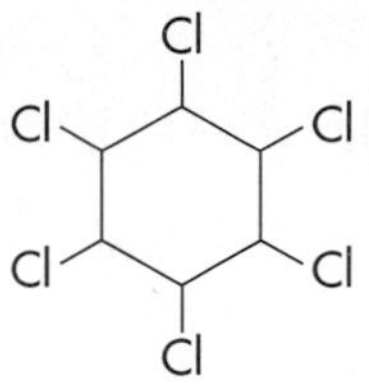

Fig. 9.25 Structure of benzene hexachloride (lindane).

in mice, resulted in it being banned for use in the United States in 1972. It is still used extensively in some tropical countries to control malaria.

- **Chlorinated cyclodienes** Four chlorinated cyclodienes have been used as pesticides (Fig. 9.24). Their pharmacologic and toxicologic properties are similar to those described for DDT, except they have caused numerous fatalities and are more readily absorbed through the skin. Their use on agricultural crops was suspended in the United States in the 1970s.

- **Lindane** Because lindane (gamma isomer of hexachlorocyclohexane) is less persistent than DDT, it is used as a pesticide (Fig. 9.25).

- **Toxaphene** The toxicology of toxaphene is similar to DDT but is less persistent in the environment.

- **Mirex and kepone** These two insecticides produce toxicologic effects similar to DDT (Fig. 9.26). However, they also produce decreases in sperm counts and liver injury. Because they are excreted into bile and undergo enterohepatic circulation, cholestyramine, which decreases the enterohepatic cycling process, enhances their elimination.

- **Organophosphorus insecticides** The chlorinated hydrocarbon insecticides have largely been replaced by organophosphate insecticides because

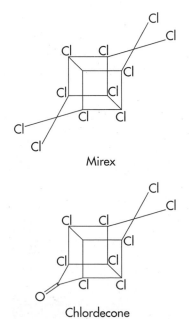

Mirex

Chlordecone

Fig. 9.26 Structure of mirex and chlordecone (Kepone).

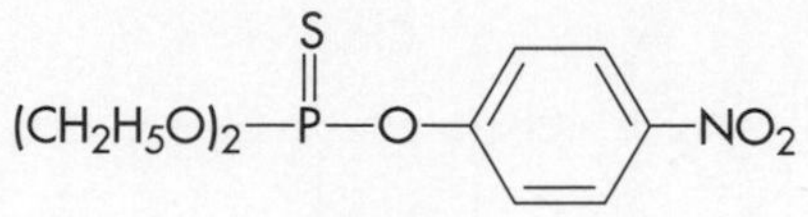

$$(CH_2H_5O)_2 - \overset{\overset{S}{\|}}{P} - O - \underset{}{\bigcirc} - NO_2$$

Parathion

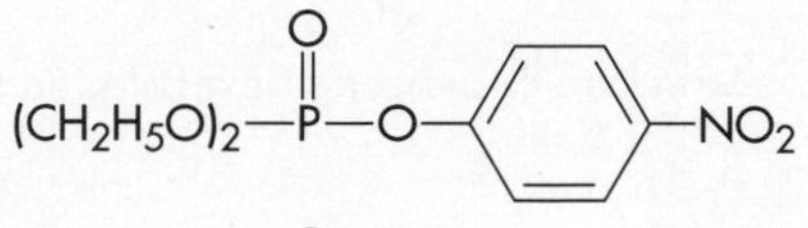

$$(CH_2H_5O)_2 - \overset{\overset{O}{\|}}{P} - O - \underset{}{\bigcirc} - NO_2$$

Paraoxon

Fig. 9.27 Structure of parathion (inactive) and paraoxon (active). Only paraoxon inhibits acetylcholine esterase (AchE).

the latter do not biomagnify and they have an extremely low carcinogenic potential.

The organophosphate insecticides are derivatives of phosphoric acid. Most are sulfur analogs that have to be transformed by cytochrome P-450 to an oxygen analog to be active (Fig. 9.27).

Some examples of organophosphates and their LD_{50} values are shown in Table 9.9.

— **Mechanism of action** The organophosphate insecticides inhibit cholinesterases by phosphorylation of the serine hydroxyl group at the esteratic site of these enzymes (Fig. 9.28).

— **Toxic effects** Organophosphate toxicity is due to an excess of acetylcholine. Muscarinic effects are most notable, including salivation, lacrimation, urination, and defecation, along with sweating, bradycardia, and hypotension. Nicotinic effects such as involuntary twitching and fasciculations, are observed, as well as CNS effects, including confusion, ataxia, and convulsions. Death is due to respiratory failure.

— **Diagnosis** In addition to the cholinergic signs and symptoms described, laboratory analysis of blood and plasma cholinesterase verifies the diagnosis of organophosphate poisoning.

Table 9.9	*Organophosphates*
EXAMPLES	LD_{50} (MG/KG)
Tetraethyl pyrophosphate	1.1
Mevinphos	6.1
Disulfoton	6.8
Azinophosmethyl	13
Parathion	13
Methylparathion	14
Chlorfenvinphos	15
Dichlorvos	80
Diazinon	108
Dimethoate	215
Trichlorfon	630
Chlorothion	880
Malathion	1375
Ronnel	1250
Abate	8000

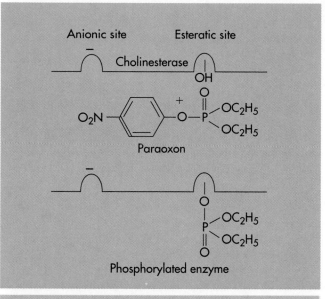

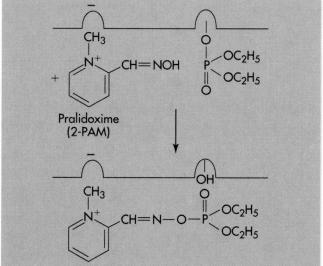

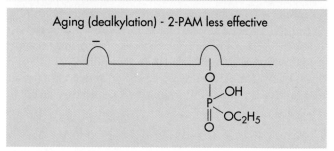

Fig. 9.28 Inactivation, reactivation, and aging of cholinesterase in the presence of paraoxon.

— *Treatment* Supportive therapy, including maintenance of respiration and administration of diazepam to control convulsions, is the primary treatment for organophosphate poisoning. Removal of the poison by decontamination of the skin, lavage, or emesis should also be attempted if possible. In addition, two specific antidotes are available for treating organophosphate poisoning. The first is atropine, which is given in large doses to block the cholinomimetic effects. Pralidoxime (2-PAM) is then given to reactivate the cholinesterase (see Fig. 9.28). However, reactivation is less effective after the phosphorylated cholinesterase has been further biotransformed, or "aged" (dealkylation) (see Fig. 9.28).

— *Delayed neurotoxicity* Most of the toxic effects of organophosphate insecticides are observed soon after exposure. Delayed neurotoxicity, characterized by paralysis and axonal degeneration, is not apparent until weeks after exposure to some organophosphates. In humans, triothocresylphosphate (TOCP), as well as the insecticides mipafox and leptophos, produce this delayed neurotoxicity.

● **Carbamate insecticides** The carbamate insecticides resemble the organophosphate insecticides in many ways, including the fact that they inhibit cholinesterase. However, they carbamylate cholinesterases rather than phosphorylate them. The carbamylated enzyme is more labile than the phosphorylated enzyme, and thus the carbamates are considered reversible inhibitors and the organophosphates are considered irreversible inhibitors of these enzymes. The carbamates are direct inhibitors of cholinesterase and do not require biotransforamtion by the cytochrome P-450, as do many of the organophosphates. Carbamate poisoning is treated with atropine; pralidoxime is not used in this case because of the lability of the carbamylated enzyme.

● **Botanical insecticides** There are three main botanical insecticides: **pyrethrums, rotenone,** and **nicotine.**

Pyrethrums are obtained from the flowers of chrysanthemums (Fig. 9.29). Because they are not very photostable, synthetic pyrethrums have been produced. They are considered the safest insecticides and display a rapid knock-down action, so they are widely used in homes. However, some people are allergic to pyrethrums. At very high doses they act on sodium channels of neurons, as does DDT, causing convulsions, which are treated with diazepam.

Rotenone comes from the roots of plants and was used for centuries to paralyze fish for capture (Fig. 9.30). Oral ingestion of rotenone produces gastrointestinal irritation, nausea, and vomiting. Conjunctivitis, dermatitis, and pulmonary irritation have been reported after exposure to this agent. At the cellular level, rotenone blocks mitochondrial respiration.

Nicotine is well absorbed from the skin. Nicotine poisoning is characterized by salivation and vomiting, from ganglionic stimulation; muscular weakness, from stimulation followed by depression at the neuromuscular junction; and ultimately convulsions and respiratory arrest from stimulation of the CNS.

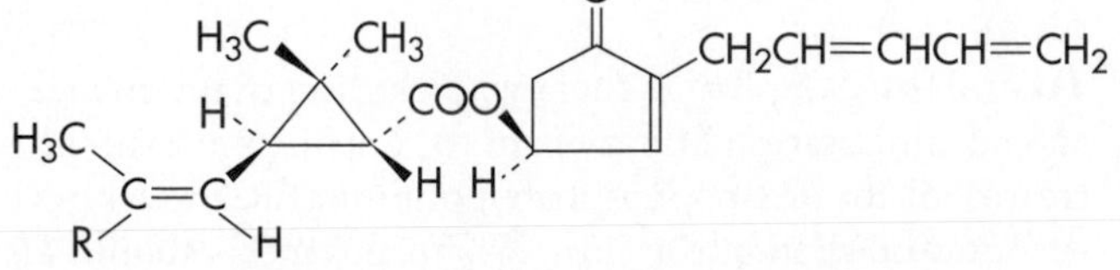

Fig. 9.29 Structure of pyrethrin I.

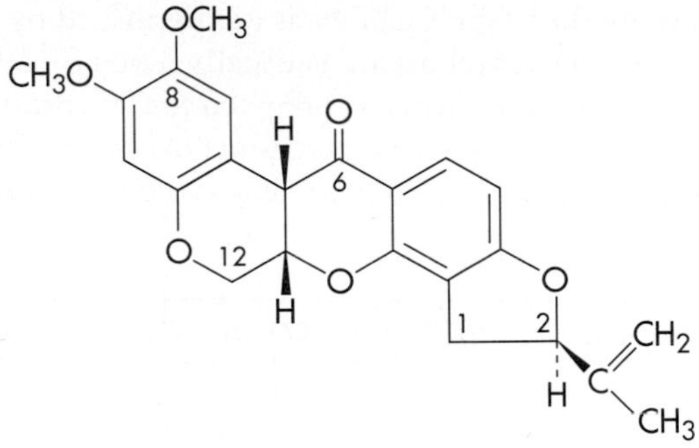

Fig. 9.30 Structure of rotenone.

■ **Fumigants** Fumigants are used to control insects, rodents, and soil nematodes. They exert their pesticide activity in a gas form and thus can penetrate into relatively inaccessible areas.

● **Cyanide** Cyanide is used as a fumigant. It is also used in metallurgy, electroplating, and metal cleaning. Because many chemical processes use cyanide, chemists are subject to accidental poisoning. Cyanides are present in silver polish, plants (cassava), and fruit seeds (apple, apricot, almond). Burning of plastic materials, such as those found in commercial aircraft, releases large amounts of cyanide. Cyanide is also used as a rodenticide.

— *Mechanism of action* Cyanide forms a stable complex with ferric iron, which keeps the metal in the high oxidation state (Fe^{3+}). It prevents iron from acting as an electron carrier in reactions involving $Fe^{3+}+e \rightarrow Fe^{2+}$ transitions. Numerous enzymes may be involved, but the most important is the trivalent ion of cytochrome oxidase in mitochondria. This impairs cellular oxygen use and therefore aerobic metabolism. This histotoxic hypoxia causes a shift to anaerobic metabolism, which results in lactic acidosis. Because tissues cannot use oxygen, venous blood becomes bright red and has an oxygen tension similar to arterial blood.

— *Toxicity* Cyanide is one of the most rapidly acting poisons, with victims often dying within minutes of exposure. One of its first effects is to increase respiration because chemoreceptors respond as they would to a decrease in oxygen. Flushing, headache, dizziness, and tachypnea are other early symptoms. Tissues most sensitive to hypoxia, such as the CNS and heart, are first affected. Eventually, all tissues become involved. Hypoxic convulsions ensue, with death from respiratory arrest. After acute exposure to cyanide, death is immediate or recovery is complete. However, neurologic sequelae, including extrapyramidal syndromes, personality changes, and memory defects, have been reported.

— *Treatment* Because cyanide is one of the most rapidly acting poisons, it is imperative that therapy be initiated as soon as symptoms appear. In addition to general supportive therapy, specific antidotes are available. Because much of cyanide toxicity results from its binding to ferric iron in cytochrome oxidase, treatment is aimed at prevention or reversal of such binding by providing a large pool of ferric iron to compete for cyanide. Therefore a fraction of the hemoglobin is oxidized to methemoglobin. This is accomplished by administering nitrite (Box 9.1). Amyl nitrite is usually given by inhalation while a solution of sodium nitrite is prepared for IV administration. Methemoglobin competes with cytochrome oxidase for the cyanide ion, cyanmethemoglobin is formed, and cytochrome oxidase is restored.

Box 9.1

USE OF NITRITE IN CYANIDE POISONING
1. Sodium nitrite + Hemoglobin (ferrous iron) $\rightarrow$ Methemoglobin (ferric iron)
2. Methemoglobin + Cyanide $\rightarrow$ Cyanmethemoglobin

Inasmuch as cobalt compounds have a high affinity for cyanide, Co_2EDTA and hydroxocobalamin are used to treat cyanide toxicity. Hydroxocobalamin combines with cyanide to form cyanocobalamin (vitamin B_{12}).

The primary mechanism for removing cyanide from the body is enzymatic conversion by mitochondrial enzyme rhodanese (transfulfurase) to thicyanate, which is relatively nontoxic (Box 9.2). Thiosulfate is administered to provide reducing sulfur so the body can more rapidly form the thiocyanate.

Box 9.2

USE OF THIOSULFATE IN CYANIDE POISONING
1. Cyanmethemoglobin $\xrightarrow[\text{dissociation}]{\text{slow}}$ Cyanide + Methemoglobin
2. Cyanide + Thiosulfate $\xrightarrow{\text{rhodanese}}$ Thiocyanate excreted in urine

- **Phosphine** Phosphine is a fumigant used on grains. When tablets of aluminum or zinc phosphide are used in the presence of atmospheric moisture, phosphine (PH_3) is released. Severe pulmonary irritation and pulmonary edema are the main toxic effects of phosphine.

- **Dibromochloropropane and ethylene dibromide** Both of these soil fumigants are used to control nematodes. They produce pulmonary edema, and dibromochloropropane has been found to decrease sperm counts in workers engaged in their manufacture. Both agents cause gastric carcinoma in rats and mice.

Rodenticides

- **Warfarin** is one of the safest and most widely used rodenticides. Its safety is largely due to the fact that its toxicity depends on repeated exposure. An anticoagulant, warfarin is an antimetabolite of vitamin K and inhibits the synthesis of prothrombin in the liver. Death from poisoning is due to hemorrhage. Overdose is treated with vitamin K.

- **Red squill** comes from the bulbs of a plant. The bulbs contain scillarin glycosides, which are similar to the digitalis glycosides. Therefore they have cardiotoxic actions and at higher doses produce cardiac irregularities, ventricular fibrillation, and convulsions. Red squill is selective for rodents because they are unable to vomit.

- **Sodium fluoroacetate** is a potent rodenticide used only by licensed pest-control operators. Fluoroacetate is metabolized to fluorocitrate, a toxic metabolite. This is sometimes referred to as lethal synthesis. Fluorocitrate inhibits the citric acid cycle. Target organs for fluorocitrate toxicity are the heart and CNS.

- **Strychnine** produces excitation of the CNS by inhibiting glycine receptors. Glycine is an inhibitory neurotransmitter, primarily in the spinal cord. The first effect noted is stiffness of the face and neck muscles, which may be followed by convulsions. During the seizure the body is arched in hyperextension (opisthotonos) so that only the crown of the head and the heels may be touching the ground.

  The objectives of therapy are to prevent convulsions and support respiration. All sensory stimuli should be minimized. Diazepam is used to control convulsions, but anesthesia or neuromuscular blocking agents may be required to treat the severely intoxicated patients.

- **Phosphorus** produces gastrointestinal irritation and vomiting. The vomitus is luminescent and has a garlic odor. The gastrointestinal injury may cause hemorrhage, cardiovascular collapse, and death within 24 hours. If the patient survives the gastrointestinal insult, severe liver injury may ensue. Long-term poisoning from phosphorus can cause anemia, bronchitis, and necrosis of the mandible, the so-called "phossy jaw."

- **Thallium** is a hazardous rodenticide because it is not selectively toxic for rodents. In addition to gastrointestinal irritation, thallium is toxic to the brain, liver, and kidney. Neurologic symptoms, especially in the legs, and psychoses and delirium are common. Characteristic signs of thallium poisoning are reddening of the skin and alopecia. Treatment includes oral administration of Prussian blue (ferric ferrocyanide), which interrupts the enterohepatic circulation and enhances fecal excretion of thallium.

■ **Herbicides** Herbicides are used to kill noxious weeds. Their use exceeds that of the insecticides. There is an increase in concern about the health effects of herbicides because of agricultural runoff and the appearance of herbicides in drinking water.

- **Chlorophenoxy compounds** Included are 2,4-dichlorophenoxyacetic acid (2,4-D) and 2,4,5-trichlorophenoxyacetic acid (2,4,5-T) (Fig. 9.31). These agents are used to control broad leaf plants and woody plants along rights-of-way. They are rapidly excreted and have a half-life in humans of about 1 day. They are relatively safe herbicides, but high doses in laboratory animals produce signs of neuromuscular involvement, including stiffness of the extremities, ataxia, and paralysis.

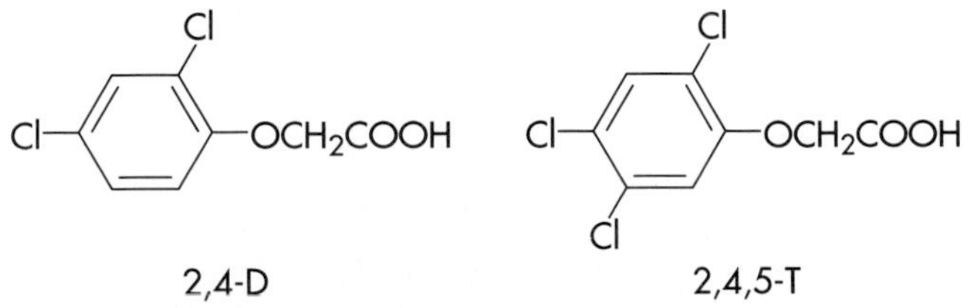

Fig. 9.31 Structure of chlorophenoxy herbicides.

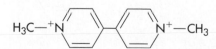

Fig. 9.32 Structure of 2,3,7,8-tetrachloro-*p*-dioxin (TCDD).

Some chlorophenoxy herbicides contain the contaminant 2,3,7,8-tetra-chloro-*p*-dioxin (TCDD) (Fig. 9.32). Whereas 2,4,5-T contains dioxin, 2,4-D does not. Extremely toxic in some species, TCDD has an LD_{50} of 0.6 μg/kg in guinea pigs, whereas its LD_{50} is 10,000 times higher in hamsters. The mechanism by which TCDD causes death is unknown. It has effects on the thymus and liver and is a potent inducer of certain cytochrome P-450s. It is also a teratogen and carcinogen in laboratory animals.

Humans appear to be much more resistant to TCDD than hamsters. An effect of TCDD in humans is chloracne, a severe form of dermatitis. During the Vietnam War, Agent Orange, a mixture of 2,4-D and 2,4,5-T (contaminated with TCDD), was used extensively. Although many adverse effects have been attributed to TCDD by some Vietnam veterans, epidemiologic data do not support their claims. With a long half-life in humans (7 years), it is possible to estimate the exposure to TCDD years later. Surprisingly, there appears to be no difference in the plasma concentration of TCDD between Vietnam veterans and the general population, suggesting that exposure during the war might not have been as extensive as thought. Several epidemiologic studies have been conducted on those exposed to high levels of TCDD by industrial exposure or from chemical explosions. These data suggest that TCDD might be carcinogenic in humans after exposure to large quantities.

● **Dinitrophenols** Dinitrophenols, such as dinitroorthocresol, uncouple oxidative phosphorylation, increasing the metabolic rate and temperature. This may result in fatal hyperthermia. Treatment consists of ice baths to reduce fever, correction of fluid and electrolyte balance, and administration of oxygen.

● **Bipyridyl compounds** Paraquat is the prototype of the class (Fig. 9.33). Several hundred people have died from accidental or intentional exposure to paraquat.

The main target organ of paraquat is the lung and is independent of the route of exposure. Paraquat undergoes a single electron reduction-oxidation with the subsequent formation of superoxide anion radical (Fig. 9.34). This radical is nonenzymatically transformed into singlet oxygen, which attacks polyunsaturated lipids in cell membranes to produce lipid hydroperoxides. The lipid hydroperoxides are unstable in the presence of iron and decompose into lipid-free radicals. This chain reaction results in pulmonary toxicity.

Treatment of paraquat toxicity involves its removal from the gastro-

$$H_3C{-}^+N \bigcirc\!\!\!-\!\!\!\bigcirc N^+{-}CH_3$$

Fig. 9.33 Structure of paraquat.

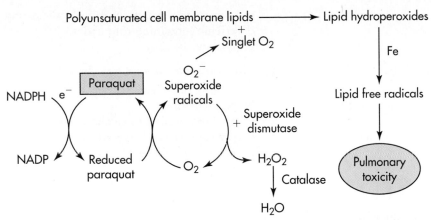

Fig. 9.34 Toxicity from redox cycling of paraquat giving rise to superoxide anion radical (O_2^-) and other reactive oxygen species, leading to lipid peroxidation.

intestinal tract before absorption. Gastric lavage, cathartics, and oral administration of Fuller's earth are used for this purpose. After absorption, hemodialysis or hemoperfusion may be helpful.

Fungicides

● **Mercurials** Mercurial fungicides have been responsible for many deaths and neurologic disabilities after consumption of treated grain. Their toxicology is discussed on p. 329.

● **Hexachlorobenzene** In the 1950s over 300 poisonings occurred in Turkey as a result of consumption of hexachlorobenzene-treated wheat. Although some deaths occurred, the major effect was cutaneous porphyria with skin lesions, porphyrinuria, and photosensitization.

● **Pentachlorophenol** Pentachlorophenol is used for a number of purposes, but particularly as a wood preservative. It uncouples oxidative phosphorylation, similar to the dinitrophenols, and therefore increases body temperature, which can be fatal. In recent years it has become apparent that pentachlorophenol is contaminated with polychlorinated dibenzodioxins and dibenzofurans. These are less toxic than TCDD but may be responsible for some of the toxic effects of pentachlorophenol.

MULTIPLE CHOICE REVIEW QUESTIONS

1. Which of the following statements about lead poisoning is most correct?

   a. Any level of lead in the body is considered to cause serious toxicity.
   b. Tolerance to lead develops with continued exposure.
   c. Most cases of lead poisoning are due to unusual susceptibility of the individuals concerned.
   d. Lead retention by the body is cumulative.
   e. Most cases of lead poisoning result from the acute accidental ingestion of lead containing drugs.

2. Carbon monoxide:

   a. accumulates in blood through an irreversible combination with hemoglobin.
   b. is taken up by the blood at a rate which is initially proportional to the CO concentration in the respired air.
   c. is detoxified by metabolism to form carbon dioxide.
   d. increases oxyhemoglobin dissociation.
   e. toxicity is due to the decreased capacity of tissue cells to absorb oxygen.

3. Chronic toxic effects are **most** likely to result when:

   a. the rate of input exceeds the excretion rate of elimination.
   b. exposure is sudden and severe and absorption is rapid.
   c. the ingested agent is inactive but metabolized to a more toxic derivative.
   d. the poison is conjugated in the liver and excreted in the bile.
   e. the route of exposure is via the skin.

4. A black line on the gums, tremors of the extremities, progressive anuria, and emotional disturbances suggest chronic poisoning by:

   a. lead.
   b. arsenic.
   c. arsine.
   d. mercury.
   e. thallium.

5. Atropine is an effective antidote for poisoning by:

   a. dichlorophenoxyacetic acid herbicides.
   b. botanical insecticides (pyrethrins).

   c. rodenticides which inhibit blood clotting.
   d. arsenic containing fungicides.
   e. none of the above.

6. Mild salicylate poisoning is characterized by:

   a. ringing of the ears.
   b. hallucinations.
   c. euphoria similar to alcoholic euphoria.
   d. slow and labored respiration.
   e. none of the above.

7. Carbon monoxide:

   a. is detoxified by biotransformation to formate.
   b. denatures hemoglobin.
   c. results from incomplete oxidation of carbon compounds.
   d. combines irreversibly with iron bearing pigments.
   e. produces methemoglobin.

8. A 32-year-old riveter who had worked for years as an automechanic was seen in the ER with severe abdominal pain, nausea, vomiting, headache, weakness, and leg cramps. He was diagnosed as having spastic constipation and given 15 ml of castor oil orally. He returned the next day with the same complaints. A blood count at this time revealed a hypochromic anemia with erythrocyte stippling. His bilirubin was increased to 1.6 mg% and his sedimentation rate was 13 mm/hr. Physical examination revealed radial nerve weakness in both forearms and moderate muscular atrophy of the left thenar muscle. The patient appeared pale and had intermittent tremors. In this case the toxic agent is most likely to be stored in the:

   a. lungs.
   b. kidney.
   c. liver.
   d. bone.
   e. gastrointestinal tract.

9. A 35-year-old man spent a week spraying his orchard with mechanical equipment. After a few days, he experienced gastrointestinal discomfort, headaches, and insomnia. One week after the last exposure, his symptoms became severe and he was brought to the ER. He has diarrhea, vomiting, jerking of the arms and legs, and is obviously ill. The patient's wife reports that the patient spilled some of the spray on his clothes and that it was very windy during the spraying period. Upon laboratory examination, the serum cholinesterase is found to be 5% of normal. The

central nervous system signs should respond best to treatment with:

a. pralidoxime (PAM).
b. methylatropine.
c. methacholine.
d. atropine.
e. physostigmine.

10. An entire family (2 adults and 2 children) developed erythema of the face, arms, and trunk about 1 hour after eating. All had tachycardia, pupillary dilatation, and dryness of the mouth. The father and mother stated that they felt disoriented. Which of the following is the most likely cause of these effects?

a. Carbon monoxide poisoning
b. Homatropine eye drops in the iced tea
c. Leaking refrigerant gas
d. Parathion contamination of their flour
e. Food poisoning (botulism)

Answers and Explanations to Multiple Choice Review Questions

CHAPTER 1: GENERAL PRINCIPLES OF PHARMACOLOGY

1. **Answer c:**

   Increasing the concentration of drug A is not able to overcome completely the effects of drug C. If both agents were merely competing for the same site, then increasing the concentration of drug A would be expected to overcome the effects of C with a resultant equal response.

   a: If drug C were a competitive inhibitor, then increasing the concentration of drug A would completely overcome the effect.

   b: As noted in the figure, drugs B and C have no agonistic effects.

   d: If drug C potentiated the effects of drug A, the dose-response curve would be shifted to the left.

   e: By definition, drug B has no agonistic effects. Therefore, one could argue that drug C would have no effect. One would have to do the experiment to be certain; this experiment is not represented in the figure.

2. **Answer a:**

   Note that the V_d = amount of drug in the body/concentration in plasma. This relationship applies and uses the 50 kg patient weight with an estimated time 0 blood concentration of 0.003 mg/ml of the drug. The range for plasma water compartments can range somewhat higher than 0.045 L/kg and the value of 0.1 L/kg is consistent with extensive protein binding that may be associated with the drug. It may also be binding to other non-plasma protein sites.

   b: The calculation result is wrong; however, if the V_d were to have been correct, the very large volume of distribution would have been consistent with strong binding to tissue.

   c: Here the calculation was based on a 70 kg patient. If 0.07 L/kg were correct, then the compartment might have been mostly plasma water.

   d: Here again the calculation was based on a 70 kg patient, but the value is quite inconsistent with the values for total body water.

   e: It is not possible to have a volume distribution less than plasma water (0.045 l/kg).

3. **Answer d:**

   Clearance = $V_d \times K_{el} = V_d \times 0.693/t_{1/2}$; note that for the units in the answer options, the volume of distribution should be expressed in milliliters and the half-life expressed in minutes. Also, the volume of distribution should be normalized for body weight. That is:

   4 L/kg × 50 kg × 1000 ml/L × 0.693 / (4 hours × 60 min/hour) = 577.5 ml/min

4. **Answer b:**

   The various formulations for estimations of creatinine clearance are inversely proportional to the steady-state serum creatine levels. For example, if the steady-state serum creatinine were to double, the creatinine clearance would be reduced by about one-half. In this case, use the following formula:

   $$G = 1 - f(1 - \tfrac{Cr'}{Cr})$$

G is the fraction by which the dose is reduced, f is the fraction of drug eliminated by the kidney; Cr′ is the creatinine clearance in the patient with renal impairment and Cr is the creatinine clearance in patients with normal renal function.

Using a creatinine rate of ⅓ normal and $f = 0.8$, the dosage would be reduced to about 45 mg.

$$G = 1 - 0.8 \times (1 - [⅓])$$

5. Answer b:

The formula is used for clearance:

$$Cl = V_d \times K_{el}$$
$$= 100 \text{ mg/kg} \times 70 \text{ kg} \times (.693/360 \text{ min})$$

Note that the answers are in the units of ml/min, requiring you to convert from L and to normalize the results for your 70 kg patient. Also, the half-life is given in hours, so you must convert to minutes.

6. Answer a:

Acetylcholine activation of the muscarinic cholinergic receptor system results in stimulation of the IP_3, diacylglycerol (DAG) cascade. There are other effects of muscarinic receptor activation including enhancement of intracellular concentrations of cGMP, changes in K^+ conductance, and inhibition of adenylyl cyclase activity.

b: The nicotinic cholinergic receptors are membrane ionic channels. Acetylcholine binding increases the membrane conductance directly by altering receptor conformation.

c: Activation of beta receptors results in an increase in cAMP concentration through enhancement of adenylate cyclase activity.

d: Diazepam effects are unrelated to the IP_3–DAG system, but rather are associated with the GABA receptor complex.

e: The insulin receptor system is not related to the IP_3–DAG system. Activation of insulin receptors results in tyrosine kinase activation and changes in cellular phosphorylation patterns.

7. Answer b:

The therapeutic response is greater than either of the other two drugs.

a: However, given the high doses required to obtained the slight increase in therapeutic response, other considerations, such as unwanted side effects, may favor selection of drug X for clinical use.

c: Y is an unlikely candidate since its therapeutic response is much smaller than the other drugs.

d: The figure shows that the drugs have different therapeutic responses.

8. Answer d:

A placebo is defined as inert or dummy medication.

a: A highly toxic drug has harmful effects at very low doses. Even more important is a drug that exerts toxic effects at doses close to its therapeutic range.

b: Penicillin induced anaphylaxis is an example of an effect mediated via immunological response.

c: A person showing an unusual reaction to a drug is said to have an idiosyncratic response.

e: Liver endoplasmic reticulum is a cellular compartment where drug transformation occurs.

9. Answer c:

The agent with the faster rate of absorption would reach a higher peak concentration and would reach that point sooner in time after administration.

a and b: Both C_{max} and T_{max} are affected by rates of absorption.

10. Answer b:

It takes 4 to 5 half-lives to reach concentration at steady-state. Since $t_{1/2} = 0.693/k_{el}$, the time to reach steady state is inversely related to the elimination rate constant of the drug.

a: Time to reach steady-state is independent of drug-dosage; however, the plateau level attained does depend on the drug dosage.

c: Time to reach steady-state does not depend on the target plasma concentration necessary for therapeutic efficacy; however, that is the level that should achieve a concentration at steady state if a proper dosage regimen is selected.

d: Time to reach steady state is independent of bioavailability but the plateau level attained with a given dosage regimen does depend on the bioavailability.

e: Only answer b is correct.

CHAPTER 2: AUTONOMIC NERVOUS SYSTEM

1. Answer c:

Atropine was administered because its anti-muscarinic effect would inhibit vagal influences at the SA node. The same anticholinergic effect could, especially at higher concentrations, induce pupillary dilation.

a: Atropine has no sympathomimetic effects; rather, it has antiparasympathetic actions.

b: Atropine would not be expected to influence ganglionic transmission, given the dominance of nicotinic receptors at the ganglion.

d: The presence of serum cholinesterases suggests that there is no reason to suspect that acetylcholine is present in any significant concentration in blood. The patient's hypotensive state is due to inadequate cardiac output secondary to severe bradycardia.

2. Answer c:

The beta-1 receptor system is activated by isoproterenol and produces the increase in heart rate and force of contraction. cAMP levels are increased by isoproterenol as is phosphorylation of troponin and phospholamban. These proteins are likely to be important in mediation of positive inotropism. Tachyarrhythmias and PVCs could occur because of increased normal automaticity in latent pacemaker fibers.

a: The beta-2 system does not predominate in the heart. Isoproterenol is active at both beta-1 and beta-2 receptors.

b: Isoproterenol would not be expected to activate alpha receptors.

d: Isoproterenol is not a cholinergic muscarinic agonist.

3. Answer c:

Reserpine depletes noradrenergic terminals of norepinephrine and dopamine. As the transmitter leaks from the vesicle, it is inactivated by intraneuronal, cytoplasmic monoamine oxidase. The hypotensive response occurs as a consequence of diminished amine levels both in the central and peripheral nervous systems.

a: Botulinum toxin diminishes release of acetylcholine by specifically interfering with the release process. Choline uptake and acetylcholine synthesis are not influenced. The symptoms listed above all results from impairment of neuromuscular transmission. This condition can progress to respiratory paralysis and death.

b: The action of nicotine results from activation of "nicotinic" cholinergic receptors in many systems and produces a variety of physiological responses. Prominent effects occur in the central and peripheral nervous systems, cardiovascular system, gastrointestinal tract, and exocrine glands. At autonomic ganglia, nicotine produces initial stimulation followed by depression of neurotransmission.

d: Prazosin acts by blocking alpha-1 receptors. This action reduces vascular smooth muscle tone and produces a hypotensive effect. Clinically, prazosin may be used in treatment of hypertension.

e: Propranolol competitively blocks beta adrenergic receptors. This action reduces heart rate and force of contraction.

4. Answer b:

Increasing the dosage of dobutamine in the presence of a beta blocker would result in the further stimulation of alpha adrenergic receptors, with an attendant increase in peripheral resistance.

a: The patient had been taking metoprolol, which is a beta-1 blocker. The positive inotropic effect of dobutamine is mediated by beta-1 adrenergic receptors in the heart. At normal therapeutic doses of dobutamine the beta-1 effects dominate and would accordingly be blocked by metoprolol.

c: The positive inotropic effects of dobutamine would be blocked by metoprolol, and increased doses of dobutamine would result in increased peripheral resistance caused by stimulation of alpha adrenergic receptors.

d: The inotropic action of dopamine would also be blocked until the beta blocking effects of metoprolol abate.

5. **Answer e:**

Hexamethonium is a ganglionic blocker. In each of the options, one must determine if the effect on the heart and systemic blood pressure is a direct influence or requires mediation through the autonomic ganglia. For the parasympathetic system, the ganglia are located close to the target site. E is correct because isoproterenol activates beta-1 and beta-2 receptor systems directly. Beta-1 activation accounts for the increase in heart rate and beta-2 receptor mediated vasodilation results in the fall in blood pressure.

a: Stimulation of the cervical vagus nerve would be at the preganglionic site, which would be blocked by hexamethonium.

b: Methoxamine is an alpha receptor agonist which would produce an increase in blood pressure by receptor activation; however, the reflex bradycardia would not occur because it depends on intact ganglionic transmission.

c: Stimulation of the cervical vagus nerve would be at the preganglionic site, which would be blocked by hexamethonium.

d: The noted effects seen subsequent to methacholine injection are autonomic reflex-mediated and therefore would not occur in the presence of a ganglionic blocker.

6. **Answer e:**

Reduced effects of adrenergic nerve activity and circulating catecholamines on the heart result in reduced rate and inotropism. Both factors reduce myocardial oxygen demand and thus may increase exercise tolerance and reduce anginal effects.

E is correct because metoprolol is a beta-1 cardioselective blocker. Enhanced adrenergic activity accompanying exertion would normally produce enhanced heart rate and force of contraction. Both of these factors significantly increase myocardial oxygen demand. By blocking the beta-1 receptor with metoprolol, these effects are attenuated.

a: Scopolamine is a muscarinic blocker. Since the heart is under parasympathetic dominance, blocking the muscarinic receptors will actually increase heart rate and myocardial work. This action is more likely to produce angina than block it.

b: Phentolamine is an alpha blocker and would reduce blood pressure; however, phentolamine causes significant reflex cardioacceleration thus increasing myocardial work. Phentolamine is known to produce myocardial ischemia.

c: Isoproterenol is a beta receptor agonist that increases cardiac work and would tend to precipitate angina.

d: Phenoxybenzamine is an alpha blocker and would reduce blood pressure; however, phenoxybenzamine causes significant reflex cardioacceleration, thus increasing myocardial work.

7. **Answer e:**

Methoxamine is a direct acting alpha receptor activator. The increase in blood pressure caused by constriction of vascular smooth muscle is countered by an autonomic nervous system-mediated decrease in heart rate.

a–d: None of these drugs produce the increase in blood pressure required to stimulate the reflex-producing bradycardia.

8. **Answer d:**

Cocaine causes a competitive block of Uptake I.

a: Tryamine is an indirect-acting sympathomimetic amine that enters the nerve terminal and displaces norepinephrine from synaptic vesicles. Tyramine enters the nerve terminal using the uptake system that can be blocked by cocaine.

Therefore, cocaine would block the pharmacologic actions of tyramine.

b: Clonidine is a centrally active alpha-2 adrenergic agonist. Clonidine reduces central sympathetic outflow and may also increase parasympathetic outflow. These effects result in lowering of blood pressure.

c: Isoproterenol is a nonselective beta agonist.

e: Oxymetazoline, which is often used as a topical decongestant in over-the-counter nasal sprays, is a direct-acting alpha receptor agonist.

9. **Answer d:**

Cocaine blocks the reuptake of epinephrine and thereby markedly potentiates the blood pressure response to epinephrine.

a: Doxazosin is a selective α_1 blocker and thereby would block the response to epinephrine.

b: Propranolol is a beta blocker that would block the cardiac effects as well as the vasodilator actions of epinephrine but probably would not markedly potentiate the pressor effects of epinephrine.

c: Phenoxybenzamine is an irreversible alpha-1 and alpha-2 blocker and would block the pressor effects of norepinephrine.

e: Acetylcholine would cause the release of EDRF and thereby causes a marked vasodilation.

10. **Answer a:**

Doxazosin is a selective alpha-1 blocker and thereby blocks the pressor response to epinephrine. The depressor response seen after alpha-1 blockade is classically referred to as epinephrine reversal (i.e., a depressor response is observed in contrast to the pressor response observed when epinephrine is given to a control subject).

b: Atropine is an antimuscarinic agent and would not block the pressor response to epinephrine.

c: Propranolol is a beta blocker and therefore would block the depressor responses but not the pressor response to epinephrine.

d: Acetylcholine would cause a depressor response itself but would not block the pressor response to epinephrine.

e: Phenylephrine is an alpha-1 agonist and would cause a marked pressor response.

11. **Answer c:**

Remember that the infusion of cocaine and doxazosin are still occurring, thus when propanolol is added, both the alpha and beta effects of epinephrine are blocked, so minimal pressor change is observed.

a: Acetylcholine would not block the depressor response to epinephrine.

b: Atropine would not block the depressor response to epinephrine.

d: Tyramine releases norepinephrine, but this effect would be blocked by cocaine since tyramine requires uptake I to get into the nerve terminal. Moreover, tyramine will not block the depressor response of epinephrine.

e: Trimethaphan blocks the ganglia and thereby would block all reflex responses but not the depressor response of epinephrine.

CHAPTER 3: ENDOCRINE PHARMACOLOGY

1. **Answer e:**

In the elderly, there may be poor nutrition. In this patient, her not eating well may be secondary to a depressive condition triggered by the loss of her husband. Perhaps her depression inhibits her interest in leaving her home, thus reducing her exposure to sunlight. Her symptoms of muscle spasms are consistent, as are the laboratory findings, with chronic hypocalcemia. Phenytoin is known to reduce calcium absorption. It also increases the activity of the microsomal liver metabolizing system which results in increasing the rate of clearance of vitamin D and its metabolites.

2. **Answer b:**

Growth stimulation is NOT directly mediated by GH. Anabolic effects of growth hormone are due to production of somatomedins.

a: True: Excessive production of growth hormone in children before epiphyseal closure results in gigantism. Therapeutic use of growth hormone after epiphyseal closure is contraindicated.

c: True: Growth hormone may produce an antiinsulin effect.

d: True: Growth hormone does stimulate the incorporation of amino acids into protein.

e: True: Growth hormone is secreted by pituitary somatotrophs.

3. **Answer e:**

L-DOPA and clonidine increase serum levels of growth hormone.

a: Both L-DOPA and clonidine increase serum levels of growth hormone. Dopamine stimulates the release of growth hormone releasing hormone (GHRH) by the hypothalamus, which results in an increase in GH released by the pituitary. L-DOPA, a dopamine precursor that crosses the blood brain barrier, results in an increase in dopamine levels. Clonidine, an alpha-adrenergic agonist, stimulates release of GHRH thus causing, indirectly, an increase in growth hormone levels.

b: Cyproheptadine is a serotonin antagonist and blocks serotonin-mediated rise in GHRH.

c: L-Dopa and clonidine increase serum levels of growth hormone.

d: Phentolamine, an alpha blocker, antagonizes alpha-agonist-mediated increases in GHRH.

4. **Answer e:**

Hypertension may occur secondary to increased fluid retention. Hyperglycemia occurs because of enhancement of gluconeogenesis and impairment of peripheral glucose utilization. Moon facies and truncal obesity are due to alterations in normal fat distribution.

a–d: Hypertension, hyperglycemia, moon facies, and truncal obesity are all effects of long term corticosteroid treatment.

5. **Answer b:**

The islets of Langerhans are innervated by both cholinergic and adrenergic nerves. Secretion of insulin from the beta-cell is regulated by blood glucose levels, together with other nutrients (e.g., amino acids), GI hormones, pancreatic hormones, and autonomic neurotransmitters, which act to stimulate, amplify, or inhibit insulin release. Glucose is the primary stimulus for insulin release, which occurs as a result of increased Ca^{2+} in the beta-cell. Eating stimulates vagal activity and also releases GU hormones; both increase beta-cell Ca^{+2} and promote insulin release. Alpha-2 receptor activation inhibits the release of insulin. Alpha-2 blockers will increase insulin release. In contrast, beta-2 receptor activation promotes release, and beta-2 adrenergic blockers reduce insulin release.

a: Phentolamine is an alpha-2 receptor blocker and may increase plasma insulin.

c: Vagal nerve stimulation affects the muscarinic receptors and results in an increase of intracellular free Ca^{+2}, causing insulin release.

d: The GI hormones, which are elaborated upon food ingestion, increase pancreatic beta-cell Ca^{+2} and result in enhanced insulin secretion.

e: Propranolol, a beta-adrenergic antagonist, may decrease insulin release. Activation of the autonomic nervous system overall results in insulin release suppression, mediated by alpha-2 receptor mechanisms.

6. **Answer b:**

Oliguria is not a presenting symptom of diabetes mellitus. As a result of hyperglycemia, polydipsia, polyuria, and polyphagia are the most common symptoms that result in a patient seeking medical attention.

a: Polydipsia is a common symptom of diabetes mellitus.

c: Polyphagia, resulting from hyperglycemia, is also a common symptom of diabetes mellitus.

d: A diabetic coma is also a possible presenting symptom.

e: Although rare, peripheral neuropathy is also a presenting symptom in diabetes mellitus.

7. **Answer d:**

Mannitol is classified as an osmotic diuretic. Mannitol is filtered but not reabsorbed. This effect results in diuresis. Similarly, delivery of glucose to the tubule in concentrations that exceed the reabsorption capacity of the nephron also results in an osmotic diuresis.

a, b, c, and e: These drugs affect sodium reabsorption or prevent the recovery of filtered bicarbonate.

8. **Answer e:**

A diabetic may experience hypoglycemia from an overdose of insulin, unaccustomed exercise, failure to eat breakfast, or over-indulgence in alcohol.

9. **Answer c:**

The total clearance is about 700-800 mL/min. Hepatic clearance accounts for 300-400 mL/min. Renal clearance accounts for 190-270 mL/min.

a: Hepatic clearance accounts for the majority but not all of insulin clearance.
b: Renal clearance accounts for some clearance of insulin.
d: Insulin is cleared through hepatic and renal systems.

10. **Answer c:**

Glipizide is a second generation sulfonylurea, oral hypoglycemic drug. The second generation sulfonylureas, glipizide and glyburide, are significantly more potent than the first generation agents, but they are not as effective as hypoglycemic agents.

a, b, d, and e: All of these drugs are first generation sulfonylureas.

11. **Answer b:**

Glyburide, a second generation compound, is more potent than tolbutamide.

a: Efficacy measures clinical effectiveness. Since glyburide and tolbutamide achieve the same therapeutic effect, their efficacy is the same.

c: Because glyburide achieves the same effect as tolbutamide, but at a lower dosage, it is more potent than tolbutamide.
d: Glyburide and tolbutamide produce the same therapeutic affect and therefore are equally efficacious.
e: The second generation compound, glyburide, is more potent but not more clinically affective.

12. **Answer e:**

Iodide inhibits the release of thyroid hormone from the overactive thyroid gland. Its effects are very rapid, more rapid than the action of the thiocarbamides agents such as methimazole and propylthiouracil that inhibit thyroid hormone synthesis. Their mechanism is through inhibition of iodination of tyrosyl residues in thyroglobulin and coupling of monoiodotyrosine (MIT) and diiodotyrosine. Hydrocortisone is used in severe thyroitoxicosis (thyroid storm).

CHAPTER 4: AUTOCOID, RENAL, RESPIRATORY, AND GI PHARMACOLOGY

1. **Answer c:**

All of the other agents can produce significant potassium loss. Spironolactone is a competitive inhibitor of aldosterone. Therefore, in the presence of mineralocorticoids, spironolactone will produce a decrease in potassium elimination.

a, b: For the loop diuretics (bumetanide and furosemide) increased potassium loss results from increased delivery of sodium and water to the distal segments of the nephron. Increased sodium delivery stimulates potassium excretion.
d: The thiazides (hydrochlorothiazide) increased potassium loss also results from increased delivery of sodium and water to the distal segments of the nephron. Increased sodium delivery stimulates potassium excretion.
e: For acetazolamide, increased luminal concentration of bicarbonate, as a result of carbonic anhydrase inhibition, results in increased sodium and potassium loss.

2. **Answer d:**

Furosemide is more effective than hydro-chlorothiazide. The "high-ceiling" or loop diuretics include bumetanide, furosemide, and ethacrynic acid. These agents produce the most significant diuretic effect. The mechanism of action is inhibition of sodium reabsorption at the ascending limb of the loop of Henle. This inhibition reduces the hypertonicity of the medullary interstitium and, as a result, reduces the amount of water extracted from the thin descending limb of the loop. Thiazides produce a lesser diuretic effect compared to the loop agents and act mainly in the early distal tubule to inhibit NaCl reabsorption.

a: Bumetanide is more efficacious than acetazolamide. Acetazolamide is less efficacious than hydrochlorothiazide.

b: Hydrochlorothiazide is less efficacious than furosemide. Furosemide is less effective than acetazolamide.

c: Acetazolamide is a carbonic anhydrase inhibitor and represents the least efficacious agent. This diuresis is accompanied by substantial loss of bicarbonate and a hyperchloremic metabolic acidosis.

3. **Answer d:**

Furosemide and bumetanide depend upon the organic acid transport system of the renal proximal tubule to gain access to their site of action in the ascending loop of Henle. Probenecid is an example of a drug that blocks this transport system. Significantly increased doses of furosemide would be required to overcome the probenecid effect. Furosemide is a powerful loop diuretic that would otherwise be expected to rapidly reduce excess fluid loads in this patient.

a: Furosemide is effective in the peripheral edematous states associated with acute pulmonary edema.

b: The amount of sodium in the diet does not affect furosemide.

c: Both furosemide and probenecid are highly protein bound. The clinical situation would not be explained to protein binding effects.

e: Options a, b, and c are false.

4. **Answer b:**

After tolerance to the asthma-inducing effects of aspirin has been increased because of desensitization, other cross-reactive drugs are no longer as likely to induce acute asthma episodes. This effect is an example of cross-tolerance. Another example of cross-tolerance is seen among sedative-hypnotic drugs. An increased tolerance to a particular agent (e.g., diazepam) is also seen for other sedative-hypnotics, such as phenobarbital or alcohol.

a: Placebo effects are used in controlled studies to determine the efficacy of medicinal studies. They describe drugs without intrinsic therapeutic value.

c: Systemic bioavailability refers to the degree to which a drug or other substance becomes available to the target tissue after administration.

d: Potency is defined as the power of a drug to produce the desired effects.

e: Efficacy is the capacity of a drug to elicit a response.

5. **Answer c:**

Bronchiolar constriction in a region of the lung results in an alveolar hypoxic state and a compensatory regional vascular constriction. Under this condition, however, some blood flows through this region and is poorly saturated with oxygen. Terbutaline activates beta-2 receptors and the ensuing bronchiolar relaxation, and improved ventilation results in a more normal ventilation-perfusion ratio.

a: Terbutaline will not affect pulmonary artery perfusion pressure in the lung. Also, increased blood flow to the lung may worsen the ventilation/perfusion (V/Q) ratio since more blood may pass through poorly ventilated lung regions.

b: The effect of terbutaline is not due to pulmonary vasodilation.

d: Supplemental oxygen may be helpful, but pharmacologic correction of the bronchiolar constriction is most important.

e: The effects of terbutaline result from bronchiolar relaxation.

6. **Answer b:**

Cromolyn is an effective prophylactic by preventing release of bronchoconstricting mediators.

a: Beclomethasone is a corticosteroid. Corticosteroids inhibit several aspects of the inflammatory response, including arachidonic acid metabolism, neutrophil and eosinophil migration, and kinin, neuropeptide, and histamine release.
c: Metaproterenol is a beta-2 selective agonist that produces bronchodilation.
d: Albuterol is also a selective beta-2 agonist and will produce bronchodilation.
e: Theophylline is classified as a phosphodiesterase inhibitor but produces a dose-related bronchodilation probably by another mechanism.

7. **Answer e:**

All treatment options are paired with their correct drug.

a: Pirenzepine is an anticholinergic agent which appears effective in healing duodenal ulcers.
b: Aluminum hydroxide is useful in treating individuals prone to develop PO_4 kidney stones.
c: Bismuth provides both cytoprotective and antibacterial properties.
d: Amoxicillin has activity against *Heliobacter pylorii,* which has been implicated in peptic ulcer disease.

8. **Answer d:**

After activation at pH values less than 5, omeprazole's active derivatives, a sulphenic acid and a sulphenamide, are concentrated in parietal cells where they inhibit secretion of protons by irreversibly blocking the hydrogen/potassium pump. Decreasing gastric acidity leads to a twofold to fourfold hypergastrinemia in some individuals and a small percentage of patients (7%) may exhibit exocrine cell hyperplasia.

a: Magnesium hydroxide is an antacid

and would not produce hyperplasia of enterochromaffin-like cells.
b: Ranitide is an H_2 receptor antagonist and would not produce hyperplasia of enterochromaffin-like cells.
c: Cimetadine is an H_2 receptor antagonist and would not produce hyperplasia of enterochromaffin-like cells.
e: Sucralfate is a mucosal protective agent and would not produce hyperplasia of enterochromaffin-like cells.

9. **Answer d:**

Most gastrinomas are pancreatic islet cell tumors, which contain gastrin. In Zollingen-Ellison syndrome, large amounts of gastrin are found in the circulation. The trophic effects of gastrin on parietal cells result in large increases (from three to six times) in cell mass. The increase in parietal cell mass results in hypersecretion of gastric acid. In studies that compare H_2 antagonists, H_2 blockers (cimetidine, ranitidine, and famotidine) are effective in decreasing gastric acid output and promoting ulcer healing. The antacids are much less effective and rarely promote healing. The most effective agent for reducing gastric acid secretion is omeprazole which is unsurpassed in reducing secretion with prolonged effectiveness.

a: Sucralfate does not inhibit the secretion of protons, and it does not have acid-buffering capacity.
b: Although famotidine, an H_2-receptor antagonist, inhibits gastrin-stimulated acid secretion, it is not nearly as effective as omeprazole.
c: Misoprostol is a prostaglandin E_1 analog that induces mucus production and bicarbonate secretion in the stomach, reducing the acid content; it does not interfere with gastrin secretion.
e: 5-Aminosalicylate is used in the treatment of chronic inflammatory bowel disease and is ineffective in the treatment of Zollingen-Ellison syndrome.

10. **Answer a:**

Diphenhydramine and other H_1 antihistamines may be markedly sedating, such as the phenothiazine derivative, promethazine.

b: Loratidine is a nonsedating H_1 blocker.

c: Terfenadine is a nonsedating H_1 blocker.

d: Astemizole is a nonsedating H_1 blocker.

e: Chlorpheniramine, found in over-the-counter cold medications, is slightly sedating, whereas pyrilamine is sufficiently sedating to be marketed as the active agent in over-the-counter sleep aids.

CHAPTER 5: CARDIOVASCULAR DRUGS

1. Answer c:

All of the arteriolar vasodilators (minoxidil, hydralazine, and diazoxide) produce significant water and salt retention secondary to decreased renal perfusion pressure and alpha adrenergic receptor activation. These effects can cause the significant edema seen in this patient. The reflex tachycardia resulting from the powerful hypotensive effects of minoxidil is sufficient to explain angina in a patient with coronary vascular disease.

a: Minoxidil does not directly affect cardiac alpha receptors.

b: Minoxidil does have direct affects on the kidney.

d: Minoxidil does not directly affect cardiac beta-1 receptors.

e: Minoxidil is not a beta blocker.

2. Answer b:

With minoxidil as well as other vasodilators, such as hydralazine, there is a very significant sodium and fluid retention. The thiazide diuretics do not produce a sufficiently profound diuresis. Loop diuretics, like furosemide, produce an adequate diuresis to handle fluid retention produced by vasodilators. Minoxidil, like hydralazine, also produces significant reflex tachycardia. This effect is mostly blocked by the nonspecific beta receptor antagonist propranolol. The tachycardia may not be completely blocked because of the contribution of reduced parasympathetic tone. Since blocking the cardiac beta receptors is of prime concern, the use of alpha blockers (phenoxybenzamine, prazosin, or tetra-

zosin) would not be indicated. Atropine would increase heart rate, which is opposite of the desired effect.

a: Chlorothiazide may not provide sufficient diuresis, and phenoxybenzamine, an alpha blocker, would not prevent possible reflex tachycardia after minoxidil administration.

c: Acetazolamide, a carbonic anhydrase inhibitor, would not provide sufficient diuresis, and prazosin, an alpha blocker, would not prevent possible reflex tachycardia after minoxidil administration.

d: Mannitol, an osmotic diuretic, has no role in treating hypertension. Atropine, an antimuscarinic, increases heart rate, which is not desirable in this patient.

e: The absence of a diuretic in this combination would render this choice inappropriate. Verapamil is a calcium channel blocker. Tetrazosin is an alpha receptor blocker.

3. Answer e:

Hexamethonium and trimethaphan are ganglionic neurotransmission blockers. The tachycardia associated with vasodilator use is reflex mediated. Therefore if ganglionic transmission is blocked, the reflex effects are blunted. Propranolol and metoprolol are beta adrenergic receptor blockers. Cardioacceleration is mediated mainly by beta-1 receptors. These agents block this effect. Since the reflex response to vasodilators results in a decrease in cholinergic tone in addition to an increase in sympathetic tone, some increase in heart rate may still be observed because of the cholinergic component.

4. Answer d:

Diltiazem, a calcium channel blocker, would be both an effective antihypertensive and antianginal agent. Diminished calcium entry in vascular smooth muscle cells will promote vasorelaxation and after-load reduction.

a: Although propranolol, a nonselective beta blocker, would lower this patient's blood pressure and assist in controlling his angina, it could precipitate an asthma attack. Propranolol diminishes bronchiolar smooth muscle relaxation and increases airway resistance.

b: Minoxidil or hydralazide would cause reflex bradycardia, which would predispose to worsening angina in this patient.

c: Propranolol is contraindicated in patients with asthma. It increases airway resistance.

e: Propranolol is contraindicated in patients with asthma. Diltiazem is more appropriate.

5. **Answer c:**

Nitroglycerin forms the reactive free radical nitric oxide. Nitric oxide activates guanylate cyclase and ultimately results in stimulation of cGMP-dependent protein kinase. Reduction in the extent of phosphorylation of the light chain of myosin causes a decrease in smooth muscle tone promoting relaxation. This effect is rather general and would include effects on bronchiolar, biliary, and esophageal smooth muscle. As a result, nitroglycerin could terminate esophageal spasm.

a: Because nitrates tend to relax almost all smooth muscle, it cannot be proven that the pain is due to myocardial oxygen insufficiency.

b: Because nitrates tend to relax nearly all smooth muscle, it cannot be concluded that the pain is due to esophageal spasm.

d: Because nitrates tend to relax almost all smooth muscle, it cannot be concluded that pain is due to myocardial oxygen insufficiency.

e: The test by itself is inconclusive.

6. **Answer b:**

This patient perhaps could be treated with a calcium channel blocker with less vasodilatory properties, such as diltiazem.

a: The calcium channel blocker nifedipine is appropriate.

c: Propranolol in combination with nifedipine would be appropriate except that this patient has significant COAD. The use of a beta blocker therefore would be contraindicated because the beta adrenergic system mediates bronchodilation

and this desired effect would be blocked.

d: Only one option is appropriate.

e: Nifedipine alone is appropriate.

7. **Answer e:**

All of the above are correct.

a: Prazosin, an alpha adrenergic receptor antagonist, produces both an arteriolar and venular vasodilation. As a consequence, both preload and afterload are reduced.

b: Captopril is an ACE inhibitor that also dilates both arteries and veins to reduce afterload and preload, respectively.

c: Hydralazine is an effective arterial dilator and significantly reduces afterload.

d: Sodium nitroprusside dilates both arteries and veins, producing a reduction in both preload and afterload.

8. **Answer c:**

Amrinone and milrinone belong to this category. They are both positive inotropic agents, although amrinone also has arterial and venous vasodilatory properties. As a result, in congestive heart failure it acts to reduce preload and afterload in addition to improving cardiac output through its positive inotropic effect.

a: Digoxin is a cardiac glycoside that increases myocardial contractility by inhibiting Na-K-ATPase.

b: Dobutamine is a beta agonist, which at low doses increases renal blood flow and causes a decrease in afterload.

d: Isoproterenol is a beta agonist and hydralazine is an arterial vasodilatory without positive inotropic properties.

e: Hydralazine is a direct acting vasodilator.

9. **Answer e:**

Lidocaine is exclusively used to treat ventricular arrhythmias, effectively suppressing premature ventricular contractions and ventricular tachyarrhythmias.

a: Procainamide is used to treat supraventricular tachycardia.

b: Nitroglycerine is used to treat angina pectoris.

c: Digoxin is used to treat congestive heart failure.

d: Quinidine is frequently used to treat atrial flutter.

10. **Answer c:**

Niacin has several side effects. Facial flushing occurs as a result of prostaglandin release and may be reduced by aspirin. Hepatotoxicity may also occur in a dose-related manner.

a: Cholestyramine may cause constipation and bloating.

b: Side effects of colestipol include constipation and bloating.

d: Probucol may cause diarrhea and nausea.

e: The side effects of clofibrate include gastrointestinal and hepatobiliary neoplasia.

CHAPTER 6: CENTRAL NERVOUS SYSTEM DRUGS

1. **Answer b:**

Buspirone is an anxiolytic that does not exhibit cross-tolerance with benzodiazepines. Compared with benzodiazepines, it is relatively nonsedating and has limited abuse potential.

a: Triazolam is a benzodiazepine that interacts with the GABA receptor system.

c: Diazepam is a benzodiazepine that interacts with the GABA receptor system.

d: Paraldehyde is a sedative-hypnotic agent, but it does not act through 5-HT systems.

e: Pentobarbital belongs to the barbiturate class of sedative-hypnotics but does not act through 5-HT systems. They may affect sodium and potassium transport and may also influence GABA effects on chloride conductance.

2. **Answer b:**

Diphenhydramine is an antihistamine used in over-the-counter sleep aids because it has significant sedative properties. Triazolam is a benzodiazepine used as a hypnotic. Trazodone is an antidepressant. Buspirone is an antianxiety agent with minimal sed-

ative properties. Chlorpromazine is used to treat schizophrenia and is sedating.

a: Triazolam is a benzodiazepine that is used as a hypnotic.

c: Trazodone is an antidepressant.

d: Chlorpromazine is used to treat schizophrenia and is sedating.

e: Buspirone is an antianxiety agent with minimal sedative properties.

3. **Answer c:**

Tranylcypromine and phenelzine are examples of MAO inhibitors that can be used in treatment of depression refractory to SSRIs, such as fluoxetine, or to first generation tricyclics. Inhibition of monoamine oxidase prevents degradation of pressor amines that may be present in certain foods. These active amines can induce hypertensive reactions and, as a result, certain foods should be avoided. Red wines, aged cheeses, and certain meats including herring, sausage, salami, and corned beef are high in tyramine content.

a: In normal use tranylcypromine should not cause hypertension.

b: Tranylcypromine is not a beta blocker.

d: Tranylcypromine is not a first-generation tricyclic antidepressant.

e: Tranylcypromine, a MAO inhibitor, could have caused the problem.

4. **Answer c:**

Buspirone does not produce side effects associated with CNS depression.

a: Buspirone is not a benzodiazepine; it is a $5HT_{1a}$ antagonist.

b: The onset of therapeutic effectiveness with buspirone may be delayed for up to four weeks.

d: Buspirone is classified as an anxiolytic.

e: Buspirone does not exhibit cross-tolerance with drugs classified as sedative-hypnotics.

5. **Answer b:**

Haloperidol is an antipsychotic agent and, as most antipsychotics, has neurologic side effects. In addition, side effect profiles include anticholinergic (e.g., dry mouth, urinary hesitancy) and anti-adrenergic (e.g., orthostatic hypotension) effects.

a: Chloral hydrate is a sedative-hypnotic devoid of significant antiadrenergic, anticholinergic, or extrapyramidal effects.

c: Meprobamate is a sedative-hypnotic devoid of significant antiadrenergic, anticholinergic, or extrapyramidal effects.

d: Tranylcypromine is a monoamine oxidase inhibitor that may be used clinically to treat endogenous and atypical depression. It does not have prominent extrapyramidal side effects.

e: Lithium is used in treating bipolar affective disorder and does not have a side effect profile similar to antipsychotic agents.

6. **Answer b:**

Agranulocytosis is a side effect of clozapine. Rapid decline of WBC is possible, although slower decline is more common. The risk of agranulocytosis is sufficient to warrant the use of clozapine only if other antipsychotics are not working or if the patient suffers from severe extrapyramidal reactions, especially tardive dyskinesia, from other antipsychotic drugs.

a: Loxapine is a high-potency, antipsychotic drug with significant extrapyramidal effects.

c: Hydralazine is a vasodilator.

d: Chlorpromazine is a phenothiazine antipsychotic drug.

e: Doxepin is an antidepressant.

7. **Answer b:**

L-DOPA is the mainstay therapeutic agent for management of moderate to severe Parkinson's disease. It is used often in combination with carbidopa, a decarboxylase inhibitor.

a: Amantadine, an antiviral, improves symptoms of Parkinson's disease, possibly by promoting dopamine release or inhibiting reuptake. It also has some anticholinergic properties, but it is not the primary medicine.

c: Selegiline is effective in treating symptoms of Parkinson's disease probably because it inhibits a major degradative pathway for dopamine, monoamine oxidase B (MAO-B). However, it is not the primary medicine.

d: Pergolide directly stimulates D1 and D2 dopamine receptors and therefore ameliorates Parkinsonian symptoms. However, it is not the primary medicine.

e: Bromocriptine stimulates D2 postsynaptic dopamine receptors, improving symptoms of Parkinson's disease. However, it is not the primary medicine.

8. **Answer c:**

Ethosuximide and valproate are top choices for treating absence seizures.

a: Primidone is effective in most seizure classes except absence.

b: Phenytoin is used to treat generalized tonic-clonic, simple partial, and complex partial seizures.

d: Thiopental would be acceptable treatment for rapid termination of generalized tonic-clonic, repetitive seizures seen in status epilepticus.

e: IV diazepam is effective treatment for status epilepticus.

9. **Answer c:**

This patient is resistant to the effects of the commonly used agents. This circumstance meets a criteria for use of clozapine. Clozapine is a very effective drug; however, it causes a life-threatening agranulocytosis in some patients. As a result, very carefully monitoring for blood disorders is a requirement when clozapine is prescribed.

a: Trifluoperazine is a phenothiazine antipsychotic agent.

b: Amoxapine is an antidepressant drug.

d: Benztropine is an anticholinergic that is sometimes given to treat extrapyramidal symptoms associated with antipsychotic therapy.

e: Molindone is a nonphenothiazine antipsychotic with very low sedative properties.

10. **Answer d:**

Most deaths from morphine toxicity are due to respiratory depression. Even small doses produce some respiratory depression. There is a decreased sensitivity to CO_2 by the brain stem respiratory centers.

a: The narcotic agonists are not considered arrhythmogenic.

b: Depression would not be commonly associated with narcotic analgesics.

c: The motility of the GI tract is depressed with narcotic agonists.

e: Convulsions may occur with high doses of certain narcotic agonists, although in children convulsions may occur at doses only slightly higher than therapeutic levels. Convulsions, although serious, are an uncommon side effect. Naloxone is effective in blocking these convulsions.

11. **Answer c:**

Naloxone is a pure antagonist that reverses effects of narcotic agonist overdosage. Another relatively pure antagonist is naltrexone. Naloxone is often used to reverse respiratory depression accompanying narcotic overdosage.

a: Fentanyl is a potent narcotic agonist.

b: Pentazocine is a narcotic partial agonist.

d: Droperidol is a neuroleptic, butyrophenone derivative.

e: Oxycodone is a narcotic agonist.

CHAPTER 7: CHEMOTHERAPY DRUGS

1. **Answer e:**

Sulfisoxazole is an example of a sulfonamide, a folate inhibitor. Sulfonamides, nitrofurantoin, furazoline, chloramphenicol, pyrimethamine and sulfones can produce hemolysis in patients with glucose-6-phosphate dehydrogenase deficiency. This is an example of a genetically-determined idiosyncratic drug response.

a: Penicillins do not produce this syndrome.

b: Neomycin, an aminoglycoside, does not produce this syndrome.

c: Augmentin, a combination of amoxacillin with a beta-lactamase inhibitor, does not produce this syndrome.

d: Cefotaxime, a third generation cephalosporin beta-lactam antibiotic, does not produce this syndrome.

2. **Answer c:**

In the abscess described, the penicillin would be ineffective against the beta-lactamase producing strains of Bacteroides; however, it would be effective against anaerobic streptococci. By contrast, metronidazole would be effective against Bacteroides but would not work against the streptococci. The drugs therefore have additive effects.

a: With drug synergism the activity of the two drugs together is greater than would be expected given the activity of each alone. An example would be the combination of a beta-lactamase inhibitor, such as sulbactam and ampicillin which is beta-lactamase sensitive.

b: An antagonistic effect would occur if drugs used in combination produce a lesser effect than would be expected if the drugs were used separately.

d: This is an example of additive drug effects.

3. **Answer b:**

Erythromycin is a macrolide antibiotic that binds to bacterial 50 S ribosomes preventing peptidyl transfer. Resistance occurs as a result of methylation of two adenine nucleotides in the 23 S component of 50 S RNA.

a: Aztreonam is a beta-lactam that is neither a penicillin nor a cephalosporin and has excellent activity against many strains of gram-negative bacilli. It is an inhibitor of cell wall synthesis.

c: Vancomycin, a glycopeptide, inhibits cell wall synthesis and is active against grampositive organisms.

d: Ceftazidime is a third generation cephalosporin and, like penicillins, is a bacteriocidal, cell wall synthesis inhibitor.

e: Primaxin is a combination of imipenem and cilastatin. Imipenem, a carbapenem, is a beta-lactam antibiotic, which must be combined with cilastatin to prevent destruction of imipenem by renal dehydropeptidases.

4. **Answer e:**

Rifampin is not combined with isoniazid for treatment of otitis media.

a: Rifampin is a macrocyclic antibiotic that inhibits DNA-directed RNA polymerase. Resistance to rifampin results from a mutation on the beta subunit of the polymerase. The altered polymerase does not bind rifampin in a similar matter.

b: Rifampin in combination with isoniazid is used in the treatment of tuberculosis.

c: In addition to staining contact lenses, rifampin produces a red coloring of the urine.

d: Rifampin has few adverse effects. Occasional flu-like symptoms have been noted and rarely, interstitial nephritis, hemolytic anemia, and thrombocytopenia.

5. **Answer e:**

Trimethoprim is easily absorbed from the GI tract.

a: Trimethoprim inhibits bacterial dihydrofolate reductase. Resistance can occur as a result of production of altered enzyme with reduced affinity for trimethoprim.

b: Trimethoprim is active against most gram-positive cocci.

c: Trimethoprim can be combined with sulfamethoxazole and the combination can be used to treat urinary tract infections, otitis media, and GI infections due to *Salmonella.* It is also active against *Shigella* and toxigenic *E. coli.*

d: High dose trimethoprim-sulfamethoxazole is used to treat *Pneumocystis carinii* infection.

6. **Answer b:**

Use of IV chloramphenicol instead of ampicillin addresses the possibility of *H. influenzae* resistance to ampicillin. Third generation cephalosporins may be preferable to this combination due to the potential toxicity of chloramphenicol.

a: There is reason to suspect that ampicillin alone is not effective, possibly because of *H. influenzae* resistance to the agent. The condition of the child constitutes a therapeutic emergency requiring action that takes into account possible ampicillin resistance.

c: Gentamicin is an aminoglycoside that might be used in treating meningitis caused by gram-negative agents. If it is used, it must be injected intrathecally and would probably not be used unless resistance to third generation cephalosporins had been demonstrated.

d: Streptomycin is an aminoglycoside that is not indicated for use in meningitis. It is effective in treating bacterial endocarditis, tularemia, and plague.

e: Streptomycin is not indicated for use in meningitis.

7. **Answer d:**

Ganciclovir is similar to acyclovir, but it has much better activity against cytomegalovirus (CMV). It is effective in the treatment of CMV retinitis. It can produce significant bone marrow depression, especially neutropenia.

a: Acyclovir is a selective inhibitor of some herpes viruses, including herpes simplex 1 (HSV-1), herpes simplex 2 (HSV-2), varicella-zoster virus (VZV) and Epstein-Barr virus (EBV). Acyclovir acts after its conversion to acyclovir monophosphate and ultimately to a triphosphate form, which inhibits viral-induced DNA polymerases.

b: Amantadine and rimantidine inhibit influenza A viral replication. These agents are effective in the prevention of influenza A in young adults with a decreased effectiveness in the elderly and children.

c: Vidarabine has activity against HSV-1, HSV-2, VZV, and EBV. Vidarabine inhibits viral DNA synthesis.

e: Zidovudine competitively inhibits HIV reverse transcriptase possibly through DNA chain termination.

8. **Answer c:**

The combination of trimethoprim/ sulfamethoxazole (TMP/SMX) given IV is now the treatment of choice for

Pneumocystis carinii pneumonia (PCP). Other agents such as trimethoprim plus dapsone or pentamidine are also effective. TMP/SMX is as effective as pentamidine, the first effective drug for PCP but has a more favorable side effect profile.

a: Penicillin G is not effective in treating the organisms responsible for this patient's infection. Penicillin is most effective against gram positive bacteria.

b: Cefotaxime is not effective in treating the organisms responsible for this patient's infection. It is useful against gram positive and gram negative bacteria.

d: Pentamidine is effective in treating PCP; however, it has a more serious side effect profile when compared with the combination of TMP/SMX. Producing insulin-dependent diabetes is an especially serious side effect of pentamidine.

e: Foscarnet, although effective for CMV retinitis, is not indicated in the treatment of PCP.

9. **Answer c:**

Pyrimethamine with sulfadiazine is an effective, synergistic treatment protocol for toxoplasmosis. It is effective in treating acute or reactivated toxoplasmosis but does not affect the tissue cyst. In the immunocompromised individual, cessation of treatment usually results in eventual relapse. Alternative treatments include the combination of pyrimethamine and clindamycin or high dose oral clindamycin.

a: The combination of trimethoprim/sulfamethoxazole (TMP/SMX) given IV is now the treatment of choice for *Pneumocystis carinii* pneumonia (PCP). It has some *in vivo* and *in vitro* effects against *Toxoplasma* but has not been verified as an effective alternative to the pyrimethamine/sulfadiazine combination.

b: Penicillin is not effective as an antiprotozoal agent in treating *Toxoplasma gondii*. It is used to treat gram positive bacteria.

d: Cefotaxime, a third generation cephalosporin, is not effective as an antiprotozoal agent in treating *Toxoplasma gondii*. It is

used to treat gram negative and gram positive bacterial infections.

e: Pyrimethamine with sulfadiazine is a treatment of choice.

10. **Answer c:**

Parenteral antibiotics are the primary treatment for epiglottitis. Since croup is viral, the only role for antibiotics would be for treatment of secondary infection.

a: Corticosteroids might be used, but with unproven benefit.

b: Humidified air may be beneficial.

d: Parenteral antibiotics are useful.

11. **Answer d:**

Gentamicin plus nafcillin plus piperacillin supports broad gram-negative coverage, a penicillinase-resistant agent covering possible *S. aureus* involvement and adds piperacillin, which is an extended spectrum drug with activity against gram-negative organisms, including *Klebsiella* and *Pseudomonas*. The addition of piperacillin provides coverage to these additional likely pathogens.

a: Gentamicin alone is not optimum, although broad spectrum aminoglycoside coverage of gram negative species is central to the treatment approach.

b: Ampicillin by itself has limited gram-negative activity compared to other antibiotics.

c: Gentamicin plus nafcillin supports broad gram-negative coverage and adds a penicillinase-resistant agent that would cover possible *S. aureus* presence.

e: Gentamicin, nafcillin, and piperacillin would be appropriate.

CHAPTER 8: HEMO/IMMUNOPOIETIC AND ANTIINFLAMMATORY DRUGS

1. **Answer c:**

Aspirin causes a sustained inhibition of platelet cyclooxygenase, which results in decreased synthesis of prothrombogenic eicosanoid, thromboxane.

a, d: Ranitidine does not activate the fibrinolytic system or induce thrombocytopenia.

b: The patient has no previous history of bleeding disorders, making hemophilia an unlikely cause of the excessive bleeding.

e: Antacids do not cause vitamin K deficiency.

2. **Answer a:**

Cimetidine inhibits the cytochrome P-450-dependent metabolism of warfarin, enhancing its anticoagulant effects, and aspirin causes a sustained inhibition of platelet cyclooxygenase, which results in decreased synthesis of prothrombogenic eicosanoid, thromboxane.

b: The major interaction between cimetidine and warfarin is at the level of cytochrome P-450, not protein binding.

c: The systemic bioavailability of warfarin is close to 100%, hence, its absorption from the gastrointestinal tract cannot be increased further.

d: Cimetidine does not activate the fibrinolytic system.

e: Aspirin and cimetidine exert no synergist antiplatelet effects.

3. **Answer b:**

Aspirin is an inexpensive and effective treatment for rheumatoid arthritis.

a: Levamisole has not been approved by the FDA for the treatment of rheumatoid arthritis and, even if it were, levamisole would be given only when aspirin or another NSAID was found to provide inadequate control of rheumatoid arthritis.

c, d: These slow-acting drugs are used only after treatment with aspirin if another NSAID was found to provide inadequate control of rheumatoid arthritis.

e: Acetaminophen is one of the few NSAIDS that lacks significant antiinflammatory effects.

4. **Answer d:**

A gold salt is one of several slow-acting drugs used to treat rheumatoid arthritis that is inadequately controlled by aspirin or other NSAIDs.

a, b: The antiinflammatory effect of ibuprofen and phenylbutazone involves inhibition of cyclooxygenase, as is the case with other NSAIDs.

c, e: Colchicine and allopurinol are used to treat acute gouty arthritis, not rheumatoid arthritis.

5. **Answer a:**

Type I drug allergies are mediated by IgE.

b, c: Type II and III drug allergies are both mediated by IgG or IgM, not IgE.

d: Type II and III drug allergies are cell-mediated allergic reactions.

e: Type I drug allergies are mediated by IgE.

6. **Answer d:**

Cyclosporin is used to treat organ transplant patients, but it is not used for cancer chemotherapy.

a, b, c: Vincristine, cyclophosphamide and methotrexate are used as cancer chemotherapeutic agents.

e: D is the correct answer.

7. **Answer d:**

A gold salt is the preferred treatment for degenerative rheumatoid arthritis that cannot be controlled adequately by aspirin or another NSAID.

a, b: Phenylbutazone and indomethacin are NSAIDs that would be expected to offer no significant advantages over aspirin in the control of rheumatoid arthritis.

c: This can be used as an adjunct to aspirin therapy, but gold salts are the preferred slow-acting drugs to treat degenerative rheumatoid arthritis that cannot be controlled adequately by aspirin or another NSAID.

e: N-acetylcysteine is used to treat acetaminophen-induced liver toxicity. It is not used to treat rheumatoid arthritis.

8. **Answer d:**

Intrinsic factor does not antagonize the effects of vitamin B_{12} but actually facilitates the intestinal absorption of vitamin B_{12} (which is also known as extrinsic factor).

a: Protamine sulfate binds to heparin and blocks its anticoagulant effects, for which reason protamine sulfate is used to treat heparin overdose.

b: Desferal is a high affinity chelator of iron that can be used to treat iron overload.

c: Vitamin K and the oral anticoagulant warfarin compete with each other for binding to the same enzyme, namely vitamin K epoxide reductase. Because vitamin K is a substrate for vitamin K epoxide reductase, whereas warfarin is an inhibitor, vitamin K is used to treat warfarin overdose.

e: Vitamin K and the oral anticoagulant bishydroxycoumarin compete with each other for binding to the same enzyme, namely vitamin K epoxide reductase. Because vitamin K is a substrate for vitamin K epoxide reductase, whereas bishydroxycoumarin is an inhibitor, vitamin K is used to treat bishydroxycoumarin overdose.

9. **Answer b:**

There is a preponderance of factors that predispose this patient to iron deficiency anemia, including increased loss of iron through menstrual and gastric bleeding (due to an antiplatelet effect and gastric irritation) and decreased iron absorption through repeated and frequent use of antacids and milk.

a: This symptom of severe aspirin intoxication is preceded by numerous other symptoms that are not apparent in this patient.

c: Aspirin rarely causes interstitial nephritis (in contrast to other NSAIDs). Furthermore, the patient's symptoms do not support a diagnosis of interstitial nephritis.

d: The patient's symptoms do not support a diagnosis of lactose intolerance.

e: Aspirin has antithrombogenic, not prothrombogenic, effects. Furthermore, the patient's symptoms do not support a diagnosis of disseminated intravascular coagulation.

Chapter 9: Toxicology

1. **Answer d:**

Lead retention is cumulative.

a: As with all chemicals, the toxicity of lead is dependent on the dose.

b: Tolerance is not observed with lead.

c: There does not appear to be a genetically susceptible subpopulation to lead; however, the fetus and newborn are more susceptible than adults.

e: Lead poisoning usually results from chronic exposure.

2. **Answer b:**

CO is taken up by the blood at a rate which is initially proportional to the CO concentration in the respired air.

a: CO has a high affinity for hemoglobin, but it is reversible.

c: CO is detoxified by exhalation.

d: CD decreases the dissociation of oxygen from hemoglobin.

e: CO poisoning is due to a lack of distribution of oxygen to the tissues.

3. **Answer a:**

The rate of input exceeds the excretion rate of elimination.

b: Acute toxicity is more likely to occur when exposure is sudden and severe and absorption is rapid.

c: Many chemicals, such as the metals, produce chronic toxicity but are not biotransformed.

d: Many chemicals, such as metals, produce chronic toxicity but are not conjugated in the liver and excreted in the bile.

e: Most chemicals that produce chronic effects do so after oral exposure.

4. **Answer d:**

The clinical presentation is most consistent with mercury poisoning.

a: Lead is not likely to produce emotional disturbances or tremors.

b: Arsenic produces dermatological changes.

c: Arsine mainly produces hemolysis.

e: Thallium produces alopecia.

5. **Answer e:**

Atropine would be an effective antidote against some organic phosphate poisonings.

a: DDT has low potential for acute toxicity, but if observed, an anticonvulsant would be employed.
b: Pyrethrins have low potential for acute toxicity. Allergy is the most likely adverse effect.
c: Vitamin K antagonists can be treated by administering Vitamin K.
d: Chelators are used to treat metal poisoning.

6. **Answer a:**

Ringing of the ears is associated with mild salicylate poisonings.

b: Salicylates are not hallucinogens.
c: Salicylates do not produce euphoria.
d: Mild salicylate poisoning stimulates respiration and produces respiratory alkalosis.
e: Ringing of the ears is associated with salicylate poisonings.

7. **Answer c:**

CO results from incomplete carbon compound oxidation.

a: Carbon monoxide is detoxified by exhalation.
b: CO binds to but does not denature hemoglobin.

d: The binding is avid, but reversible.
e: It produces carboxyhemoglobin.

8. **Answer d:**

Bone.

a, b, c, e: Lead is stored in bones.

9. **Answer d:**

Atropine penetrates the CNS.

a: PAM does not readily enter the CNS.
b: Methylatropine does not readily enter the CNS.
c: There is too much cholinergic stimulation so one would not give a cholinergic stimulant.
e: The problem is cholinesterase inhibition, so further inhibition of cholinesterase is not desired.

10. **Answer b:**

Antimuscarinic agents in the tea.

a: CO does not cause dryness of the mouth.
c: Ammonia was extensively used as a refrigerant and its main toxicity is to the lung. Freons are presently used, and they have very few biological effects.
d: Parathion inhibits cholinesterase and then produces cholinergic effects such as salivation, lacrimation, urination, diarrhea, and muscle fasciculations.
e: Botulism symptoms begin after a longer incubation period. A characteristic descending paralysis is seen.

APPENDIX
INTERNATIONAL SYSTEM OF UNITS (SI)

SI Derived Units with Special Names

FORMULA	SYMBOL	SPECIAL NAME	PHYSICAL QUANTITY
$1 \text{ kg} \cdot \text{m/s}^2$	$= 1 \text{ N}$	1 newton	force
1 N/m^2	$= 1 \text{ Pa}$	1 pascal	pressure or stress
$1 \text{ N} \cdot \text{m}$	$= 1 \text{ J}$	1 joule	work, energy, or quantity of heat
1 J/s	$= 1 \text{ W}$	1 watt	power or radiant energy flux
1 W/A	$= 1 \text{ V}$	1 volt	electric potential, potential difference, or electromotive force
1 A/V	$= 1 \text{ S}$	1 siemens	electric conductance
1 V/A	$= 1 \text{ } \Omega$	1 ohm	electric resistance
$1 \text{ A} \cdot \text{s}$	$= 1 \text{ C}$	1 coulomb	quantity of electricity or electric charge
1 C/V	$= 1 \text{ F}$	1 farad	electric capacitance
$1 \text{ V} \cdot \text{s}$	$= 1 \text{ Wb}$	1 weber	magnetic flux
1 Wb/A	$= 1 \text{ H}$	1 henry	inductance
1 Wb/m^2	$= 1 \text{ T}$	1 tesla	magnetic flux density or magnetic induction
$1 \text{ cd} \cdot \text{sr}$	$= 1 \text{ lm}$	1 lumen	luminous flux
1 lm/m^2	$= 1 \text{ lx}$	1 lux	illuminance
1 J/kg	$= 1 \text{ Gy}$	1 gray	absorbed dose (of ionizing radiation)
1 (disintegration)/s	$= 1 \text{ Bq}$	1 becquerel	activity (of a radionuclide)
1 (cycle)/s	$= 1 \text{ Hz}$	1 hertz	frequency (of a periodic phenomenon)

SI Prefixes

FACTOR	PREFIX	SYMBOL	FACTOR	PREFIX	SYMBOL
10^{-18}	atto	a	10	deca	da
10^{-15}	femto	f	10^2	hecto	h
10^{-12}	pico	p	10^3	kilo	k
10^{-9}	nano	n	10^6	mega	M
10^{-6}	micro	μ	10^9	giga	G
10^{-3}	milli	m	10^{12}	tera	T
10^{-2}	centi	c	10^{15}	peta	P
10^{-1}	deci	d	10^{18}	exa	E

From Brody TM, Larner J, Minneman KP, New HC: *Human pharmacology*, ed 2, St. Louis, 1994, Mosby.

INDEX

Pages in italics indicate figures; pages with *t* indicate tables.

Mosby's Review Series
Copyright © 1996,
Mosby–Year Book, Inc.

How to install this program—Windows users

1. Place the disk in Drive A: (or B:)
2. From Program Manager, select File, then Run, then enter:
   A:SETUP (or B:SETUP if your disk drive is B:)
3. Follow the instructions on screen.

How to run this program—Windows users

Open the MOSBY Program Group and select the ACE program.

How to install this program—Macintosh users

1. Create a new folder on your hard disk called MOSBY, then open it.
   If you already have a MOSBY folder, you may use any other name.
2. Insert the disk into your floppy drive and open it.
3. Drag all items from the disk to the new folder.
4. If more than one disk is included, perform steps 2 and 3 for each disk.

How to run this program—Macintosh users

Open the MOSBY folder and select the ACE program.

For complete instructions on using the program, please read the "How to use this Program" file.

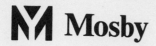 **Mosby**

Dedicated to Publishing Excellence

WE WANT TO HEAR FROM YOU!

To help us publish the most useful materials for students, we would appreciate your comments on this book. Please take a few moments to complete the form below, and then tear it out and mail to us. Thank you for your input.

Mosby's reviews: PHARMACOLOGY

1. What courses are you using this book for?

___medical school   ___1st year
___pharmacy school   ___2nd year
___physician assistant program   ___3rd year
___nursing school   ___4th year
___dental school   ___other
___osteopathic school
___undergrad
___other _____

2. Was this book useful for your course? Why or why not?

___yes ___no _____

_____

3. What features of textbooks are important to you? (*check all that apply*)

___color figures
___summary tables and boxes
___summaries
___self-assessment questions
___price
___other _____

4. What influenced your decision to buy this text? (*check all that apply*)

___required/recommended by instructor
___recommendation by student
___bookstore display
___other _____

5. What other instructional materials did/would you find useful in this course?

___computer-assisted instruction
___lab time   ___slides
___case studies book
___other _____

Are you interested in doing in-depth reviews of our basic science textbooks? If so please fill out the information below.

NAME:_____

ADDRESS:_____

_____

TELEPHONE:_____

THANK YOU!

◥◣ **A Times Mirror**
◣◢ **Company**

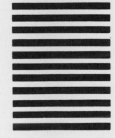

NO POSTAGE
NECESSARY
IF MAILED
IN THE
UNITED STATES

BUSINESS REPLY MAIL
FIRST CLASS MAIL   PERMIT No. 135   St. Louis, MO.

POSTAGE WILL BE PAID BY ADDRESSEE

CHRIS REID
MEDICAL EDITORIAL
MOSBY–YEAR BOOK, INC.
11830 WESTLINE INDUSTRIAL DRIVE
ST.LOUIS, MO 63146-9987

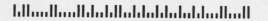